CONJUNCTIVITIS – A COMPLEX AND MULTIFACETED DISORDER

Edited by **Zdenek Pelikan**

Conjunctivitis – A Complex and Multifaceted Disorder
Edited by Zdenek Pelikan

Published by InTech

Janeza Trdine 9, 51000 Rijeka, Croatia

Publishing Process Manager Marina Jozipovic

Technical Editor Teodora Smiljanic

Cover Designer InTech Design Team

Additional hard copies can be obtained from orders@intechopen.com

Conjunctivitis – A Complex and Multifaceted Disorder, Edited by Zdenek Pelikan
p. cm.
ISBN 978-953-307-750-5

For EU product safety concerns:
IN TECH d.o.o., Prolaz Marije Krucifikse Kozulić 3, 51000 Rijeka, Croatia, info@intechopen.com or visit our website at intechopen.com.

Meet the editor

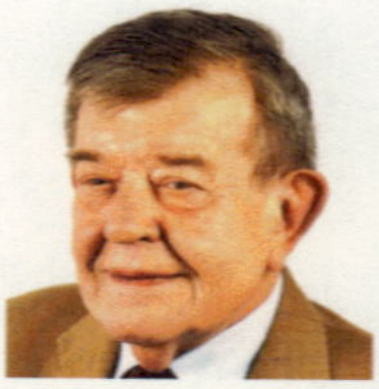

Dr. Z. Pelikan, MD, PhD, allergologist, graduated from the Medical School MU (Brno) in 1961 (MD, PhD). He accomplished the training and certified qualification in the internal medicine, ophthalmology, clinical immunology and allergology. In 1996 he finished the second Thesis (PhD) at the Free University in Amsterdam. In 1975 he has, together with his spouse Dr. Marta Filipek, pediatrician, founded the Department of Allergology and Immunology (CAI/DAI) of the Institute of Medical Sciences "De Klokkenberg " (Breda, The Netherlands). In 1976 he became a Director of the CAI/DAI. In 1996 he has been nominated an associated professor in the Clinical Immunology of the Masaryk's University (Brno, Czech Republic). His current affiliation is Director of the Allergy Research Foundation (ARF) in Breda (The Netherlands). He is the author of more than 300 scientific publications. He is a member/fellow of 23 national and international medical, allergology, immunology and scientific societies, a.o. EAACI, AAAAI, ACAAI.

Contents

Preface

Conjunctivitis, a group of inflammatory disorders of the conjunctiva and often also in conjunction with cornea, lacrimal ways and eyelids, is very common condition affecting large adult as well as pediatric population.[1-3] These disorders, especially their chronic forms, can be a source of relatively extensive discomfort for the patients, which can negatively influence their professional carriers as well as their private lives.

Conjunctivitis can be classified by various manners and according to various parameters. However, the classification according to the causal aspects might be preferred.[1-7]

Conjunctivitis can be divided into two basic groups, with respect to the localization of the primary pathophysiologic process and involved mechanisms [8-11]; (A) *Primary conjunctivitis,* including all primary and independent forms/disorders whose underlying pathophysiologic processes are initiated and localized in the conjunctival tissue, eventually in conjunction with the adjacent tissues, such as cornea, sclera, lacrimal ways or eyelid skin. (B) *Secondary conjunctivitis,* including all conjunctivitis forms, in which the primary pathophysiologic process is localized outside the conjunctivae, in another organ. This group can further be divided into two sub-groups; (B_1) *Secondarily induced conjunctivitis* including conjunctivitis forms induced by factors (mediators, cytokines, chemokines, neuropeptides,activated cells) released during the primary pathophysiologic and/or immunologic process in another tissue, e.g. nasal mucosa, middle ear, paranasal sinus mucosa, bronchial mucosa, eyelid skin, and reaching secondarily the conjunctivae; (B_2) *Secondary conjunctivitis forms,* being a part of a complex and multifaceted pathophysiologic processes, such as systemic diseases, metabolic disorders, some infectious and parasitic diseases, (auto)-immune disorders, immunodeficiencies, angio-neurotic (Quincke) edema, some malignancy forms, etc.

Regarding the cause, the conjunctivitis can be divided into a number of categories.[1-7]

[1] **Allergic conjunctivitis**
Disorders of the conjunctiva, and sometimes also cornea, where an allergic component plays an important causal role, summarized by a term "allergic conjunctivitis", are very common conditions affecting 15-25% of the adult and pediatric populations. This group includes: Seasonal allergic conjunctivitis (SAC), perennial allergic conjunctivitis (PAC), vernal keratoconjunctivitis (VKC), atopic

keratoconjunctivitis (AKC) and giant papillary conjunctivitis (GPC). All these disorders can occur in a acute, recurrent or a chronic feature as well as in a primary or a secondarily induced form. With respect to the involved immunologic mechanisms and underlying hypersensitivity type, various types of the primary conjunctival response (immediate, late or delayed) can be recorded after the conjunctival provocation tests with allergen as well as the various types of the secondarily induced conjunctival response (immediate, late and delayed) can be measured after the nasal provocation tests with allergen. [1-14]

The allergens causing the allergic conjunctivitis include various inhalant (aero) allergens, several food allergens, contact allergens, various drugs and a relatively high number of occupational allergens. [1-14]

Allergic conjunctivitis due to the foods and food allergy represents a special sub-group of this entity. Various foods and/or their parts/ingredients, being ingested, can act as allergens causing either the primary or the secondarily induced conjunctival response. Moreover, various foods, in a powder, fluid or vapor form, can act as contact allergens, causing usually the primary form of allergic conjunctivitis or they can act as non-specific agents causing a conjunctival response through the non-specific hyperreactivity mechanism. [8, 11]Additionally, the same powdered, vaporized or liquid food, affecting the nasal mucosa, may cause a secondarily induced conjunctival response.

The various drugs can also cause both the (allergic) conjunctivitis by means of the similar multi-facet pathophysiologic and immunologic mechanisms and the non-specific conjunctival response (=irritation). [15, 16]

[2] **Bacterial conjunctivitis** may usually be caused by bacteria from the families Staphylococcus, Streptococcus, Gonococcus, Neisseria, Chlamidia, Haemophilus, Pneumococcus, Pseudomonas, Escherichia, Klebsiella, Proteus, Enterobacter, Mycobacterium, Meningococcus, Moraxella and Spirochetes.[4-7, 17-20]
A special sub-groups of bacterial conjunctivitis are represented by conjunctival inflammation processes caused by *Chlamydia trachomonas,* occurring as a part of the complex ocular disorders termed "Trachoma", and those due to a number of zoonoses.[4-7, 17-20]

[3] **Viral conjunctivitis** is caused by a number of viruses, such as adenovirus (APC) virus, coxackie, herpes simplex , herpes zoster, influenza, measles, variola, varicella, enteroviruses, echo-virus and HIV.[4-7, 17-19]

[4] **Parasitic conjunctivitis** is caused by amebae, trypanosomae, leishmaniae, toxoplasmae, nematodes, Rickettsiae.[4-7, 21-23]

[5] **Mycotic conjunctivitis** is caused by various kinds of actinomycetes, molds, fungi and yeasts and/or their spores, such as Aspergillus, Alternaria, Cladosporium, Penicillium, Fusarium, Actinomycetes, Zygomycetes, Candida albicans.[4-7, 24]

[6] **Chemical conjunctivitis** (=conjunctival irritation) is usually caused by volatile, liquid or vaporized chemical compounds.[4-7]

[7] **Reactive conjunctivitis** due to the non-specific hyperreactivity, upon involvement of various mechanical, physical and simple (small-molecular) chemical stimuli.[4-8] Some kinds of post-traumatic conjunctival response would belong to this sub-category as well.

[8] **Toxic conjunctivitis** and/or toxic conjunctival reaction caused by some chemical or biological toxins.

[9] **Conjunctivitis neonatorum** is caused by *Chlamidia trachomatis* and sometimes by *Neisseria gonorrhoeae* [4-7]

[10] **Varia**, such as as Sjögren's syndrome, Keratoconjunctivitis sicca (Dry eye syndrome), Contact lens syndrome, Ocular cicatrical pemphigoid, Stevens-Johnson syndrome and various forms of occupational diseases, in which a multifactor, although not always clear, etiology is suspected.[4-7, 25]

Diagnostic procedure of conjunctivitis should include all facets of this condition and all main aspects related to the possible causes of these disorders, basic and if necessary supplementary laboratory and bacteriological examinations (including the blood, tears, conjunctival, nasal and throat swab), complete ophthalmological examination (including the slit lamp examination, ophthalmoscopy, intraocular pressure measurement, cytologic examination of the tears, and if indicated also conjunctival biopsy, ultrasound biomicroscopy, confocal scanning laser ophthalmoscopy), basic allergological examination, such as skin testing and determination of the serum immunoglobulins (PRIST, RAST, ImmunoCap) and if necessary supplementary tests, such as conjunctival provocation tests with allergens (and non-specific hyperreactivity agents, e.g. histamine, cold air,etc) and/or nasal provocation tests with allergens (and non-specific hyperreactivity agents), and if indicated also appropriate roentgen and/or imaging examination.[1-16]

The therapeutic management of the conjunctivitis should be: (a) motivated and derived from the results of diagnostic procedure; (b) focused on the causal aspects, as far as possible; (c) as complex as possible, including all principal as well as additional facets of this condition; (d) administered for a sufficiently long period of time, and finished by a final control examination. The only symptomatic and/or empiric treatment is insufficient and not more acceptable. An additional and very important remark concerns the treatment of bacterial (and exceptionally also viral) conjunctivitis by means of antibiotics and sulphonamides. The treatment with these drugs should not be routinely limited only to the topical (intraconjunctival) administration, but a combination of the topical and simultaneous systemic (e.g. oral) administration of these drugs may always be considered, to prevent the possible development of the antibiotic/sulphonamide resistant bacterial strains. Also the therapeutical capacity and position of the Disodium cromoglycate (Cromolyn) and Nedocromil sodium in the pharmacologic repertoire and control of the allergic conjunctivitis should be re-evaluated and up-graded, especially with respect to the growing limitation of the use of glucocorticosteroids regarding their side-effects and limited effectiveness of the H_1–receptor antagonists in several cases of this condition.[8, 11] The conjunctivitis may be considered and accepted as a serious medical problem and it should not be underestimated either by the patients or by the doctors, since this entity could lead under certain circumstances to the serious, permanent and sometimes irreversible, limitation of the ocular function and/or ocular damage.

This book/monograph is an attempt of a team of international experts to present a survey on the current knowledge of this condition, in its various facets and from various point of views.

The editor would like to express his acknowledgment not only to all authors contributing to this monograph, but also to the Publisher "InTech", and its associates/collaborators, for taking the initiative to realize, process and produce this monograph.

Dr. Zdenek Pelikan,
Director of Allergy Research Foundation, Breda
The Netherlands

References

[1] McGill JI, Holgate ST, Church MK, Anderson DF, Bacon A. Allergic eye disease mechanisms. Br J Ophthalmol 1998; 82: 1203-1214
[2] Bielory L. Ocular allergy overview. Immunol Allergy Clin N Am 2008; 28: 1-23
[3] Barney NP, Graziano FM, Cook EB, Stahl JL. Allergic and immunologic diseases of the eye. In: Adkinson NF, Bochner BS,Busse WW, Holgate ST, Lemanske RF, Simons FE, eds. Middleton's Allergy, principles & practice (7th Ed). Philadelphia: Elsevier Inc. 2009: 1117-1137
[4] Easty DL, Sparrow JM. Oxford book of ophthalmology (1st Ed). Oxford (UK): Oxford University Press 1999
[5] Crick EP, Khaw PT. A textbook of clinical ophthalmology (3rd Ed). Singapore: World Scientific Publishing Co.Ltd. 2003
[6] Kanski JJ. Kanski's Clinical Ophthalmology: A systemic approach (5th Ed). Oxford (UK): Butterworth-Heinemann-Elsevier Ltd. 2003
[7] Agarwal S, Agarwal A, Apple DJ. Textbook of Ophthalmology. New Delhi (India): Jaypee Brothers Publishers 2002
[8] Pelikan Z. The late nasal response. Thesis. Amsterdam: The Free University of Amsterdam 1996
[9] Pelikan Z. The possible involvement of nasal allergy in allergic keratoconjunctivitis. Eye 2009; 23: 1653-1660
[10] Pelikan Z. Seasonal and perennial allergic conjunctivitis: the possible role of nasal allergy. Clin Exp Ophthalmol 2009; 37:448-457
[11] Pelikan Z. Allergic conjunctivitis and nasal allergy. Curr Allergy Asthma Rep 2010; 10: 295-302
[12] Sheppard JD, Scoper SV. Ocular allergy in clinical practice. In: Garg A, Sheppard JD, Meyer D (Eds). Step by step, Clinical diagnosis and management of ocular allergy. New Delhi (India): Jaypee Brothers Medical Publishers Ltd. 2007: 245-278

[13] Adeuwala A. Clinical features of ocular allergy. In: Garg A, Sheppard JD, Meyer D (Eds). Step by step, Clinical diagnosis and management of ocular allergy. New Delhi (India): Jaypee Brothers Medical Publishers Ltd. 2007: 31-46

[14] Bacon AS, Ahluwalia P, Irani AM, Schwartz LB, Holgate ST, Church MK, McGill JI. Tear and conjunctival changes during the allergen-induced early- and late-phase responses. J Allergy Clin Immunol 2000; 106: 948-954

[15] Ferreira PC, Rodrigues NJ, Deschenes J. Ocular allergy and hypersensitivity to ophthalmic drugs. In: Garg A, Sheppard JD, Meyer D (Eds). Step by step, Clinical diagnosis and management of ocular allergy. New Delhi (India): Jaypee Brothers Medical Publishers Ltd. 2007: 279-294

[16] Garg A. Allergic ocular surface disorders due to drug toxicity. In: Garg A, Sheppard JD, Meyer D (Eds). Step by step, Clinical diagnosis and management of ocular allergy. New Delhi (India): Jaypee Brothers Medical Publishers Ltd. 2007: 173-244

[17] Baron S et al. Medical Microbiology (4th Ed).Galveston (TX): The university of Texas Medical Branch at Galveston 1996.

[18] Levinson WE. Medical Microbiology & Immunology (8th Ed). New York: MacGraw-Hill/ Appleton & Lange 2004

[19] Ryan K, Ray C, Ray CG. Sherris Medical Microbiology (E-book). New York: MacGraw-Hill Comp. 2003

[20] Gorbach SL, Bartlett JG, Blacklow NR (Eds). Infectious diseases (3rd Ed). Philadelphia: Lippincott Williams & Wilkins (A Wolters Kluwer Company) 2004

[21] Fauci AS, Braunwald E, Kasper DL, Hauser SL, Longo DL, Jameson JL, Loscalzo J (Eds). Harrison's Principles of Internal Medicine (17th Ed). New York, Chicago, San Francisco, Lisbon, London, Madrid, Mexico City, New Delhi, San Juan, Seoul, Singapore, Sydney, Toronto: MacGrow-Hill Medical Comp. Inc 2008

[22] John DT, Petri WA. Markell and Voge's Medical Parasitology (9th Ed). Philadelphia: W.B. Saunders 2006

[23] Najarian HH. Textbook of Medical Parasitology. Baltimore: Williams & Wilkins Comp. 1967

[24] Dismukes WE, Pappas PG, Sobel JD (Eds). Clinical Mycology. Oxford (UK): Oxford University Press, Inc. 2003 -5-25. Sheppard J, Bodner BI. Ocular allergy and contact lenses. In: Garg A, Sheppard JD, Meyer D (Eds). Step by step, Clinical diagnosis and management of ocular allergy. New Delhi (India): Jaypee Brothers Medical Publishers Ltd. 2007: 165-172

Part 1

Epidemiology of Conjunctivitis

1

Epidemiological Aspects of Infectious Conjunctivitis

Herlinda Mejía-López[1], Carlos Alberto Pantoja-Meléndez[2], Alejandro Climent-Flores[1] and Victor M. Bautista-de Lucio[1]
[1]*Institute of Ophthalmology "Fundación Conde de Valenciana" I.A.P. Research Unit, Mexico City*
[2]*Faculty of Medicine, National Autonomous University of Mexico Public Health Dept. Mexico*

1. Introduction

Conjunctivitis can be broadly classified into two groups, infectious and noninfectious. Infectious conjunctivitis is mainly caused by bacteria (60%), followed by viruses (20%), with the remaining cases caused by Chlamydia, fungi and parasites. Infectious conjunctivitis tends to present during the summer months.

Non-infectious conjunctivitis includes allergic causes, often during the flowering period in spring. However, nosocomial outbreaks and work related conditions, as well as mechanical and functional causes are not associated with any particular time of year.

Conjunctivitis can also be divided into epidemic and non-epidemic, associated with risk factors, immunological factors, and mechanical-functional causes. This classification allows professionals to tailor patient care more effectively.

1.1 Epidemic conjunctivitis

There are several pathogens reported to be able to affect large groups and cause greater or wider than expected epidemics. However, conjunctivitis has caused several epidemics in the past and although most cases are benign and self-limiting, many underestimate its impact on the population and its ability to spread rapidly.

Epidemic types of conjunctivitis, especially hemorrhagic types, are subject to surveillance by world health systems. They are more common in the summer and one of their main features is the rapid spread and numbers of cases that occur in short periods of time. Some serotypes are widely distributed, and these are usually those which show this epidemic capability.[1,2]

Conjunctivitis can be transmitted efficiently by virtually all known methods of transmission (see Modes of transmission), which partly explains the rapidity of its spread.

It is known that acute hemorrhagic conjunctivitis occurs in tropical areas due to high temperatures and high relative humidity, which prolongs the survival of viruses. Other viral intrinsic factors, such as in adenovirus, allow viral establishment in adverse environments, and these factors are associated with epidemics. It is increasingly becoming clear that medical staff also participate in the spread of an epidemic, as the handling of patients without appropriate risk management can make medical personnel a disease vector.

Cases of epidemic hemorrhagic conjunctivitis are mainly caused by adenovirus. However, coxsackie A24 is currently responsible for the reported worldwide epidemic. It was first identified in Ghana in 1969, later spread to Asia and Oceania, and at the end of the twentieth century regular reports of events caused by several strains of coxsackievirus had been published.[3-9] This epidemic affected several countries in all continents including Australia, where an acute conjunctivitis caused by coxsackie A24 in a non-.hemorrhagic form was identified.[10-12] (Figure 1).

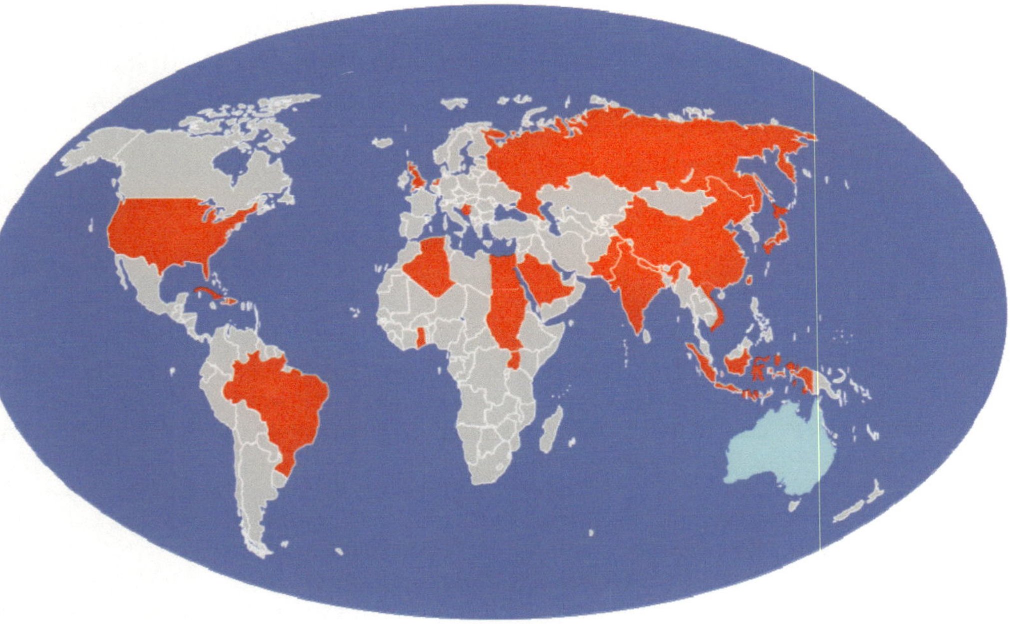

Fig. 1. Distribution of epidemic hemorrhagic conjunctivitis caused by coxsackie A24. In red, countries that presented with hemorrhagic conjunctivitis; in blue, countries that presented with non-hemorrhagic conjunctivitis.

1.2 Non-epidemic conjunctivitis

Conjunctivitis is a disease that represents a significant proportion of ophthalmologist consultations. Usually, non-epidemic forms of this condition do not have the potential to affect large populations, but its impact is on medical spending, temporary disability and in rare cases, steps to contain a possible outbreak.

The main cause of non-epidemic conjunctivitis is allergic conjunctivitis. As a group, they represent the main reason for consultation for conjunctivitis in developed countries and have also shown an increase in prevalence and incidence.

Allergic conjunctivitis is a very common disorder in adults as well as in children. The estimations of its incidence, reported in the literature, vary from 15 to 25 % of the general population.[13]

Allergic conjunctivitis includes 5 clinical entities (classes), such as Seasonal Allergic Conjunctivitis (SAC), occurring most frequently, followed by Atopic Keratoconjunctivitis (AKC), Vernal Keratoconjunctivitis (VKC), Perennial Allergic Conjunctivitis (PAC) and

Giant Papillary Conjunctivitis (GPC). The SAC and PAC occur in relatively mild forms, while VKC and AKC, in which also cornea is affected, and represent more severe, often bilateral, forms. The GPC appears only sporadically.[14]

Allergic conjunctivitis is associated with common allergens; is common to find that sufferers also have atopy and a family history of allergy. This type of conjunctivitis occurs most often between 10 and 40 years of life, peaking in the second decade.

The most frequently involved allergens are: I. Various inhalant allergens, such as pollen species, *Dermatophagoides pteronyssinus, Dermatophagoides farinae*, various moulds (*Aspergillus fumigatus, Aspergillus niger, Alternaria* family, *Cladosporium* family, *Penicillium* family, *Candida albicans, Thermopolyspora polyspora*), animal danders (hairs, feathers, squamae), organic dusts, some foods in powder form (flour kinds, spices); II. Some drugs (e.g. in powder form, ointments, etc); III. Digested foods; IV. Contact allergens.[15]

Some cases of conjunctivitis are associated with chemical or physical agents inherent in patients' work conditions and occupational hazards. Among these chemicals, the most common causes of work-related conjunctivitis are mepacrine, ammonia and vanadium, mainly linked to the metalworking industry. In the case of physical agents, ultraviolet light received in outdoor occupations such as police and construction work is the main cause of conjunctivitis.

Another type of occupational hazard associated with conjunctivitis is the handling of infected secretions. This can present a high risk to medical staff that provides care to patients if appropriate hygiene measures are not taken.

The remaining conjunctivitis cases can be attributed to bacteria, parasites, fungi and viruses (non-epidemic serotypes), which are also an important cause of daily ophthalmic consultations. However, these should be tackled depending on the causative factor. These types of conjunctivitis can be considered as nosocomial outbreaks, as they are mainly acquired in hospitals (e.g. *Staphylococcus* sp., adenovirus, herpes virus and *Candida* spp., among others).

2. Risk factors

2.1 Environmental risk factors, host susceptibility and pathogen factors

Conjunctivitis is not distributed randomly; cases manifest when increasing risk factors converge. Like other diseases that affect humans, it occurs on the conjunction of three factors: the causative agent, the environment and host specific factors.

Allergic conjunctivitis requires both a significant interaction of the environment and the individual's susceptibility to develop allergic conditions. The major known risk factors are a history of asthma or multiple allergies, smoking, contact lenses and environmental pollution.[13]

On the other hand, infectious conjunctivitis depends on the specific capabilities of the infective agent, though the human factor is also important as humans can often act as a disease reservoir.

Theoretically, we are all susceptible to conjunctivitis, but its presentation may depend more on risks associated with patient contact or contaminated materials. It has, however, been observed that age and sex are important factors, with children, young adults and women being the main groups affected.

There are 2 basic forms of allergic conjunctivitis with respect to the localization of the initial allergic reaction (antigen-antibody or antigen-sensitized Th1-cells interaction with subsequent steps). In the primary form of allergic conjunctivitis, the allergic reaction, due to direct exposure of Conjunctiva to an external allergen, occurs in the conjunctival mucosa. In this case, the conjunctiva is the primary and solely site of the allergic reaction with all subsequent steps, resulting in the development of the primary (classical) form of allergic conjunctivitis. In the secondary form of allergic conjunctivitis, the initial allergic reaction takes place in other (related) organ, mostly in the nasal mucosa, due to the direct exposure of nasal mucosa to an external allergen, leading to release of various factors (mediators, cytokines, chemokines and other factors), which can then reach conjunctiva by various ways, such as lacrimal system, blood, lymphatic or neurogenic network, and induce there the secondary conjunctival response (secondarily induced allergic conjunctivitis). In principle, all five clinical classes of allergic conjunctivitis can occur either in a primary or in a secondary form.[14,16]

Various hypersensitivity (immunologic) mechanisms can be involved in all five clinical classes of allergic conjunctivitis, both in their primary and in their secondary forms. The immediate (IgE-mediated) hypersensitivity mechanism, upon participation of the IgE antibodies, mast cells, eosinophils, epithelial cells and Th2-cells also designated as atopy, having been often studied and well documented, has been confirmed as the most frequent mechanism underlying the allergic conjunctivitis.

However, the evidence for involvement and causal role of other so-called non-immediate (non-IgE-mediated) hypersensitivity mechanisms, such as late (Type III) and delayed (Type IV, cell-mediated) in the allergic conjunctivitis of all five classes, is growing and became to be recognized.[17-19] The existence of the primary and secondary form of the allergic conjunctivitis as well as particular types of conjunctival response can only be demonstrated by provocation tests with allergen.

The conjunctival provocation tests with allergen confirm the primary allergic conjunctivitis form, whereas the nasal provocation tests with allergen upon monitoring of objective conjunctival signs and subjective symptoms confirm the secondary (secondarily induced) conjunctivitis form. Patients with both the forms of allergic conjunctivitis can develop various types of conjunctival response to allergen challenge, such as immediate (early), late or delayed response, depending on the type of hypersensitivity mechanism(s) involved.[19-21]

2.2 Immune response and risk factors

Epidemic keratoconjunctivitis caused by adenovirus induces a strong acute inflammatory response. Efforts have been made to identify host factors that promote and influence the severity of the clinical picture, with the purpose of generating an idea of prognosis. Among the factors to be studied, the immune response is important, as this may influence the damage done by the disease. The mechanisms that decide the initial response of the host depends on the innate immune response mediated by proinflammatory cytokines. These are essential in establishing the adaptive immune response, which provides long term protection.

Recently, the study of receptors in the cells involved with the innate immune response has received particular attention. The early interactions between pathogens and host cells are critical in the establishment of the infection. These receptors, known as Pattern Recognition Receptors (PRRs), recognize molecular patterns of pathogens (PAMP) that are highly conserved, and manage the effectiveness of the adaptive immune response that may limit or exacerbate the infection.[22] It has been shown that human Toll-like receptors (TLRs) play an essential role in triggering the innate immune response, recognizing a variety of PAMPs associated with bacteria, viruses, protozoa and fungi. The signals initiated by the interaction of TLRs with specific antigen ligands direct the inflammatory response, which attempts to eliminate the pathogen and start the adaptive response. In humans, eleven TLRs have been identified (TLR1-TLR11).[22,23]

The TLR2 receptor is particularly important, as it has a unique mechanism of ligand recognition where it cooperates with other TLR family members, particularly TLR1 and TLR6.[24] There are several studies showing that herpes simplex virus type 1 (HSV1), type 2 (HSV2), cytomegalovirus (CMV) and respiratory syncytial virus (RSV) induce TLR2-dependent proinflammatory cytokines in an attempt to induce cell protection.[25-27]

On the other hand, single nucleotide polymorphisms (SNPs) in genes encoding TLRs have also been reported. The TLR2 Arg677Trp and Arg753Gln SNPs are associated with susceptibility and severity of viral infections.[25-28] In our laboratory we found the Phe707Phe polymorphism in the Mexican population, with an allelic frequency of 7.5% and this suggests that this SNP not affect our population.[29]

The first line of defense against viruses is interferons. However, proinflammatory cytokines and antimicrobial peptides also promote the cell-mediated immune response, which is essential for the resolution of infection.[30] Beta-defensins (HBDs) act as antimicrobial peptides in humans and are also effective against a variety of microorganisms.[31]

In immunoprivileged tissue such as the cornea, the complex mechanisms that prevent the induction of inflammation and the behavior of cytokines and peptides of the innate immune response must be tightly regulated. An infection may then upset this microenvironment and cause damage to the ocular surface. Adenovirus infections induce expression of IP-10 and I-TAC, defense peptides against Ad5 and Ad3 respectively. It is suggested that epidemic strains of adenovirus (Ad8 and Ad19) could be resistant to these defensins. Interestingly, HBDs have also been suggested to possess an additional protective effect that contributes to the corneal healing process.[32,33]

Genetic variants at the promoter region of the beta defensin-1 (DEFB-1) gene are uncommon, however recent reports showed three SNPs that affect gene expression.[34,35] These -20A/-44C/-52G haplotypes have all been associated with chronic lung infection with P. aeruginosa.[36] The -44C allele also predisposes to infection by HIV[37,38] and *Candida* spp.[39] Moreover, Carter et al also found that it strongly associated with endophthalmitis.[40] In a recent study in our laboratory, we found a significantly higher frequency of -44C and -52G DEFB-1 polymorphisms in a cohort of 30 samples taken from patients with adenovirus infection. These showed an increased risk of infection of 2.86 for -44C allele and 2.44 for allele -52 G. These findings indicate that genotypes -44C/G and -52G/G may be associated with adenovirus infection (data not reported). The results obtained in the works above represent preliminary studies that require analysis of larger populations worldwide to determine whether these polymorphisms can be used as marker of infection susceptibility.

3. Transmission

Infectious conjunctivitis has a transmission capability dependant on the etiological agent involved.

Bacterial conjunctivitis is highly contagious and is associated with close contact between patients, a situation common in kindergartens and childcare. This predisposes to constant outbreaks, but these are rarely identified as children gradually leave the disease area.

Viruses, particularly respiratory adenovirus, which produces pharingoconjunctivitis also have a high capability of infection and is often confused with *Streptococcus pneumoniae*.

Fungi have a low transmission capability, but can be transmitted more efficiently amongst the sick or immunocompromised.

4. Forms of transmission

Conjunctivitis is most commonly transmitted by direct contact with secretions from a sick patient. However, air droplet transmission is also common, as well as via vehicles such as *Hyppelates* spp., which act as a vector for bacterial transmission.

4.1 Contact transfer

Transmission by contact with a contaminated body surface is the usual transfer mechanism for staphylococci, streptococci and enterobacteria. This is also the classic mechanism of transmission of nosocomial infections. Hand washing and use of protective barriers such as gloves and lab coats are sufficient to prevent transmission, as well as changing the dose of medication. Despite the fact that protective measures are simple, compliance is difficult and may become costly. However, contact transmission is responsible for a large proportion of cases, which implies that control of basic hygiene may reduce the case load significantly.

4.2 Droplet transmission

This transmission occurs through close contact with a patient. The droplets have a diameter greater than 5µm and are generated by coughing, sneezing, talking and during certain health care procedures.

Transmission occurs when droplets are deposited on the Conjunctiva or nasal mucosa of a susceptible host. The droplets travel an average distance of one meter from the patient and quickly fall to the ground. Therefore, transmission does not occur at greater distances and drops are not kept in the air for long periods, so special air handling is not required to prevent transmission by this mechanism.

4.3 Air transmission

This occurs through close or medium range contact with a patient. The droplets in this case have a diameter less than 5µm and are generated from an infected person during breathing, speech, coughing and sneezing.

Transmission occurs when microorganisms containing droplets generated by an infected person dry and remain airborne for long periods of time. These organisms (usually viruses) can be dispersed widely by air currents and inhaled by a susceptible host within the same room or even at distance depending on environmental factors, so in this case air handling and ventilation are important to prevent contagion. This type of transmission is less common but control is more expensive and complex.

4.4 Transmission by vectors

Transmission by vector is not considered widely relevant, but it is well known that *Chlamydia* can be transmitted by flies.

In the case of trachoma, which starts as a follicular conjunctivitis, it has been documented that the housefly (*Hyppelates* spp.) facilitates the transfer of infected secretions from patients to others.

5. Outbreaks

Conjunctivitis has high potential for nosocomial outbreaks depending on the causative agent, and has the capability to affect a large number of people. One of the most important features of these outbreaks is the speed of propagation, but with the appearance of a benign condition. Its importance lies in allowing us a panoramic view of the strengths and weaknesses of the systems of epidemiological surveillance in hospitals.

5.1 Microorganisms involved in outbreaks

5.1.1 Bacterial

5.1.1.1 Acute infections

The most common outbreaks are produced by *Staphylococcus* spp., *Streptococcus* spp., and *Haemophilus* sp. Some patients may be positive in culture for *Pneumococcus* sp.

Crum et al. described an outbreak of *Streptococcus pneumoniae* in 92 of 3500 soldiers.[41] Martin et al also reported an outbreak affecting 698 college students with this organism.[42] In another report, *Haemophilus influenzae* was shown to be responsible for 428 cases in Israel.[43]

5.1.1.2 Hyperacute infections

Hyperacute bacterial conjunctivitis is most frequently caused by *Neisseria gonorrhoeae*, related to oculopharingeal disorders in neonates and in sexually active young people. In 1987 and 1988, there were over 9,000 cases of conjunctivitis caused by *N. gonorrhoeae* in Ethiopia and children under 5 years were the group primarily affected.[44] The aboriginal population of central Australia has also has been frequently affected, with 447 cases reported in 1997.[45]

5.1.1.3 Chronic infections

Staphylococcus aureus is the bacteria most commonly reported in the literature as causing chronic conjunctivitis.

5.1.1.4 Chlamydial conjunctivitis

Conjunctivitis is considered chronic after 4 weeks and the best known cases of chronic follicular conjunctivitis are caused by *Chlamydia trachomatis*. This bacterium also causes cervicitis in women and urethritis and epididymitis in men. Unfortunately, these clinical manifestations may occur as subclinical infections, preventing the detection of the bacteria.

The newborn of women carrying *Chlamydia trachomatis* have a high incidence of conjunctivitis and pneumonia. In adults, conjunctivitis appears to be transmitted primarily by contact with infected genital discharge and usually occurs as isolated individual episodes, with few progressing to eye symptoms.[46,47]

On the other hand, in areas endemic for trachoma the first contact with *C. trachomatis* is related to the prevalence of infection in the community. Trachoma is clinically characterized by the presence of papillae and follicular inflammation of the tarsal conjunctiva and is referred to as active trachoma.[48] Trachoma can be produced by serovars A-C (A, B, Ba and C) of *C. trachomatis* and is endemic in 55 countries around the world.[49] Serovars D-K (genitals) may also affect the neonatal conjunctiva. It has also been reported that the species *Chlamydophila pneumoniae* and *Chlamydophila psittaci* may also cause trachoma, and may cause polyinfection with *C. trachomatis*.[50] However, as trachoma is a chronic infection, it does not usually cause epidemics.

5.1.2 Viral infections

Viruses are the principal cause of conjunctivitis worldwide, with adenovirus and coxsackievirus being the most frequent. It is reported that follicular conjunctivitis can occur as part of the pharynx and respiratory syndrome, or as a separate entity.

5.1.2.1 Pharyingoconjunctival fever caused by adenovirus

This disease is often accompanied by lymphadenopathy and most commonly associated with genotypes of the subgenera B and E (Ad3, Ad7 and Ad4).[51-53]

5.1.2.2 Epidemic keratoconjunctivitis

This severe form of conjunctivitis caused by adenovirus can incapacitate the patient for several weeks. The aftermath of the infection can leave subepithelial infiltrates that may affect the visual field. Outbreaks are caused by subgenus D (AD8, and AD37 Ad19).[54,55]

5.1.2.3 Acute hemorrhagic conjunctivitis

The coxsackieviruses, which are subtypes of enterovirus from the family *Picornaviridae* are usually responsible for this infection. (See Epidemic conjunctivitis). The greatest number of reports of conjunctivitis worldwide is shown on this webpage (http://www.promedmail.org). This page shows that since 2003, coxsackievirus A24 has been responsible for most outbreaks, followed by avian influenza conjunctivitis (H1N1).

5.1.2.4 Herpes conjunctivitis

Herpes (HSV) conjunctivitis produces insidious and recurrent forms, and therefore can be very difficult to eradicate. HSV1 causes the typical forms of herpetic keratitis but HSV2 conjunctivitis has also been reported in infants or adults with sexual herpes. In 1989, an outbreak of HSV1 in a school population in Minneapolis in Minnesota, USA affected 175 children, of which HSV1 was isolated in 35%.[56]

5.2 Prevention and control of outbreaks

Prevention and control of outbreaks of conjunctivitis are subject to support by the work in hospitals, community and laboratories.

Initially, it is essential to have a formal or informal surveillance (epidemiological work) to monitor infections that can commonly affect the health of a group. For example, causes of hemorrhagic conjunctivitis are subject to surveillance by national health systems of many countries.

One of the most important components in the presentation of any outbreak is medical and nursing staff who may become a source of contagion. This failure is due to widespread use of antibiotics and insufficient cleaning of surfaces and equipment due to reduced vigilance by medical staff and unsafe risk management. Hence, the use of preventive measures is necessary to cut the chain of transmission. Contact isolation is also critical to preventing outbreaks in institutions and should be strictly executed.

During epidemics, emphasis should be put on preventing the spread of infection, which is achieved by careful hand washing, cleaning and meticulous handling of objects that have been in contact with eye or respiratory secretions. It is also critical to consider that patients are contagious until the symptoms disappear completely.

The following is highly recommended:

- Wash hands immediately after treating or handling secretions from a patient diagnosed with probable or confirmed conjunctivitis. Hand washing should be performed even when latex gloves were used.
- Use gloves and lab coat if in contact with a patient or their body fluids.
- Use of personal protective measures when conducting procedures that may generate splashes to mucous membranes of the staff.
- Restrict access of health staff only to those who have direct patient responsibility.

- Medical equipment (apparatus and instruments) as well as chairs and tables of should be scrupulously disinfected to prevent contamination of other patients and/or health personnel.
- Patients should be isolated or grouped with other patients with an active infection with the same pathogen. It is important to restrict access to family, particularly in the case of neonates, infants or immunocompromised individuals. The material used with patients should be disposable equipment, or if that is not possible the equipment should be disinfected.

5.3 Outbreak vigilance

Preventive measures have the effect of decreasing the frequency and severity of outbreaks, however, personnel should be prepared to efficiently deal with them should they arise.
It is necessary to follow a methodology to reach containment of the outbreak to contain the damage to the population by: identifying risk factors, controlling sources of infection, implementation of interventions to prevent additional cases and breaking the chain of transmission.
The outbreak vigilance involves four phases (Figure 2):

i. Knowledge of the problem
ii. Critical phase (decision making)
iii. Care phase
iv. Resolution phase

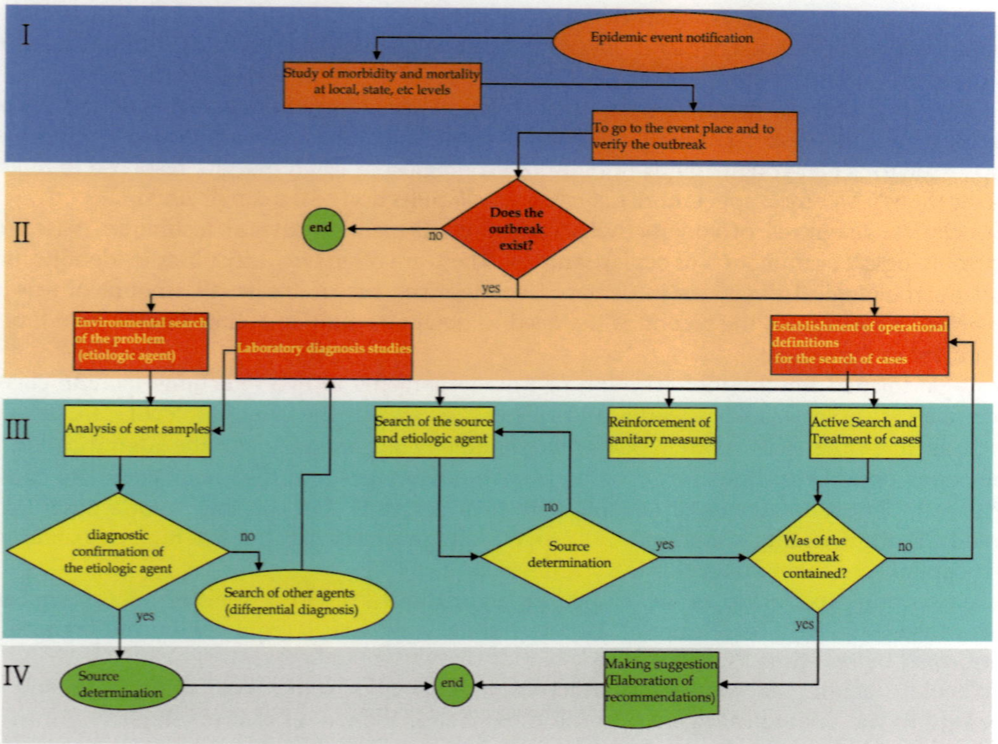

Fig. 2. Outbreak vigilance algorithm: I) Knowledge of the problem, II) Decision making, III) Attention of the outbreak and IV) Problem resolution.

Stage I requires detection of conjunctivitis cases and confirmation either in the hospital or the community. In Stage II, decisions are made to deal with extreme conditions and guide further action. The critical phase is essential, as it is necessary to react to suspected cases and identify the infectious agent in order that efficient control measures can be undertaken. This also allows the search for the pathogen in the environment or community (particularly in cases with contact transmission), as well as establishment of accurate diagnostic tests.[57-61]

5.4 Laboratory assays

The clinical manifestations of conjunctivitis suggest the possible etiology of infection, but the diagnosis should be confirmed by laboratory testing.

The type of inflammatory response (papillary, follicular, membranous, pseudomembranous or ulcerative granulomatous), time of onset, intensity and duration of inflammation (acute or chronic), type of discharge (mucoid, purulent or watery) and associated symptoms (itching, foreign body sensation) should be carefully evaluated and taken into consideration to establish a presumptive diagnosis.

Generally, bacterial conjunctivitis presents with diffusing conjunctival injection, conjunctival chemosis, papillary hypertrophy (in areas of conjunctiva firmly attached, such as the tarsus and semilunar fold) and purulent discharge.

The most frequent causative organisms with this pathology are *Staphylococcus* spp, *Neisseria gonorrhoeae or N. meningitidis, Streptococcus pneumoniae, Pseudomonas aeruginosa* or *Escherichia coli.*

Follicular conjunctivitis is characterized by tearing, mucopurulent discharge, redness, conjunctival follicles and cellular infiltration. It can be diagnosed as acute or chronic according to onset and duration of inflammation. Causes of acute follicular conjunctivitis include: acute adenovirus infection (pharyngoconjunctival fever), epidemic keratoconjunctivitis, herpes simplex, varicella zoster, and viral influenza. In contrast, chronic cases are caused by *Chlamydia* spp., toxic follicular conjunctivitis (molluscum contagiosum of lid margin, response to topical medications), *Moraxella* spp. and *Actinomyces israelli* (infection of the canaliculus).

The clinical diagnosis of conjunctivitis can be confirmed by several techniques based on microbiological examination of ocular samples. There are often two difficulties in identification and microbiological diagnosis in ocular infections. The first is the small amount of sample obtained from the eye; the second is the need to obtain a result in a short time to give timely treatment to the patient.

Tests performed for the identification of microorganisms in eye infections include classic microbiological tests, such as stains and cultures, as well as the use of molecular techniques such as real-time PCR. Both types of methodology are suitable for the identification of infectious organisms; however, they both have advantages and disadvantages. The classic tests can identify infectious organisms with near certainty, but can take a long time. Real-time PCR offers results in a short time, as well as high sensitivity, but has high costs and not all hospitals are able to offer this test routinely.

Based on our experience, we developed an algorithm for identification of microorganisms that cause conjunctivitis (Figure 3). Here we show how a presumptive clinical diagnosis is confirmed by real-time PCR.

Molecular techniques to identify microorganisms at species level allow tailoring of therapy to the etiological agent. On the other hand, the use of microbiological culture is not ruled out completely, as these can be used for confirmatory studies. Automated sequencing of 16S ribosomal genes to identify bacterial species may also be important for epidemiological studies.

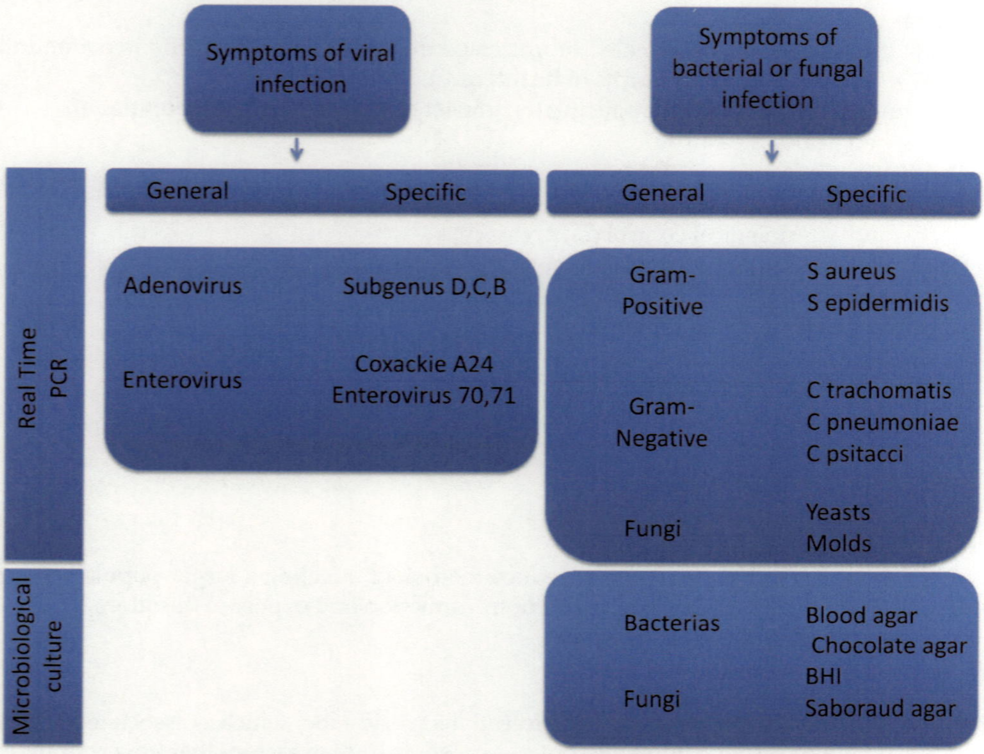

Fig. 3. Algorithm for identification of the causative agent of conjunctivitis.

5.5 Knowledge phase

- Formal notification sources: Weekly reporting of new cases, cases with poor outcomes, case study reporting, etc.
- Informal notification sources: Radio, television and other communication media.
- Comparison of the observed and expected incidence, mortality and morbidity statistics from affected area, as well as national and international spread.
- Information gathering: go to the affected area to verify the existence of outbreak.
- Confirm the diagnosis to ensure that the problem has been properly assessed (medical and laboratory assessment etc.).
- Association of two or more cases in time, place and person.
- Verify the presence or not of "artifacts" that could give false positive or negatives (intentional awareness campaigns, changes in case definition, implementation of new diagnostic tests, etc.).
- Standardize criteria for deciding the criteria for determining if a suspected patient is involved in the outbreak.
- Construct an operational definition of a case with:
  - Syndromic approach
  - Simple and clear
  - Broad enough to include all cases (sensitive) but restricted enough to capture only the affected group (specific).

5.6 Critical phase

- Know the number of cases treated or untreated by health staff (especially in community cases where there are other forms of health care).
- Give immediate attention to reducing the impact of the disease in the population.
- Strengthen health measures.
- Conduct a syndromic approach.
- Focus on known risk factors with measures to cut the chain of transmission.
- Carry out bacteriological control (if necessary).
- Determine and characterize the source of the outbreak.
  - Common
  - Propagated
  - Mixed
- Search the environment for propagating agents.
- Apply diagnostic battery for potential agents.
- Differential diagnosis.
- Analysis of environmental samples.

5.7 Resolution phase

This stage should give health advice to reduce the risk of affecting a larger population, and this should be tailored to the source, mode of transmission and exposure duration.

6. Conclusions

Conjunctivitis is one of the most common infections worldwide, which is associated with its significant potential for infection and spread as well as human factors that govern inherent susceptibility to infection.
Infectious conjunctivitis is responsible for many nosocomial and community outbreaks, as it may be transmitted by virtually all known routes. It is also responsible for epidemics and pandemics, such as the current hemorrhagic conjunctivitis outbreak caused by coxsackie A24.
Conjunctivitis, like many conditions, is not randomly distributed and requires a convergence of risk factors: genetic, immunological, environmental and pathogen-related. These risk factors are very broad in the case of conjunctivitis and there is the additional complication of fly vector transmission of trachoma and follicular conjunctivitis.
Epidemiological knowledge of conjunctivitis allows us to identify and react promptly to control outbreaks based on the determination of the source and the re-establishment of sanitary measures and basic hygiene.

7. Acknowledgements

We acknowledge the Institute of Ophthalmology "Fundación Conde de Valenciana" IAP for sponsoring this chapter and QBP Diana Gabriela Ponce Angulo, for his technical contributions to this paper. This work was support partially by CONACyT-126779.

8. References

[1] Moura, F. E., Ribeiro, D. C., Gurgel, N, da Silva Mendes, A. C., Tavares, F. N., Timóteo, C. N. and daSilva, E. E. (2006). Acute haemorrhagic conjunctivitis outbreak in the city of Fortaleza, northeast Brazil. *Br J Ophthalmol*, 90, 1091-1093.

[2] Wright, P. W., Strauss, G. H. and Langford, M. P. (1992). Acute hemorrhagic conjunctivitis. *Am Fam Physician*, 45, 173-178.

[3] Cabrerizo, M., Echevarria, J. E., Otero, A., Lucas, P. and Trallero, G. (2008). Molecular characterization of a coxsackievirus A24 variant that caused an outbreak of acute haemorrhagic conjunctivitis in Spain. *J Clin Virol*, 43, 323-327.

[4] Jun, E. J., Nam, Y. R., Ahn, J., Tchah, H., Joo, C. H., Jee, Y., Kim, Y. K. and Lee, H. (2008). Antiviral potency of a siRNA targeting a conserved region of coxsackievirus A24. *Biochem Biophys Res Commun*, 376, 389-394.

[5] Katiyar, B. C., Misra, S., Singh, R. B. and Singh, A. K. (1981). Neurological syndromes after acute epidemic conjunctivitis. *The Lancet*, 318, 866-867.

[6] Khan, A., Sharif, S., Shaukat, S., Khan S. and Zaidi, S. (2008). An outbreak of acute hemorrhagic conjunctivitis (AHC) caused by coxsackievirus A24 variant in Pakistan. *Virus Res*, 137, 150-152.

[7] Oberste, M. S., Maher, K., Kilpatrick, D. R., Flemister, M. R., Brown, B. A. and Pallansch, M. A. (1999). Typing of human enteroviruses by partial sequencing of VP1. *J Clin Microbiol*, 37, 1288-1293.

[8] Park, S. W., Lee, C. S., Jang, H. C., Kim, E. C., Oh, M. D. and Choe, K. W. (2005). Rapid identification of the Coxsackievirus A24 variant by molecular serotyping in an outbreak of acute hemorrhagic conjunctivitis. *J Clin Microbiol*, 43, 1069-1071.

[9] Wu, D., Ke, C. W., Mo, Y. L., Sun, L. M., Li, H., Chen, Q. X., Zou, L. R., Fang, L., Huang, P. and Zhen, H. Y. (2008). Multiple outbreaks of acute hemorrhagic conjunctivitis due to a variant of Coxsackievirus A24: Guangdong. *J Med Virol*, 80, 1762-1768.

[10] Goh, K. T., Ooi, P. L., Miyamura, K., Ogino, T. and Yamazaki, S. (1990). Acute haemorrhagic conjunctivitis: seroepidemiology of coxsackievirus A24 variant and enterovirus 70 in Singapore. *J Med Virol*, 31, 245-247.

[11] Lim, K. H., & Yin-Murphy, M. (1971). An epidemic of conjunctivitis in Singapore in 1970. *Singap Med J*, 12, 247-249.

[12] Oh, M., Park, S., Choi, Y., Kim, H., Lee, K., Park, W., Yoo, Y., Kim, E. and Choe, K. *(2003). Acute hemorrhagic conjunctivitis caused* by *coxsackievirus A24 variant. Emerg Infect Dis, 9, 1010-1012.*

[13] Bielory, L. (2008). Ocular allergy overview. *Immunol Allergy Clin North Am*, 29, 1-23.

[14] Pelikan, Z. (2009). Seasonal and perennial allergic conjunctivitis:the possible role of nasal allergy. *Clin Exp Ophthalmol*, 37, 448-457.

[15] Pelikan, Z. (2009). The possible involvement of nasal allergy in allergic keratoconjunctivitis. *Eye*, 23, 1653-1660.

[16] Bacon, A. S., Ahluwalia, P., Irani, A. M., Schwartz, L. B., Holgate, S. T., Church, M. K. and McGill, J. L. (2000). Tear and Conjunctival changes during the allergen-induced early- and late-phase responses. *J Allergy Clin Immunol*, 106, 948-954.

[17] Anderson, D. F. (1996). The conjunctival late-phase reaction and allergen provocation in the eye. *Clin Exp Allergy*, 26, 1105-1111.

[18] Pelikan, Z. (2010). Allergic conjunctivitis and nasal allergy. *Curr Allergy Asthma Rep*, 10, 295-302.

[19] Calder, V. L. (2002). Cellular mechanisms of chronic cell-mediated allergic conjunctivitis. *Clin Exp Allergy*, 8, 814-817.

[20] Leonardi, A., Fregona, I. A., Plebani, M., Secchi, A. G. and Calder, V. L. (2006). The1- and Th2-type cytokines in chronic ocular allergy. *Graefe's Arch Clin Exp Ophthalmol*, 244, 1240-1245.

[21] Bielory, L. and Friedlaender, M. H. (2008). Allergic conjunctivitis. *Immunol Allergy Clin North Am*, 28, 43-57.

[22] Sandor, F. and Buc, M. (2005). Toll like receptors. I Structure function and their ligands. *Folia Biologica (Praha)*, 51, 148-156.

[23] Du, X., Poltorak, A., Wei, Y. and Beautler, B. (2000). Tree novel mammalian toll-like receptor: gene structure, expression and evolution. *Eur Cytokine Netw*, 11, 362-371.

[24] Hajjar, A. M., O'Mahony, D. S., Ozinsky, A., Underhill, D. M., Aderem, A., Klebanoff, S. J. and Wilson, C. B. (2001). Cutting edge: Functional interaction between Toll-like receptor (TLR) 2 and TLR1 or TLR6 in response to phenol-soluble modulin. *J Immunol*, 166, 15-19.

[25] Morrison, L. A. (2004). The Toll of herpes simplex virus infection. *Trends Microbiol*, 12, 353-356.

[26] Murawski, M, R., Bowen, G. N., Cerny, A. M., Anderson, L. J., Haynes, L. M., Tripp R. A., Kurt-Jones, E. A. and Finberg, R. W. (2009). Respiratory syncytial virus activates innate immunity through Toll-like receptor 2. *J Virol*, 83, 1492-1500.

[27] Texereau, J., Chiche, J. D., Taylor, W., Choukroun, G., Comba, B., and Mira, J. P. (2005). The importance of Toll-like receptor 2 polymorphisms in severe infections. *Clin Infect Dis*, 41, 408-415.

[28] Bochud, P. Y., Magaret, A. S., Koelle, D. M., Aderem, A., and Wald, A. (2007). Polymorphisms in TLR2 are associated with increased viral shedding and lesional rate in patients with genital herpes simplex virus Type 2 infection. *J Infect Dis*, 196, 497-498.

[29] Amato-Almanza, M., Bautista-de Lucio V. M., Pérez-Cano, H. J. and Mejía-López, H. (2009). Polimorfismo del gen TLR2 como factor de riesgo en la infección oftálmica por adenovirus. *Rev Mex Oftalmol*, 83, 381-384.

[30] Rehaume, L. M. and Hancock, R.E. (2008). Neutrophil-derived defensins as modulators of innate immune function. Crit Rev Immunol, 28, 185-200.

[31] Yang, D., Chertov, O., Bykovskaia, S. N., Chen, Q., Buffo, M. J., Shogan, J., Anderson, M., Schröder, J. M., Wang, J. M., Howard, O. M. and Oppenheim, J. J. (1999). Beta-defensins: Linking innate and adaptive immunity through dendritic and T cell CCR6. *Science*, 286, 525-528.

[32] Harvey, S. A., Romanowski, E. G., Yates, K. A. and Gordon, Y.J. (2005). Adenovirus-directed ocular innate immunity: The role of conjunctival defensin-like chemokines (IP-10, I-TAC) and phagocytic human defensin-alpha. Invest Ophthalmol *Vis Sci*, 46, 3657-3665.

[33] Li, J., Raghunath, M., Tan, D., Lareu, R. R., Chen, Z. and Beuerman, R. W. (2006). Defensins HNP1 and HBD2 stimulation of wound-associated responses in human conjunctival fibroblasts. *Invest Ophthalmol Vis Sci*, 47, 3811-3819.

[34] Milanese, M., Segat, L. and Crovella, S. (2007). Transcriptional effect of DEFB1 gene 5' untranslated region polymorphisms. *Cancer Res*, 67, 5997.

[35] Sun, C. Q, Arnold, R., Fernandez, C., Parrish, A. B., Almekinder, T., He, J., Ho, S. M., Svoboda, P., Pohl, J., Marshall, F. F. and Petros, J. A. (2006). Human beta-defensin-

1, a potential chromosome 8p tumor suppressor: Control of transcription and induction of apoptosis in renal cell carcinoma. *Cancer Res*, 66, 8542-8549.

[36] Tesse, R., Cardinale, F., Santostasi, T., Polizzi, A., Manca, A., Mappa, L., Lacoviello, G., De Robertis, F., Logrillo, V. P. and Armenio, L. (2008). Association of beta-defensin-1 gene polymorphisms with *Pseudomonas aeruginosa* airway colonization in cystic fibrosis. *Genes Immun*, 9, 57-60.

[37] Braida, L., Boniotto, M., Pontillo, A., Tovo, P. A., Amoroso, A. and Crovella, S. (2004). A single-nucleotide polymorphism in the human beta-defensin 1 gene is associated with HIV-1 infection in Italian children. *AIDS*, 18, 1598-1600.

[38] Milanese, M., Segat, L., Pontillo, A., Arraes, L. C., De Lima Filho, J. L. and Crovella, S. (2006). DEFB1 gene polymorphisms and increased risk of HIV-1 infection in Brazilian children. *AIDS*, 20, 1673-1675.

[39] Jurevic, R. J., Bai, M., Chadwick, R. B., White, T. C. and Dale, B. A. (2003). Single-nucleotide polymorphisms (SNPs) in human beta-defensin 1: High-throughput SNP assays and association with Candida carriage in type I diabetics and nondiabetic controls. *J Clin Microbiol*, 41, 90-96.

[40] Carter, J. G., West, S. K., Painter, S., Haynes, R. J. and Churchill, A. J. (2009). Beta-Defensin 1 haplotype associated with postoperative endophthalmitis. Acta Ophthalmol, 88, 786-790.

[41] Crum, N. F, Barrozo C. P., Chapman,F. A. , Ryan, M. A. and Russell, K. L. (2004). An outbreak of conjunctivitis due to a novel unencapsulated *Streptococcus pneumoniae* among military trainees. *Clin Infect Dis*, 39, 1148-1154.

[42] Martin, M., Turco, J. H., Zegans, M. E., Facklam, R. R., Sodha, S., Elliott, J.A., Pryor, J. H., Beall, B., Erdman, D. D., Baumgartner, Y. Y., Sanchez, P. A., Schwartzman, J. D., Montero, J., Schuchat, A. and Whitney, C. G. (2003). An outbreak of conjunctivitis due to atypical Streptococcus pneumoniae. *N Engl J Med*, 348, 1112-1121.

[43] Buznach, N., Dagan, R. and Greenberg, D. (2005). Clinical and bacterial characteristics of acute bacterial conjunctivitis in children in the antibiotic resistance era. *Pediatr Infect Dis J*, 24, 823-828.

[44] Mikru, F.S., Molla, T., Ersumo, M., Henriksen, T. H., Klungseyr, P., Hudson, P.J. and Kindan T. T. (1991). Community-wide outbreak of Neisseria gonorrhoeae conjunctivitis in Konso district, North Omo administrative region. *Ethiop Med J*, 29, 27-35.

[45] Mak, D. B., Smith, D. W., Harnett, G. B. and Plant A. J. (2001). A large outbreak of conjunctivitis caused by a single genotype of *Neisseria gonorrhoeae* distinct from those causing genital tract infections. *Epidemio Infect*, 126, 373-378.

[46] Kakar, S., Bhalla, P., Maria, A., Rana, M., Chawla, R. and Mathur, N. B. (2010). Chlamydia trachomatis causing neonatal conjunctivitis in a tertiary care center. *Indian J Med Microbiol*, 28, 45-47.

[47] Krasny, J., Tomasova-Borovanska, J. and Hruba D. (2005). The Relationship between Chlamydia trachomatis and Chlamydia pneumoniae as the cause of neonatal conjunctivitis (ophthalmia neonatorum). *Ophthalmologica*, 219, 232-236.

[48] Thylefors, C., Dawson, C. R., Jones, B. R., West, S. K. and Taylor, H. R. (1987). A simple system for the assessment of trachoma and its complications. *Bull World Health Organ*, 65, 477- 483.

[49] Burton, M.J. and Mabey, D. C. W. (2009). The global burden of trachoma: A Review. *PloS Negl Trop Dis*, 3(10): e460.

[50] Dean, D., Kandel, R. P., Adhikari, H. K. and Hessel, T. (2008). Multiple Chlamydiaceae species in trachoma: implications for disease dathogenesis and control. *PLoS Med*, 5(1/e14):0057-0068.

[51] Cooper, R. J., Yeo, A. C., Bailey, A.S. and Tullo, A. B. (1999). Adenovirus polymerase chain reaction assay for rapid diagnosis of conjunctivitis. *Invest Ophthalmol Vis Sci*, 40, 90-95.

[52] Horwitz, M. S. (1996). Adenoviruses Chapter 68. In: Fields BN, Knipe DM, Howley, PM, et al. Fields Virology. Third Ed. *Lippincott Raven Publishers Philadelphia* p 2149.

[53] Shepetiuk, S. K., Norton, R., Kok, T. and Irving, L. G. (1999). Outbreak of adenovirus type 4 conjunctivitis in South Australia. *J Med Virol*, 41, 316-318.

[54] Jernigan, J. A., Lowry, B. S., Hayden, F. G., Kyger, S. A., Conway, B. P., Gröschel, D. H. M. and Farr, B. M. (1993). Adenovirus type 8 epidemic keratoconjunctivitis in an eye clinic: risk factor and control. *J Infect Dis*, 167, 1307-1313.

[55] Takeuchi, S., Itoh, N., Uchio, E., Tanaka, K., Kitamura, N., Kanai, H., Isobe, K., Aoki, K. and Ohno, S. (1999). Adenovirus strain of subgenus D associated with nosocomial infection as new etiological agents of epidemic keratoconjunctivitis in Japan. *J Clin Microbiol*, 37, 3392-3394.

[56] Belongia, E. A., Goodman, J. L., Holland, E. J., Andres, C. W., Homann, S. R., Mahanti, R. L., Mizener, M. W., Erice, A. and Osterholm, M.T. (1991). An outbreak of herpes gladiatorum at a high-school wrestling camp. *N Engl J Med*, 325, 906-910.

[57] Aoki, K. and Sawada, H. (1992). Long-term observation of neutralization antibody after enterovirus 70 infection. *Jpn J Ophthalmol*, 36, 465-468.

[58] Jun, E. J., Won, M. A., Ahn, J., Ko A., Moon, H., Tchah, H., Kim, Y. K. and Lee, H. (2011). An antiviral small-interfering RNA simultaneously effective against the most prevalent enteroviruses causing acute hemorrhagic conjunctivitis. *Invest Ophthalmol, Vis Sci*, 52, 58-63.

[59] Langford. M.P., Ball, W. A. and Ganley, J. P. (1995). Inhibition of the enteroviruses that cause acute hemorrhagic conjunctivitis (AHC) by benzimidazoles, enviroxime (LY 122772) and enviradone (LY 127123). *Antiviral Res*, 27, 355-365.

[60] Nigrovic, L. E. and Chiang, V. W. (2000). Cost analysis of enteroviral polymerase chain reaction in infants with fever and cerebrospinal fluid pleocytosis. *Arch Pediatr Adolesc Med*, 154, 817-821.

[61] Xiao, X. L., Wu, H., Li, Y. J., Li, H. F., He, Y. Q., Chen, G., Zhang, J. W., Yang, H., Li, X. F., Yang, X. Q. and Yu, Y. G. (2009). Simultaneous detection of enterovirus 70 and coxsackievirus A24 variant by multiplex real-time RT-PCR using an internal control. *J Virol Meth*, 159, 23-28.

Part 2

Clinical Aspects and Features of Conjunctivitis

2

Clinical Features of Infectious Conjunctivitis

Udo Ubani
Dept of Optometry, Abia state university, Uturu
Nigeria

1. Introduction

Conjunctivitis is the inflammation of the conjunctiva, a thin, translucent, relatively elastic tissue layer with bulbar, forniceal and palpebral portions (figure1). The bulbar portion lines the outer aspect of the globe, whiles the forniceal which is loose and redundant swells easily and is thrown into folds. The palpebral portion covers the inside of the eyelids firmly adherent to the tarsal plates.

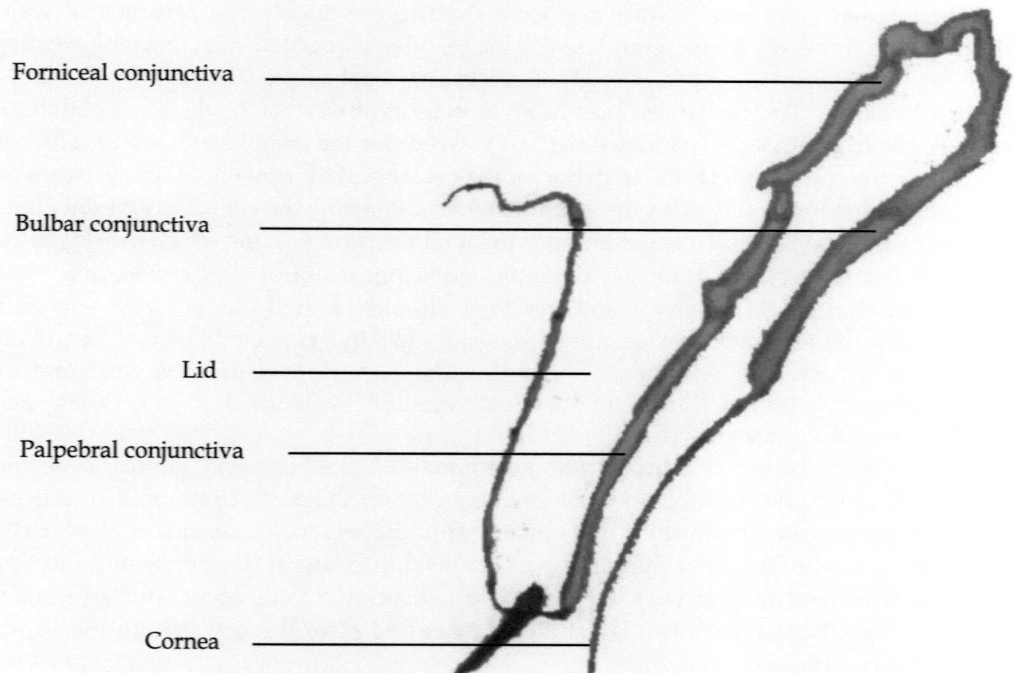

Fig. 1. Portions of the conjunctiva

Conjunctivitis usually presents with eye itching, burning and a sensation of foreign body. The others symptoms are blurred vision, photophobia and ocular pain. While the signs could be hyperaemia, injection, chemosis, hyperlacrimation, discharges, palpebral edema,

follicular and papillary hypertrophy, membrane formation and reactions of lymphatic system. On the cornea there is diminished sheen, transparency and reflexion; Horner-Trantas dots, corneal epithelial defects and scars. These signs and symptoms participate to varying degrees in the differential diagnosis of the various forms of conjunctivitis.
The forms of conjunctivitis are basically 1)Irritant- with a non-specific substance from an eyelash that got stuck to a chemical; 2) allergic- when an allergen comes into contact with the eye, such as dust mites, pollen or animal fur and; 3)Infectious - caused by a bacteria or virus. Others are forms associated with disorders of the ocular adnexia - the lacrimal system, the palpebral (skin, lashes and glands); and disorders of adjacent organs like nasal mucosa, paranasal sinuses and middle ear.
Infectious conjunctivitis accounts for 35% of all eye-related problems recorded by the health service schemes worldwide. This chapter focuses on the clinical features of infectious conjunctivitis

2. Ocular discharges

Ocular discharge can be divided into two main types, serous discharge or the 'wet eye', and purulent discharge. With the terms mucoid (stringy or ropy) or mucopurulent further used to describe purulent discharge. A serous discharge is most commonly associated with viral or allergic ocular conditions. While a mucoid discharge is highly characteristic of toxic, Chlamydial or dry eyes. A mucopurulent discharge, often associated with morning crusting and difficulty opening the eyelids, strongly suggests a bacterial infection.
Serous discharge: The ocular surface receives sensory innervation via the ophthalmic branch of the trigeminal nerve (cranial nerve V), except for the lateral canthal area which is supplied by the maxillary branch. Irritation of the ocular surface trigeminal nerve causes an increased production of the reflex tear volume which augments the conjunctival epithelium basal cells tear production. This will increase the total tear film volume which overloads the capacity of the nasolacrimal drainage apparatus and is thus manifested as a 'wet eye'.
Purulent discharge: Bacteriology and cytology should be performed in an eye with purulent discharge; with bacteriology samples ideally collected before antibiotic treatment is started. Differentiation of normal ocular flora from pathogenic flora may be difficult, however normal flora tend to be represented by more than one isolate and usually appear in lighter growth.
The most frequent causes of mucopurulent conjunctivitis are Neisseria. gonorrhoeae and Neisseria meningitidis, with N. gonorrhoeae being by far the more common. Gonococcal ocular infection usually presents in neonates (ophthalmia neonatorum) and sexually active young adults. Affected infants typically develop bilateral discharge three to five days after birth. Transmission of the Neisseria organism to infants occurs during vaginal delivery. In adults, the organism is usually transmitted from the genitalia to the hands and then to the eyes.

3. Conjunctival reaction

The stroma or substantia propria layer of the conjunctiva is a richly vascularized connective tissue, divided into the deep thicker fibrous subconjunctival, which is continuous with the tarsal plates and the superficial adenoid lymphoid tissue.

Follicles consist of hyperplasia of the lymphoid tissue of the stroma. Follicular conjunctival responses appear as smooth, rounded nodules. These nodules are avascular at their apices and are surrounded by fine vessels at their bases (figure 2). They are usually most prominent in the forniceal conjunctiva. The main causes of follicular conjunctivitis include adenoviral infection, primary herpes simplex viral infection, molluscum contagiosum infection, enteroviral infection, chlamydial infection, and toxicity from certain medications.

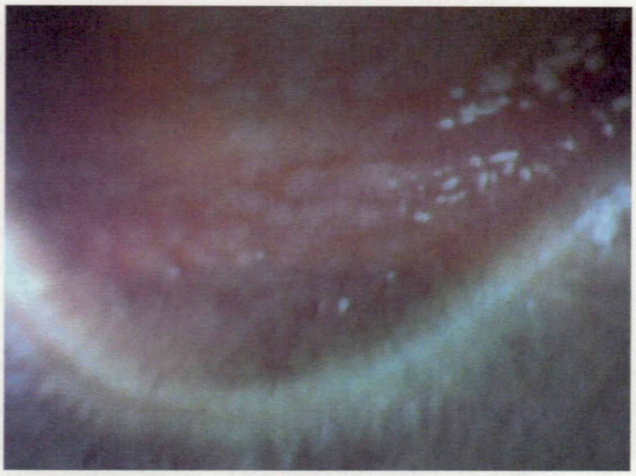

Fig. 2. Follicles at the lower fornix

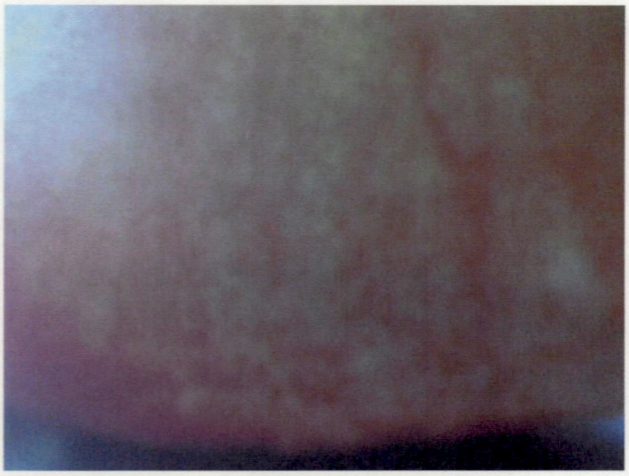

Fig. 3. Papillae reaction of the upper palpebral conjunctiva

In contrast to a follicular conjunctival response, a papillary conjunctival response is nonspecific and can be caused by many agents. It can occur in any nonspecific conjunctival inflammation, including mechanical irritation and allergic eye disease. It is usually seen on the upper tarsal conjunctiva, a papillary response is a fine mosaic pattern of dilated, telangiectatic blood vessels (figure 3). Papillae vary in size from tiny red dots to polygonal elevations. Each papilla has a central fibrovascular core that gives rise to a vessel branching outward in a spoke like pattern. The connective tissue septa surrounding the papillae are anchored in the conjunctival stroma, resulting in hyperemic areas surrounded by pale tissue when papillary hypertrophy occurs. With prolonged inflammation, the septa may rupture, leading to either papillary confluence, as in infections of bacteria or giant papillae of vernal conjunctivitis.

4. Regional lymphadenopathy

Lymph via afferent lymphatic vessels circulates to and drains into the lymph node; a small ball or an oval-shaped organ ranging in size from a few millimeters to about 1-2 cm in their normal state. Lymph nodes are important in the proper functioning of the immune system. A lymph node can be very well described as a garrison of B, T and other immune cells. In this, during an infection, the lymph nodes function to monitor the lymph for foreign particles, filtering and catching viruses, bacteria, and other unknown materials which they then destroy. With this, the lymph nodes have the clinical significance of becoming inflamed or enlarged (lymphadenopathy) primarily because there is an elevated rate of trafficking of lymphocytes into the node, exceeding the efferent lymphatic vessel rate of outflow from the node, and secondarily as a result of the activation and proliferation of antigen-specific T and B cells.

Humans have approximately 500-600 lymph nodes distributed widely throughout the body, with clusters in the neck, armpits and groin regions. The lymphatic drainage of the conjunctiva is to the preauricular and the submandibular nodes (figure 4). In conjunctivitis, the patient is examined in a well-lit room for this regional lymphadenopathy.

Regional lymphadenopathy often coexists with follicular conjunctivitis representing a similar lymphoblastic proliferation.

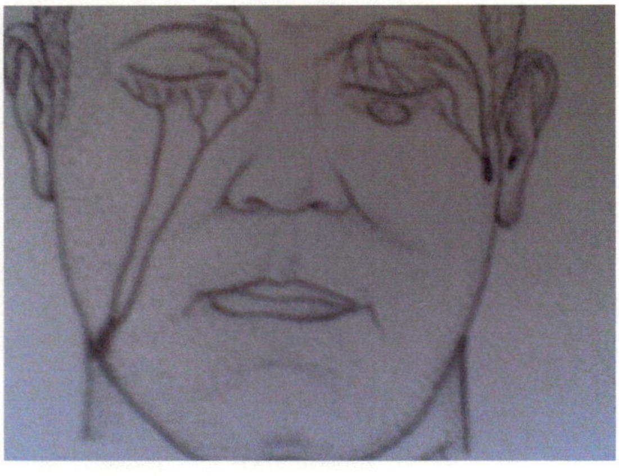

Fig. 4. Lymphatic drainage of the conjunctiva

Viral or chlamydial inclusion conjunctivitis typically presents with a small, tender, preauricular or submandibular lymph node. Toxic conjunctivitis secondary to topical medications can also produce a palpable preauricular node. Palpable adenopathy is rare in acute bacterial conjunctivitis. The exception is hyperacute conjunctivitis caused by infection with Neisseria species.

Other facial clues to the etiology of conjunctivitis include the presence of herpes labialis or a dermatomal vesicular eruption suggestive of shingles. Either of these findings may indicate a herpetic source of conjunctivitis.

5. Membrane formation

Pseudomembranes consist of coagulated exudates which adhere loosely to the inflamed conjunctiva. They are typically not integrated with the conjunctival epithelium and can be removed by peeling, leaving the conjunctival epithelium intact (figure 5). Their removal produces little if any bleeding. Epidemic keratoconjunctivitis (EKC), ligneous conjunctivitis (a rare idiopathic bilateral membranous/pseudomembranous conjunctivitis seen in children with thick, ropy, white discharge on the upper tarsal conjunctiva), allergic conjunctivitis, and bacterial infections are the primary causes.

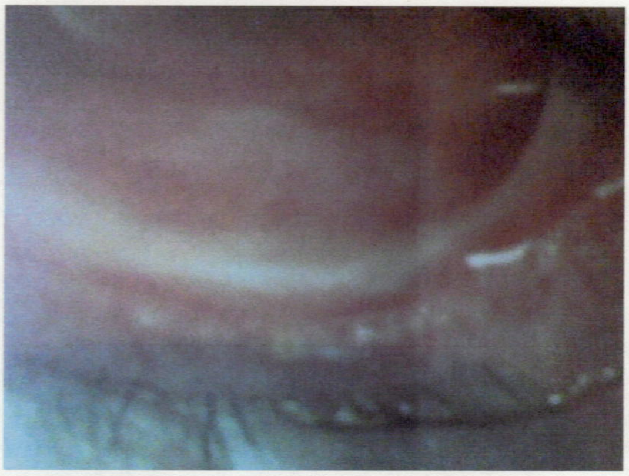

Fig. 5. Conjunctival pseudomembrane

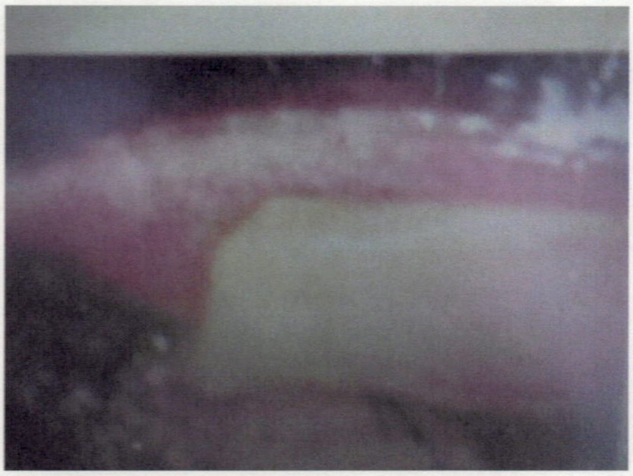

Fig. 6. Tarsal conjunctival True membrane

A **true membrane** forms when the fibrinous excretory or inflammatory exudate that is secreted by invading microorganisms or ocular tissues permeates the superficial layers of the conjunctival epithelium. True membranes become interdigitated with the vascularity of the conjunctival epithelium. They adhere firmly; tearing and bleeding often result when removed (figure 6). B-hemolytic streptococci, Neisseria gonorrhoeae, Corynebacterium diphtheriae, Stevens-Johnson syndrome (severe systemic vesiculobullous eruptions affecting the mucous membranes-erythema multiforme) and chemical or thermal burns are among the common etiologic sources.

5.1 Ecchymosis or subconjunctival haemorrhage

A subconjunctival hemorrhage is a bleeding underneath the conjunctiva. This varies in extent from small petechial hemorrhage to an extensive spreading under the bulbar conjunctiva; as a flat sheet of homogeneous bright red colour with well defined limits (figure 7). As the condition doesn't cause any pain or discomfort, the condition might be noticed by a collaegue before the patient spots it. subconjunctival hemorrhage can look extremely ugly. However, like a bruise, it will start to fade, turning bluish, green, and yellowish before disappearing entirely. Petechial subconjunctival haemorrhages are usually associated with acute picornavirus and pneumococcal infections.

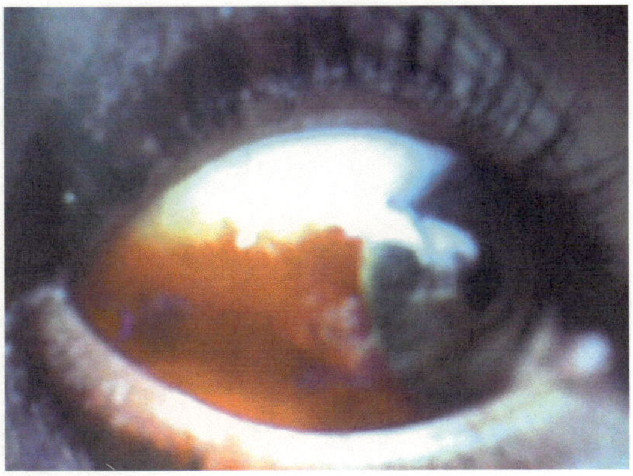

Fig. 7. Conjunctival hemorrhage

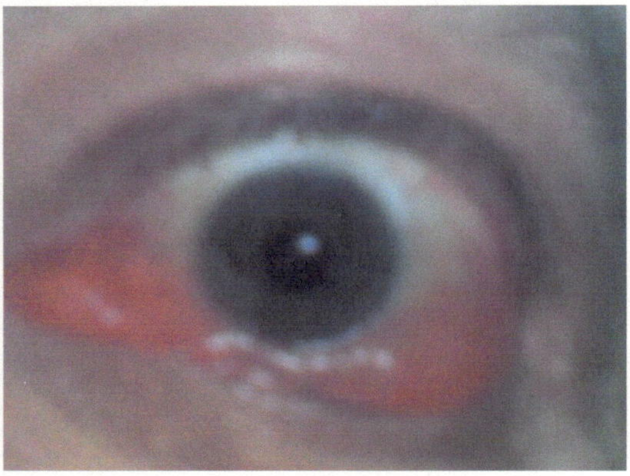

Fig. 8. Chemosis

5.2 Conjunctival injection

Conjunctival injection is an intense focal hyperemia that can outline the overlying rectus tendon.

5.3 Chemosis

Chemosis is an oedema of the conjunctiva that appears as a fold of redundant conjunctiva hanging over the mucocutaneous junction of the lowerlid (figure 8)

5.4 Corneal involvement

A complication of infectious conjunctivitis is the involvement of the layers of the cornea. The study is usually by staining with flourescein [which stays outside the cells] and rose bengal [which has affinity for dead and degenerating cells]. Observation with slit lamp biomicroscope can describe some features-

5.5 Puuctate epithelium keratitis

Punctate epithelium keratitis is characterized by a breakdown or damage of the epithelium of the cornea in a pinpoint pattern. Lesions stain well with Rose Bengal and poorly with flourscein. It usually marks a viral infection.

5.6 Dendritic ulcer

Still on the epithelium a dendrite ulceration which is usually single or multiple can be described as an earlier opaque cells arranged in a dendritic, punctuate or stellate pattern. Later a linear branching ulcer begins to form following desquamation. The center of the ulcer stain with fluorescein and the virus laden cells of the margin of the ulcer stain with Rose Bengal. Occasionally, the continual enlargement of the dendritic leads to a larger epithelial defect termed geographical.

In the subepithelial space an ingrowth of fibrovascular tissue from the limbus may develop, this is called **Pannus.**

5.7 Interstitial keratitis

In the stroma, a cellular infiltration of leucocytes into the stroma layer of the cornea without involving the epithelium or endothelium is known as interstitial keratitis. It is most notably associated with congenital syphilis and tuberculosis.

5.8 Disciform keratitis

Deep on the posterior layer, disciform keratitis also called endothelitis describes a fold in the descements membrane. It is either caused by a reactivated viral infection of the corneal endothelium or a hypersensitive reaction to antigen.

5.9 Diagnostic procedures of infectious conjunctivitis

Cultures usually are not required in patients with mild conjunctivitis. But in patients who have severe inflammation (e.g., hyperacute purulent conjunctivitis), chronic or recurrent conjunctivitis and who do not respond to treatment; cytology and specimens for cultures are obtained by scraping the conjunctiva. This helps to diagnose allergic, chlamydial, other infectious conjunctivitis and certain atypical forms of conjunctivitis in which the clinical diagnosis is not immediately apparent.

In **hyperacute bacterial conjunctivitis** which is a sight-threatening, severe infection with abrupt onset and characterized by a copious yellow-green purulent discharge that reaccumulates after being wiped away an immediate ophthalmic work-up and management is needed.

The most frequent causes are N. gonorrhoeae and Neisseria meningitidis, with N. gonorrhoeae being by far the more common. These two infections have similar clinical presentations, and can be distinguished only in the microbiology laboratory.

Gonococcal conjunctival infection usually presents in neonates (ophthalmia neonatorum) and sexually active young adults. Affected infants typically develop bilateral discharge three to five days after birth if delivery was vaginal. In adults, the organism is usually transmitted from the genitalia to the hands and then to the eyes.

If a gonococcal ocular infection is left untreated, rapid and severe corneal involvement is inevitable. The resulting ulceration and, ultimately, perforation lead to profound and sometimes permanent loss of vision. Infected infants may also have other localized gonococcal infections, such as rhinitis or proctitis, or they may have disseminated gonococcal infection, such as arthritis, meningitis, pneumonia or sepsis.

The diagnostic work-up for a gonococcal ocular infection includes immediate Gram staining of specimens for gram-negative intracellular diplococci, as well as special cultures for Neisseria species. All patients should be treated with systemic antibiotics supplemented by topical ocular antibiotics and saline irrigation.

Over 30 percent of patients with gonococcal conjunctivitis have concurrent chlamydial venereal disease. For this reason, it is advisable to treat patients with supplemental oral antibiotics that are effective against Chlamydia species.

Acute bacterial conjunctivitis typically presents with burning, irritation, tearing and, usually, a mucopurulent discharge.

Patients with this condition often report that their eyelids are matted together on awakening in the morning. Conjunctival swelling and mild eyelid edema may be noted. The symptoms of acute bacterial conjunctivitis are less severe, less rapid in onset, and progress at a slower rate than hyperacute conjunctivitis.

The three most common pathogens in bacterial conjunctivitis are Streptococcus pneumoniae, Haemophilus influenzae and Staphylococcus aureus. Infections with S. pneumoniae and H. influenzae are more common in children, while S. aureus most frequently affects adults.

Acute bacterial conjunctivitis is usually self-limited and does not cause any serious harm; but there are several reasons for which treatment should be given. These include decreasing patient morbidity by shortening the course of the disease, reducing person-to-person spread, lowering the risk of sight-threatening complications such as corneal ulceration, and eliminating the risk of more widespread extra ocular disease.

Cultures need be obtained in young children and debilitated persons and empiric treatment with a topical medication is a safe and cost-effective approach in most patients with clinically mild acute bacterial conjunctivitis.

Chronic bacterial conjunctivitis is mostly caused by Staphylococcus species. This type of conjunctivitis often develops in association with blepharitis, which is often unrecognized. Some cases of chronic bacterial conjunctivitis are also associated with facial seborrhea.

The symptoms of chronic bacterial conjunctivitis vary and can include itching, burning, a foreign-body sensation and morning eyelash crusting. Signs of this conjunctival condition include flaky debris, erythema and warmth along the lid margins, as well as eyelash loss and bulbar conjunctival injection. Some patients with chronic bacterial conjunctivitis also have recurrent styes and chalazia of the lid margin.

Meibomian is the sebaceous glands that line the posterior lid margin behind the eyelashes. They secrete an important oily component of the tear film. When inflamed, the meibomian glands malfunction, producing chronic inflammation of the eyelid margins and the conjunctiva, as well as irritating dry-eye symptoms. This condition is referred to as meibomianitis.

Blepharoconjunctivitis and meibomianitis are common in patients with acne rosacea.

The work-up of patients with chronic conjunctivitis and blepharoconjunctivitis involves culturing the conjunctiva and the eyelid margins to identify the predominant bacterial pathogen. Treatment includes the establishment of good eyelid hygiene using warm compresses and eyelid margin scrubs and the application of appropriate topical antimicrobials

Chlamydia trachomatis ocular infection occurs in two distinct clinical forms: - trachoma (associated with serotypes A through C) and inclusion conjunctivitis (associated with serotypes D through K).

Trachoma, a chronic keratoconjunctivitis, is the most common cause of ocular morbidity and preventable blindness throughout the world. It is a public health concern in the rural areas of developing countries. Patients who have emigrated from regions in which trachoma is endemic frequently present to with cicatricial ocular and eyelid changes secondary to previous recurrent infections.

Inclusion conjunctivitis is primarily a sexually transmitted disease that occurs in both adults (adult inclusion conjunctivitis) and newborns (ophthalmia neonatorum) exposed during vaginal delivery to C. trachomatis from the mother's infected cervix.

Neonatal inclusion conjunctivitis usually responds to topical antibiotics. However, this condition can be associated with otitis media, and respiratory and gastrointestinal tract infections. Adult inclusion conjunctivitis typically presents in young, sexually active persons between 18 and 30 years of age. Transmission most often occurs by self inoculation from infected genital secretions. The usual presentation is subacute or chronic infection characterized by unilateral or bilateral redness, mucopurulent discharge, a foreign-body sensation and preauricular adenopathy.

Laboratory tests are indicated in neonates and adults with suspected inclusion conjunctivitis. Most affected adults have concurrent, possibly asymptomatic chlamydial urethritis or cervicitis. There is also coinfection with pathogens that cause other sexually transmitted diseases like syphilis and gonorrhea. Therefore, once a diagnosis has been established, a genital work-up of the patient and his or her sexual contacts is indicated before antibiotic treatment is initiated.

Adenovirus is by far the most common cause of viral conjunctivitis. **Viral conjunctivitis** often occurs in community epidemics, with the virus transmitted in schools, workplaces and physicians offices. The usual modes of transmission are contaminated fingers, medical instruments and swimming pool water. Proper hand and instrument washing following patient contact can help to reduce the spread of this highly contagious infection.

Patients with viral conjunctivitis typically present with an acutely red eye, watery discharge, conjunctival swelling, a tender preauricular node, and, in some cases, photophobia and a foreign-body sensation. Occasionally, patients also have subconjunctival hemorrhage. Both eyes may be affected simultaneously, or the second eye may become involved a few days after the first eye. Some patients have an associated upper respiratory tract infection.

Since the ocular infection is contagious for at least seven days, patients should be instructed to avoid direct contact with other persons for at least one week after the onset of symptoms. Treatment is supportive. Cold compresses and topical vasoconstrictors may provide symptomatic relief. Topical antibiotics are rarely necessary, because secondary bacterial infection is uncommon.

Differential diagnosis of conjunctivitis	
Type of Conjunctivitis	**Clinical features**
Allergic	
Seasonal allergic	Bilateral. Conjunctival injection, chemosis, watery discharge, mild mucus discharge.
Vernal	Bilateral. Giant papillary hypertrophy of superior tarsal conjunctiva, bulbar conjunctival injection, conjunctival scarring, watery and mucoid discharge, limbal Trantas dots, limbal "papillae," corneal epithelial erosions, corneal neovascularization and scarring, corneal vernal plaque/shield ulcer.
Atopic	Bilateral. Eczematoid blepharitis; eyelid thickening, scarring; lash loss; papillary hypertrophy of superior and inferior tarsal conjunctiva; conjunctival scarring; watery or mucoid discharge; boggy edema; corneal neovascularization, ulcers, and scarring; punctate epithelial keratitis; keratoconus; subcapsular cataract.
Viral	
Adenoviral	Abrupt onset. Unilateral or bilateral. Varies in severity. Bulbar conjunctival injection, watery discharge, follicular reaction of inferior tarsal conjunctiva, chemosis.
	Distinctive signs: preauricular lymphadenopathy, petechial and subconjunctival hemorrhage, corneal epithelial defect, multifocal epithelial punctate keratitis evolving to anterior stromal keratitis, membrane/pseudomembrane formation, eyelid ecchymosis.
Herpes simplex virus	Unilateral. Bulbar conjunctival injection, watery discharge, mild follicular reaction of conjunctiva. May have palpable preauricular node.
	Distinctive signs: vesicular rash or ulceration of eyelids, pleomorphic or dendritic epithelial keratitis of cornea or conjunctiva.
Molluscum contagiosum	Typically unilateral but can be bilateral. Mild to severe follicular reaction, punctate epithelial keratitis. May have corneal pannus, especially if longstanding.
	Distinctive signs: Single or multiple shiny, dome-shaped umbilicated lesion(s) of the eyelid skin or margin.
Bacterial	
Nongonococcal	Unilateral. Bulbar conjunctival injection, purulent or mucopurulent discharge.
Gonococcal	Unilateral or bilateral. Marked eyelid edema, marked bulbar conjunctival injection, marked purulent discharge, preauricular lymphadenopathy.
	Important sign to detect: corneal infiltrate.

Differential diagnosis of conjunctivitis	
Type of Conjunctivitis	**Clinical features**
Chlamydial	Unilateral or bilateral.
Neonate/Infant	Eyelid edema, bulbar conjunctival injection, discharge may be purulent or mucopurulent, no follicles.
Adult	Bulbar conjunctival injection, follicular reaction of tarsal conjunctiva, mucoid discharge, corneal pannus, punctate epithelial keratitis, preauricular lymphadenopathy.
	Distinctive sign: bulbar conjunctival follicles.

Table 1.

Herpes simplex virus keratoconjunctivitis closely resemble the presentation of ocular adenovirus infection. In such patients, topical corticosteroid therapy can lead to severe ocular complications as a result of uncontrolled virus proliferation. Therefore, topical corticosteroids should not be used in the management of infectious conjunctivitis unless under the directive of a physician. Viral conjunctivitis is generally benign and self-limiting. Treatment with corticosteroids can prolong the course of the disease and also place the patient at risk for other steroid-induced ocular complications, such as glaucoma and cataracts.

Ocular infections due to herpes simplex and herpes zoster are becoming more prevalent as the incidence of human immunodeficiency virus infection continues to increase. Ocular herpes simplex and herpes zoster are managed with topical and/or systemic antiviral agents.

Conjunctivitis caused by an allergic reaction clears up once the allergen is removed. However, allergic conjunctivitis will likely recur if the individual again comes into contact with the particular allergen.

Ocular allergy encompasses a spectrum of distinct clinical conditions characterized by itching. The common of ones are seasonal allergic rhinoconjunctivitis, also called hay fever rhinoconjunctivitis and vernal in which a small, white, calcareouslike cellular infiltrates occurring on the edge of the conjunctiva (Horners trantas dot).

Seasonal allergic rhinoconjunctivitis is an IgE-mediated hypersensitivity reaction precipitated by small airborne allergens. The condition is usually, seasonal. Patients typically experience intermittent itching, tearing, redness and mild eyelid swelling. The personal or family history is often positive for other atopic conditions, such as allergic rhinitis, asthma or eczema.

Treatment measures for seasonal allergic rhinoconjunctivitis include allergen avoidance, cold compresses, vasoconstrictors, antihistamine drops, topical nonsteroidal anti-inflammatory agents and mast-cell stabilizers. Immunotherapy is also beneficial in some patients with allergic conjunctivitis.

6. References

American Academy of Ophthalmology Corneal/External Disease Panel. Preferred Practice Pattern: Conjunctivitis. San Francisco, Ca: AAO; 2003.

Baum J, Barza M. The evolution of antibiotic therapy for bacterial conjunctivitis and keratitis: 1970-2000. Cornea. 2000;19:659-672.

Block SL, Hedrick J, Tyler R, et al. Increasing bacterial resistance in pediatric acute conjunctivitis (1997-1998). Antimicrob Agents Chemother. 2000;44:1650-1654.

Borel JF, Baumann G, Chapman l. In vivo Pharmacological Effects of Cyclosporin and Some Analogues. PharmacoL 1996;35:115-246.

Greenberg MF, Pollard ZF. The red eye in childhood. Pediatr Clin North Am. 2003;50:105-124.

Kanski JJ. Disorders of the conjunctiva. Clinical ophthalmology: A systematic approach. 3rd edition Butterworth-Heinemann. Oxford 1998; pp71-74

Langley JM. Adenoviruses. Pediatr Rev. 2005;26:238-242.

Rietveld RP, ter Riet G, Bindels JE. Predicting bacterial cause in infectious conjunctivitis: cohort study on informativeness of combinations of signs and symptoms. Br Med J. 2004;329:206-208.

Rose PW, Harnden A, Brueggemann AB, et al. Chloramphenicol treatment for acute infective conjunctivitis in children in primary care: a randomized double-blind placebo-controlled trial. Lancet. 2005;8:37-43.

Stem ME, Beuerman RW, Fox Rl. The pathology of dry eye: The interaction between the ocular surface and lacrimal glands. Cornea. 1998;17:584-589.

Wald ER. Periorbital and orbital infections. Pediatr Rev. 2004;25:312-319.

Warwick, Roger; Peter L. Williams "Angiology (Chapter 6)". *Gray's anatomy*. illustrated by Richard E. M. Moore (Thirty-fifth ed.). London: Longman.1973; pp. 588–785.

3

Allergic Conjunctivitis: An Immunological Point of View

Atzin Robles-Contreras and Concepción Santacruz et al.*
Research Unit and Department of Immunology
Institute of Ophthalmology "Fundación Conde de Valenciana", Mexico City
Laboratory of Molecular Immunology, National School of Biological Sciences
IPN Mexico City
México

1. Introduction

Allergic conjunctivitis (AC) is an inflammation of the conjunctiva secondary to an immune response to external antigens, usually called allergens. This inflammation could be IgE-mediated and non-IgE mediated and atopy could play a significant role in clinical evolution. (Johansson et al., 2004) AC is not a single disease; in fact it is a syndrome affecting the entire ocular surface, including conjunctiva, lids, cornea, and tear film. The signs and symptoms of allergic conjunctivitis have a meaningful effect on comfort and patient health, and are influenced by genetics, environment, ocular microbiota, and immune regulation mechanisms, all of which work together in a complex immunological response. Dysregulation in such immune homeostasis could turn into a variety of allergic ocular diseases (AOD). This chapter describes the current understanding of cellular and molecular pathways involved in different AOD, the clinical characteristics of ocular allergies, the new therapies related to control of immune activation, and the importance of basic research to generate new types of immunotherapy to treat allergic conjunctivitis

2. Immunological mechanisms of allergic conjunctivitis

Two stages have been defined in AC immune pathophysiology. The first stage is named sensitization phase reaction, and is initiated by preferential activation and polarization of the immune response to environmental antigens, that culminates with a generation of a predominant Th2 immune response and production of IgE antibodies; the second stage, named effector phase reaction, is initiated with a second encounter with antigen (Ag)

*Julio Ayala[1], Eduardo Bracamontes[2], Victoria Godinez[1], Iris Estrada-García[3], Sergio Estrada-Parra[3], Raúl Chávez[4], Mayra Perez-Tapia[3], Victor M. Bautista-De Lucio[1] and Maria C. Jiménez-Martínez[1,4]**
[1]*Research Unit and Department of Immunology, Institute of Ophthalmology "Fundación Conde de Valenciana", Mexico City, Mexico*
[2]*ETN Department, "Clínica de Especialidades con CECIS Churubusco", ISSSTE, Mexico City, México*
[3]*Laboratory of Molecular Immunology, National School of Biological Sciences, IPN, Mexico City, México*
[4]*Department of Biochemistry, Faculty of Medicine, UNAM, Mexico City, México*
**Corresponding Author

leading to activation of effector mechanisms, such as degranulation of granulocytes and release of histamine (Abelson et al., 2003).

2.1 Sensitization phase reaction

It has been reported in patients with asthma (Takhar et al., 2007) and allergic rhinitis (Takhar et al., 2005), that both, bronchial and nasal mucosa, have the ability to capture Ag trough Langerhans cells (LC). LC could process and present Ag in the context of MHC-II molecules and stimulate specific CD4+T cells to induce secretion of interleukin (IL)-4, IL-13 and expression of CD154; this process activates genetic recombination in B cells and class switching to IgE. Similar mechanism could be involved in ocular mucosa, since it has been reported that IgE could be detectable in human tears (Allansmith et al., 1976) and B cells located in the conjunctival lymphoid follicles are CD23+ CD21+ CD40+, suggesting that they might be precursors of IgE-producing B cells and contribute to local IgE synthesis (Abu El-Asrar et al., 2001).

2.2 Effector phase reaction

Allergen-induced cell degranulation is the key event in allergic inflammation and leads to early-phase symptoms. Early phase reaction (EPR) has been studied extensively in both humans and animals; EPR is initiated with a second encounter with the antigen by IgE previously attached to IgE receptors (FcεRI, FcεRII or CD23). Cross-linking of IgE receptors induces: a) release of preformed mediators such as histamine, proteases and chemotactic factors; b) activation of transcription factors and cytokine gene expression, and c) production of prostaglandins and leukotrienes by phospholipase A2 pathway. Activation of mast cells by IgE in conjunctiva is relevant since it is well known that there are up to 6000 cell/mm^3 in conjunctiva (Bielory, 2000) and mast cell density is increased in acute and chronic conjunctivitis patients (Anderson et al., 1997; Morgan et al., 1991). Activated mast cells can release several cytokines such as IL-4, IL-6, IL-13, and Tumor Necrosis Factor (TNFα) contributing to increase local inflammatory Th2 response (Anderson et al., 2001; Cook et al., 1998), and also are able to increase FcεRI density in chronic keratoconjunctivits (Matsuda et al., 2009). On the other hand, cellular infiltration is the main feature of the late phase reaction (LPR). LPR begins 4-24 hr after EPR, and involves the infiltration of inflammatory cells, basophils, neutrophils, T Lympocytes, and mainly eosinophils (Choi & Bielory, 2008). Animal models of AC have shown that inflammatory migration is directed by T cells; recently, a relevant role for γδ T cells have been suggested since TCRγδ (-/-) mice have shown a decreased clinical manifestations and eosinophilic infiltration compared with wild type mice (Reyes et al., 2011); however, involvement of γδ T cells in human AC is still unknown. Once initiated, LPR can proceed in the presence of little or no detectable allergen-specific IgE antibody. LPR can also be induced by adoptively transference of T cells from allergen-sensitized donors to naïve recipients prior to challenging the ocular surface with the specific antigen (Fukushima et al., 2005). LPR could lead to corneal complications secondary to eosinophil infiltration. Eosinophils are attracted to ocular surface due to ligation of eotaxin-CC-chemokine receptor (CCR) 3 or RANTES-CCR1 (Heath et al., 1997). Notably, CCR3 chemotaxis induced by culture supernatant from corneal keratocytes and tear samples from severely allergic patients, could be inhibited by specific monoclonal antibodies against CCR3 (Fukagawa et al., 2002). Basophil infiltration could also be associated with AC because these cells express CCR3 and contribute with direct damage through FcεRI degranulation. Interestingly in a mice model of AC basophil activation could also be induced by IL-33, resulting in IL-4 and IL-13 expression, and potentiation of IgE-mediated degranulation (Matsuba-Kitamura et al., 2010). However, during the active inflammatory phase of the disease, multiple Th1-type and Th2-type cytokines are over expressed and produced (Leonardi, et al., 2006; Aguilar-Velazquez et al., 2009), including the typical Th1-type cytokine, interferon (IFN)-γ and TNFα, which might probably contribute to increase ocular inflammation similarly to animal models (Stern et al., 2005; Fukushima et al., 2006). The Th1-cells could also play a pivotal role in the delayed hypersensitivity ocular damage, through cell-mediated mechanisms, acting as a counter-balance factor to the Th2-cells, during antigen presentation and in the activation/inhibition of other cell types. Delayed hypersensitivity damage has also been suggested in asthma and nasal allergy (Pelikan, 2010; Pelikan, 2011)

2.3 Different cell populations and its impact in ocular allergy

Despite the role of dendritic cells (DC) have been extensively studied in animal models, other antigen presenting cells (APC) are still in research. Recently it has been suggested that macrophages could be needed in the development of experimental AC, since it appears they are able to take up antigen-labeled and act as APC (Ishida et al., 2010); nevertheless, further research in human patients is needed to know the real role of macrophages in AC. In addition, fibroblasts, conjunctival and corneal epithelial cells may contribute to human allergic inflammation by expressing and producing cytokines, chemokines, adhesion molecules and factors that maintain local inflammation and lead to tissue remodeling (Bonini et al., 2000; Leonardi et al., 2006).

2.4 T regulatory cells (Tregs)

An increasing number of reports have demonstrated that Tregs suppress allergic specific response (Akdis et al., 2004). In support of the important role of Tregs in controlling allergic diseases, it was demonstrated that CD4+CD25+ T cells protect against experimentally induced asthma, diminishing airway inflammation and hyper-reactivity after *in vivo* transfer of CD4+CD25+ regulatory T cells in IL-10 dependent manner (Lewkowich et al., 2005). In animal models of AC it has been suggested that induction of CD4+CD25+Foxp3+ T cells suppress the development of experimental allergic conjunctivitis through stimulation of alpha-galactosylceramide (Fukushima et al., 2008). Unfortunately research about involvement of Tregs in human AC is not enough yet.

2.5 Other T cell populations

Although in other allergies is well known the involvement of Th9, Th17, Th22, and NKT cells in effector responses, a long way in research is still pending in AC in both, human and animal models. Additionally, other molecules such as Toll like receptors (TLR) and Nucleotide Olimerization Domain (NOD) receptors that are expressed in epithelial cells, DC and T cell subsets (Bauer et al., 2007) could be modulating the immune response in unexpected ways depending of ocular microbiota, thus AC must be a field of extensive research.

3. Clinical aspect of allergic conjunctivitis

3.1 Classification of allergic ocular diseases

Allergic conjunctivitis includes a spectrum of a number of traditional overlapping conditions that range from intermittent to persistent symptoms and signs, variable in severity and presentation. These forms include seasonal (SAC) and perennial allergic conjunctivitis (PAC), vernal keratoconjunctivitis (VKC) and atopic keratoconjunctivitis (AKC). Giant papillary conjunctivitis (GPC), and contact or drug-induced dermatoconjunctivitis (CDC) are considered as subtypes of allergic conjunctivitis, due to their mechanism of allergy. (Leonardi et al., 2007).

Patients with mild forms of AC report symptoms with active signs not always seen at the time visit. Some of these symptoms include runny nose, sneezing, and or/wheezing. Classic reports describe allergic rhinitis and symptoms of watery (88%), itchy (88%), red (78%), sore (75%), swollen (72%) and stinging eyes (65%) (Dykewicz & Fineman, 1998). The main symptom of ocular allergy is itching, without itching; a condition should not be considered ocular allergy. Clinical manifestations of the effects of eye rubbing include injection of conjunctival vascular bed due to vascular dilation evoked by vasoactive amines released during mast cell degranulation, accompanied by an influx of water from the intravascular space, to the extravascular space, resulting in tissue edema and eyelid swelling, progressing from a milky or pale conjunctiva aspect to conjunctival swelling or chemosis. Swelling appears 15-30 minutes after antigen exposure and slowly diminished; a small quantity of white mucus secretion may form during the acute phase which can later becomes thick strands in the chronic form. In chronic forms a remodeling process is induced in conjunctiva tissue as fibrosis with vascularization that can be easily identified with slit lamp (Ono & Abelson, 2005)

There are numerous classifications for AOD according to the underlying pathophysiology and clinical findings. Common signs and symptoms exist in the different types of allergic disorders with frequent overlapping between SAC, PAC (acute forms of allergic conjunctivitis), VKC and AKC (chronic forms of conjunctivitis); therefore, classifications are recommended to standardize disease based on signs and symptoms, (mild, moderate or severe), (Abelson et al., 1990; Uchio et al., 2008; Pelikan, 2009) length of the disease (acute *vs* chronic disease), mechanism of immunopathogenesis (EPR and LPR stages), and duration of episodes activity (quiescent, intermittent and persistent), only suggested to VKC and AKC (Bonini et al., 2007; Calonge & Herreras, 2007), since they impact the quality of life. Such matter is important and should be consider in AOD diagnosis, similar to other allergic diseases (Del Culvillo et al., 2010). Although it has been suggested that SAC and GPC are milder and there is not involvement of the cornea, PAC and CDC might have a moderate risk of sight threatening, while VKC and AKC are the most serious forms of AC (Tanaka et al., 2004; Foster & Calonge, 1990). Therefore a grade of severity, in terms of signs and symptoms, is crucial to establishment of ocular clinical status, and possible vision compromise in AC patients.

3.2 Evaluation of grade of severity for allergic ocular diseases

The most common way to identify severity based mainly on conjunctiva, palpebral or cornea inflammation are mild, moderate or severe; however to better assess clinical characteristics in AOD groups, and to evaluate possible evolution of AC, the authors propose here, besides to take all recommendations mentioned above, a grading system based on a scale of 0 to 4, when 0=absent, 1=mild, 2=moderate, 3=moderately severe, and 4=severe, for both signs and symptoms. Taking in consideration, frequency in symptoms (itching, tearing, light sensitivity, gritty sensation, and burning sensation), (Table 1) and repercussion of signs implicated on alterations accompanying the inflammation at the ocular surface, such as eyelid position and skin aspect, eyelid margin state of mucocutaneous junction (MCJ) with involvement of meibomian gland disease (MGD), discharge aspect, implication of limbal stem cell deficiency and even keratoconus involvement. (Figure 1 and Table 2) The total score of signs and symptoms following grade of severity scale would give a total amount of 48 points, twenty of them corresponding to symptoms, and twenty eight of them corresponding to signs. According to this statement, we propose an objective grading system to recognize progress of allergic ocular disease, which could be defined as follows: 0 points= Absent, 1-12 points (mild), 13-24 points (moderate), 25-36 points (moderately severe) and 36-48 points (severe). The score of the more severe side in bilateral cases could be used as a clinical score.

Evaluation of Grade of Symptoms Severity for Allergic Ocular Diseases					
	0 None of the time	1 Some of the time	2 Half of the time	3 Most of the time	4 All of the time
Itching	☐	☐	☐	☐	☐
Tearing	☐	☐	☐	☐	☐
Light Sensitivity	☐	☐	☐	☐	☐
Gritty Sensation	☐	☐	☐	☐	☐
Burning Sensation	☐	☐	☐	☐	☐

Table 1. Evaluation of Grade of Symptoms Severity for Allergic Ocular Diseases

Evaluation of Grade of Severity for Allergic Ocular Diseases

Signs / Grades	Eyelid Position and Skin aspect	Eyelid Margin Marx's Line (MGD)	Conjunctiva hyperemia and swelling	Conjunctiva discharge	Tarsal conjunctiva Inflammation Response	Limbus Involvement	Cornea Involvement
0	No eyelid edema	No displacement of MCJ	No hyperemia or edema	No discharge	No papillary hyperplasia or visible follicles	No visible limbus nodules or dots	No SPK
1	Localized superior or inferior eyelid margin edema without Dennie Lines.	1/3 displacement of MCJ inferior or superior eyelid margin	hyperemia 1+ - 2 + with 1/3 pink edema aspect in conjunctiva. No conjunctiva plica formation in sac fundus	Clear watery discharge and/or slight debris within	Less than 1/3 tarsal papillae size 0.3 with visible uniform conjunctiva tarsal vessels	Less than one quadrant with dot Trantas	Slight SPK without central involvement
2	Generalized superior and/or inferior eyelid edema with slight pseudoptosis and Dennie Lines	2/3 displacement of MCJ inferior or superior eyelid margin	Hyperemia 2+ - 3+ with 2/3 redness edema aspect in conjuctiva, and/ or slight conjunctiva plica formation in sac fundus	White-gray mucoid discharge in sac fundus or adherent 1/3 to limbus or tarsal conjunctiva	1/3 to 2/3 moderate tarsal papillae 0.3-0.5 size with thin visible tarsal conjunctiva vessels.	One ¼ to one half of dot trantas on limbus with slight pigment	One quarter to one half of SPK without compromise of visual axis.
3	Unilateral or bilateral moderate pseudoptosis and several Dennie Lines	Generalized displacement of MCJ	Hyperemia > 3+ with more than 2/3 conjuctiva edema with localized engorgement of ciliary vessels Moderate plica formation in sac fundus	White, gray or yellow thick copious mucoid strands in sac fundus or adherent 2/3 to limbus or tarsal conjunctiva	Cobblestone papillae presentation. More than 2/3 tarsal papillae 0,75 size.with or without fibrosis. fairly irregular tarsal vessels.	More than one half of dot trantas on limbus with slight to moderate pigment or ¼ to one half of LSCD	Generalized SPK with compromise of visual axis, or epithelial defects. Indolent corneal Ulcer on superior quadrants.
4	Uni or Bilateral severe Pseudoptosis with Dennie Lines and changes on skin texture and pigmentation. Hertoghe´s sign present.	Scarring or keratinized changes	Same as grade 3 + generalized engorgement of ciliary vessels. Severe plica or conjunctiva folding formation in sac fundus	Thin copious farely strands adherent mainly to cornea surface	Few tarsal papillae > 0.75 with fibrosis or Macro Papillae extrusion and possible fornix foreshortening (symblefaron) or Generalized pale tarsal conjunctiva aspect without normal visible tarsal vessels.	Generalized dot trantas on limbus with fibrosis and pigment or more than one half of LSCD	Keratoconus with or without central leucoma

Hyperemia Grading: 0 = Absence of hyperemia, 1+ = mild (1/3 localized sector engorgement of bulbar conjunctival vessels), 2+ = moderate (2/3 diffuse engorgement of bulbar conjunctival vessels), and 3+ = severe (significant generalized engorgement of bulbar conjunctival vessels)
SPK (Superficial punctuate Keratopathy)
LSCD (Limbal Stem Cell Deficiency)
MGD (Meibomian Gland Disease)
MCJ (Mucocutaneous junction)

Table 2. Evaluation of Grade of Signs Severity for Allergic Ocular Diseases

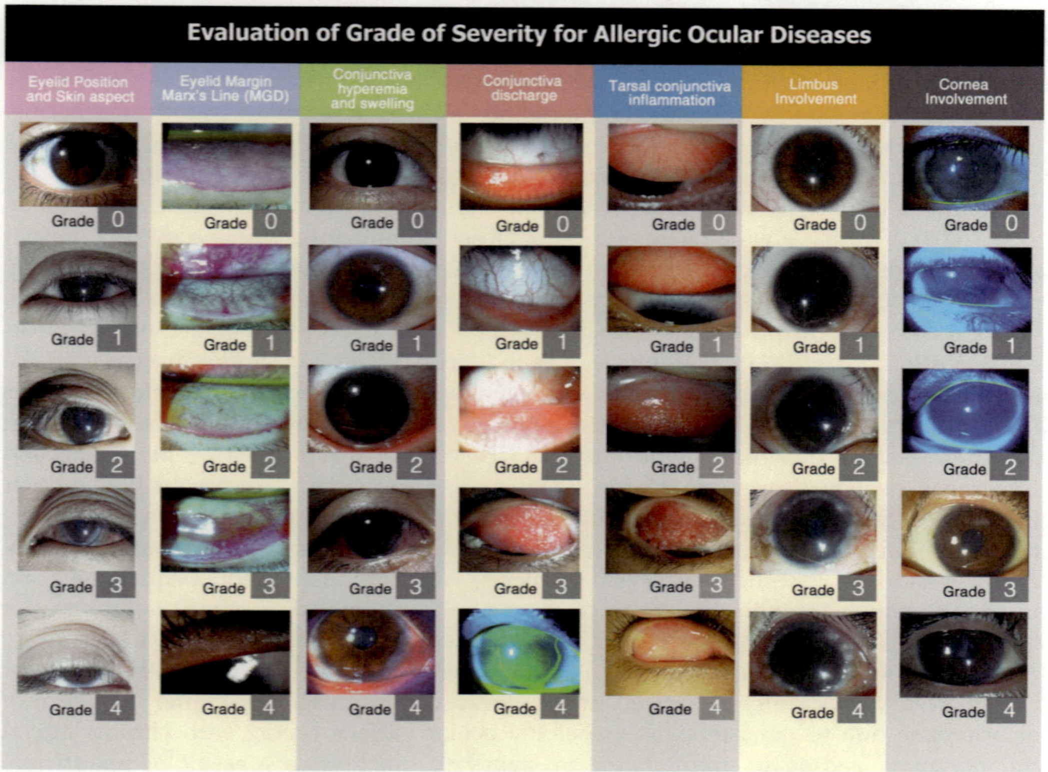

Fig. 1. Evaluation of Grade of Signs Severity for Allergic Ocular Diseases.

3.3 Acute forms of allergic conjunctivitis

3.3.1 Seasonal allergic conjunctivitis and perennial allergic conjunctivitis

Mild forms of SAC and PAC are entities which often go undiagnosed, as well as the ocular component of allergic rhinoconjunctivitis that can go also untreated. Both are acute forms of presentation and are mainly non-sight threatening conditions. Symptoms associated with SAC condition, such as ocular itching and redness, are often accompanied with tearing and nasal congestion (Wormald etal., 2004). Both, SAC and PAC patients, can also manifest symptoms of irritation, burning and foreign body sensation that might be related to increased tear film lipid layer thickness or even alterations of the lipid secretions, causing tear instability with diminished break up time (Suzuki et al., 2006). Eosinophilic activation and concomitant release of inflammatory mediators, which are thought to be detrimental to conjunctival epithelia and globet cells, are considered the cause of tear film instability (Lobefalo et al., 1999). It has been suggested that PAC patients are sensitized to house dust mite, animal dander and moulds, which are present all year round (Dart et al., 1986). However, we have observed that in our patients (Mexican mestizo population) both, SAC and PAC patients, are sensitized to house dust mite. The clinical characteristics of SAC and PAC patients can be seen on figure 1 and table 2 and correspond mainly to grade 1 and 2.

3.4 Chronic forms of conjunctivitis

3.4.1 Vernal keratoconjunctivitis

VKC is a chronic ocular surface inflammatory condition most commonly observed in young males before puberty living in dry, warm climates. VKC is bilateral and characterized by seasonal or perennial symptoms that exacerbate with recurrences in 60% during spring, early autumn and winter. Prolonged inflammation, more than 3 years, leads to a greater chance of developing perennial symptoms. During exacerbations, intense itching is the predominant feature, followed by photophobia, tearing, and sticky mucus discharge (Bonini et al., 2000). VKC has a wide range of conditions and all of them are not necessarily present at the time of visit, and could be a manifestation of disease evolution. The disease may primarily involve the tarsal or limbal conjunctiva leading to different forms of VKC: tarsal, limbal or mixed forms. In tarsal VKC, there is important hyperemic conjunctiva, chemosis and hypertrofic papillae 0.5-0.75 mm size with a cobblestone appearance representing the hallmark of disease. Typical Maxwell-Lyons sign is recognized for thick strands of mucus over papillaes. In limbal VKC gelatinous yellow-gray infiltrates are observed on the limbus, the circumference of which might appear thickened and opaque, with a peripheral and superficial neovascularization. Horner-Trantas dots are white, calcareous-like cellular infiltrates with eosinophil reaction occurring on the edge of limbal conjunctiva and also on top of nodules. Cornea involvement consider superficial punctate keratopathy, corneal erosions, indolent superficial ulcer (shield ulcers) which develops with opaque edges and plaque formation through deposition of mucus and cells, mainly located at the superior quadrants. VKC is also associated with keratoconus, which in fact should be a mandatory condition to search, because there are a 6% of patients that might end up with permanent reduction in visual acuity as a result of the cornea compromise. The higher incidence of compromise due to persistent disease at the ocular surface occurs with chronic limbal inflammation leading to gradual loss of stem cell function as a result of insufficient stromal support, ending up with limbal stem cell deficiency, and conjunctival fibrosis (Sangwan et al., 2005). Fibrosis could be associated with high immunostaining of positive mast cells to TGF, bFGF, and PDGF (Leonardi et al., 2000). Characteristic signs of VKC patients correspond to grade 2 and mainly 3. (Figure 1 and Table 2)

3.4.2 Atopic keratoconjunctivitis

AKC is a chronic ocular surface inflammatory response in men aged 30 to 50 years (Leonardi et al., 2007), however we have identified onset as earlier as in the first decade of life (Mexican mestizo population). It might be depending on severity a sight-threatening condition. The primary symptom of AKC is intense bilateral itching of the lid skin, periorbital area, and conjunctiva. Ocular symptoms also include photophobia, burning and foreign body sensation. Atopic blepharitis is evident, with tylosis and swollen eyelids that have a rugosity aspect with indurated appearance and associated with meibomian gland disease and concomitant dry eye (Onguchi et al., 2006). Infraorbital skin of the eyelid is frequently affected by single or double infraorbital creases known as Dennie-Morgan lines, which are caused by edema or thickening of the skin. Absence of the lateral eyebrow (Hertoghe sign) is present in many older patients and may be due to extensive chronic eye rubbing (Rich & Hanifin, 1985) and in the most severe cases conjunctival scarring with subepithelial fibrosis, fornix foreshortening, symblepharon, corneal ulceration and neovascularization may occur. Manifestations involving other tissues in the context of atopic dermatitis (episcleritis, scleritis, uveitis, keratoconus, cataract, and retinal detachment) must be considered. AKC is related with an increased risk of secondary infections, including bacterial, herpetic keratitis and *Chlamydia trachomatis* infections (Forte et al., 2009). There is discrepancy of evolution among AKC, the main reason for this is the overlapping of clinical pictures due to possible shift from VKC to AKC in those VKC patients that allergy did not disappear during puberty or adulthood as typical VKC does. These patients usually have at the beginning signs of AKC when they transform into adults, but most probably conserve giant papillary reaction at the upper tarsal conjunctivas. Characteristic signs of AKC patients correspond to grade 3 and mainly 4. (Figure 1 and Table 2)

3.5 Subtypes of allergic conjunctivitis

3.5.1 Giant papillary conjunctivitis (GPC)

It is not a true ocular allergic reaction, as is the case with SAC, PAC, VKC, and AKC. It is a mild ocular allergy caused by repeated mechanical irritation (contact lens wearers, ocular prosthesis, exposed sutures) and is aggravated by concomitant allergy, with an increase of symptoms during spring pollen season. (Leonardi et al., 2007) It is present during the 2nd to 5th decade of life. Symptoms of blurred vision, foreign body sensation, itching and tearing are present. Signs of mucus production with abnormal thickening of conjunctiva and visible white appearance on papillae with white or clear exudates, thick and stringy on awakening become a particular picture, in a chronic manner. Upper tarsal papillary hypertrophy has been described in 5% to 10% of soft and 3% to 4% of hard contact lens wearers. GPC is associated with the infiltration of basophils, eosinophils, plasma cells, and lymphocytes, which suggest a mixed mast cell- and lymphocyte-mediated process. (Chang & Chang, 2001)

3.5.2 Contact blepharitis or dermatoconjunctivitis

This type of reaction implies the eyelid skin and surrounding orbital limits. It is related to contact T- cell-mediated delayed hypersensitivity reaction to haptens-carrier complex such as cosmetics, metals, and chemicals as well as topical preparations with drugs or preservatives involved. Symptoms of eyelid itching, eczema, conjunctival redness and punctate keratitis might be seen. There is a participation of Langerhans cells of the eyelid skin or conjunctiva and presented to T-helper lymphocytes in the regional lymph nodes , which in turn sensitized cells react with cytokines resulting in recruitment and activation of inflammatory cells and resident cells. (Leonardi et al., 2007)

3.6 Other clinical allergic conditions and its impact in allergic ocular diseases

3.6.1 Ear nose and throat (ENT) co-morbilities

It is well known that allergic rhinitis could be present during allergic conjunctivitis. Specific nasal symptoms includes nasal congestion, nasal discharge or rhinorrhea, sneezing, hyposmia, breathing alterations, nasal voice, nose bleeding, and in some cases turbinate hypertrophy, and polypoid degenerations (De Groot et al., 2007). Mucosal edema of the upper airways induces changes in the nasal physiological equilibrium (Al-Rawi et al., 1998). Causes related to exacerbation of mucosal reactivity comprise intrinsic and extrinsic factors. Intrinsic factors include allergies, metabolic disorders, and anatomical alterations; while extrinsic factors encompass relative humidity, temperature, pollution, barometric pressure, among others. All of these alterations induce an inflammatory process that could be self limited or persistent, leading to more inflammatory responses (Nacleiro et al., 2010). Mucosal inflammation also stimulates mucin hypersecretion (Yuta et al., 1997), and if inflammatory process continues, drainage system fails and retrograde complications develops, such as paranasal sinus

dysfunction, nasolacrimal duct occlusion and middle ear alterations. Paranasal sinus dysfunction generates stasis of nasal secretions, edema and sinus infection (Ryan & Brooks, 2010). Severe ocular complications due to sinus infection include periorbital cellulitis, and cavernosus sinus thrombosis (Moubayed et al., 2011). Nasolacrimal duct occlusion is related with persistent epiphora and ocular infections. (Annamalai et al., 2003) Middle ear alterations include inflammation of Eustachian tube, generating low pressure in the middle ear. Changes in middle ear pressure develops in "glue ear" (middle ear fluid with increased viscosity), decreased audition, and in some cases mechanical vertigo (Pelikan, 2009).
Complications mentioned above can be prevented if the treatment of the rhinitis is just on time. Diagnostic management requires analysis of symptoms, physical examination, searching for eosinophilia in nasal secretions, and total IgE determination. Computerized tomography scan is a mandatory to study paranasal sinus complications (Lee et al., 2008). Treatment depends of each patient and if complications are present or not. The core of treatment must be directed to restructure the physiological nasal function. In this context, we have observed that treatment of AOD gets very favorable results in nasal symptoms; similarly, control of allergic rhinitis induces a better ocular outcome.

3.6.2 Skin co-morbidities

Patients with allergic ocular disease may have, among other systemic allergic co-morbidities, immune-mediated skin disorders. While AKC has been commonly associated with atopic dermatitis (AD), other types of AC may also be associated with conditions such as contact dermatitis (CD), urticaria and angioedema (Calonge, 2000). Early onset of AD is commonly regarded as the first manifestation of the so-called "atopic march", where asthma and allergic rhinoconjunctivitis arise eventually in patients previously suffering from AD (Spergel & Paller, 2003) (Figure 2). Conjunctival and corneal involvements among patients with AD are common signs in AKC. It has been speculated that AD with ocular involvement could be the most severe end of the spectrum of this chronic relapsing cutaneous disease characterized by erythematous pruritic vesicles that may evolve into chronic lichenified lesions (Spergel & Paller, 2003). AD and AKC may not run parallel courses; in some cases the only manifestations of AD may be limited to the eyelids with eczema and keratinization, as well as chronic blepharitis (Tuft et al., 1991). Interestingly, it has been demonstrated that AD patients have a marked deficiency of IgA in sweat and tear samples, which could account, at least in part, for the increased susceptibility to *Staphylococcus aureus* and Herpes simplex virus infections in the skin and ocular surface (Guglielmettia et al., 2010). Patients with AD may also have a higher tendency to present CD, and so do patients with allergic ocular disease (Calonge, 2000). CD may respond to allergic or irritant mechanisms that cause the development of scaly eczematous lesions. In patients with dermatoconjunctivitis, these lesions may be limited to the periorbital skin and be secondary to the application of cosmetics or topical ophthalmologic medications; lesions usually self resolve after discontinuing the offending agent. In patients with AC, acute urticarial lesions characterized by migrating edematous, pruritic plaques with serpiginous borders may develop. Likewise, patients may also develop angioedema, presenting with well-demarcated, non-pruritic areas of deeper cutaneous edema in the eyelids or perioral zone. When mediated by IgE, both urticaria and angioedema, are frequently encountered in atopic individuals, and therefore in patients with AOD.
CD, urticaria and angioedema tend to be self limited in patients with AC, patients with AKC usually have relapsing chronic courses of AD. Hence, these patients could possibly benefit from therapies capable of simultaneously targeting the ocular and cutaneous aspects of their

disease. One such approach could be the use of topical tacrolimus applied to the eyelids and subsequently spread over the conjunctiva in patients with skin involvement limited to the periorbital zone (Zribi et al., 2009). Other promising therapeutic possibilities could include the use of systemic immunosuppressive agents, such as cyclosporine, azathioprine and mycophenolate mofetil (Guglielmettia et al., 2010). Finally, immunobiological therapies such as infliximab (anti TNF-α), alefacept (T-cell inhibition) or rituximab (anti CD20) have proven to be effective in patients with AD, and could be of benefit in patients with AKC (Guglielmettia et al., 2010).

Actinic Conjunctivitis. It has been described in the dermatologic literature as part of a condition termed Actinic Prurigo. Is thought to be a photosensitive reaction to ultraviolet light in susceptible individuals; rather than primarily an allergic response. Begins in childhood and involves mainly the skin, oral mucosa and the conjunctiva. It has been described in Indian or Mestizo heritage located in Mexico or the Andean Regions of South America and in the American Indian population in the southwestern of United States. Typical characteristics consist of localized redness on the temporal side of bulbar conjunctiva advanced lesions becoming thicker and more congested with pigmentary changes, until invasion of limbus causing a linear leukoma. (Figure 2) Actinic conjunctivitis

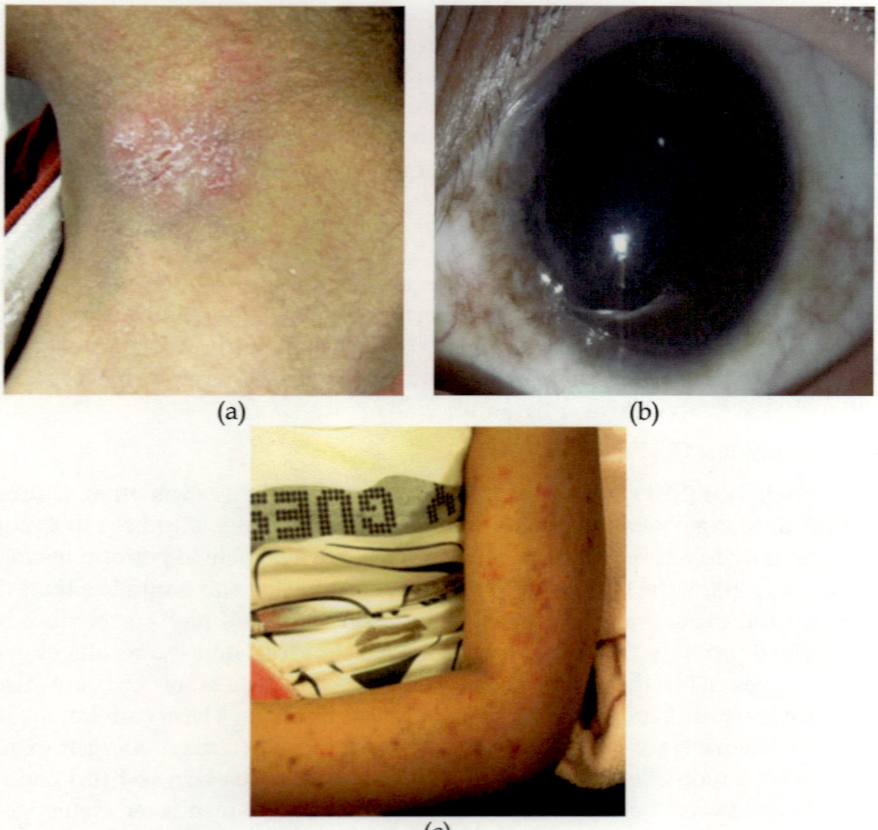

(a) (b) (c)

Fig. 2. Skin co-morbilities in patients with AC. Clinical pictures of Atopic Dermatitis in neck (a); Actinic Conjunctivitis (b); and Actinic Prurigo in forearm (c)

has infiltration of epithelium by inflammatory cells and stromal changes with plasmacytic infiltrate, vascular congestion and varying numbers of eosinophils as the source of the lesion. Children with actinic conjunctivitis frequently complain of a burning itchy sensation and relief is gained with the use of steroids. Actinic conjunctivits, in its earliest stages, is frequently misdiagnosed as vernal conjunctivitis but without papillary reaction (Engel et al., 2009). Despite that actinic conjunctivitis could be considered as a differential diagnosis, authors have observed that in some cases could coexist with AOD.

4. *In vivo* diagnostic and research procedures

Provocation tests are used to know the immediate or delay immune response against several allergens; these tests have high specificity and positive predictive value, and are the most important *in vivo* diagnostic and research procedures, some of these allergy examinations include:

Conjunctival provocation test (CPT)

CPT is used to determine the extent of conjunctival reaction to allergens. A drop of antigen to evaluate is applied to one eye, whereas a drop of balanced salt solution (BSS) is applied to the other eye as a control. Eyes must be examined using slit-lamp at different times. To control and degrade allergic eye reaction, a drop of topical antihistamine is applied at the end of CPT. CPT could be used as a model of ocular allergy to study ocular response to allergenic stimuli, and to evaluate antiallergic therapy. Considerable useful information has been gained on the ocular allergic response and drug efficacy using the CPT and naturally occurring seasonal allergic conjunctivitis. (Mortemousque, 2007; Kasetsuwan et al., 2010).

Nasal provocation test (NPT)

NPT is used to determine nasal and/or conjunctival reaction to allergens. NPT has been used primarily as a research tool for the investigation of allergic and nonallergic rhinitis with a wide variety of techniques depending on the specific scientific purposes. NPT could be a valuable supplementary diagnostic parameter for late nasal response (Pelikan & Pelikan-Filipek, 1989; Litvyakova & Baraniuk, 2001)

Epicutaneous skin test (EST)

EST or Skin Prick Test (SPT) provides a pivotal role in the allergy evaluation, is used to aid establishment of allergic symptoms and specific allergic triggers, and help to evaluate the degree of sensitivity to a specific agent. Many devices are available to perform testing. These devices attempt to allow the performer to achieve reproducible and accurate skin test results when standardized extracts are employed. It has been suggested high correlations between positive results to properly performed epicutaneous skin tests and the results of eye, nose, or lung challenges with the homologous allergen. The results of EST are also higly correlated with the results of *in vitro* tests and clinical histories. These correlations between the tests and challenges are highest when potent, well-characterized allergen extracts are used. For most common allergens, the results of Intracutaneous skin test (IST) add little if anything to correlations between skin test results and the results of challenges or to predicting clinical histories. The extra sensitivity of IST valuable when high potency of extracts are not available or when the test risk of a falsely negative test is high, as with drug or insect venom allergies. All physicians caring for patients with histories suggestive of allergic disorders must be keenly aware of the strengths and limitations of all available methods. (Ownby, 2001)

Atopy patch test (APT)

This test is able to identify triggering factors and consist of the epicutaneous application of allergens for 48 hours, with an evaluation of eczematous lesions induced after 48 and 72 hours, according to the reading criteria of the European Task Force on Atopic Dermatitis (ETFAD). APT show a higher specificity in atopic dermatitis than skin prick and specific IgE tests, since the pathophysiological mechanism of the reaction induced is very similar to that which occurs in AD lesions. (Nosbaum et al., 2010) Thus, optimization of APTs and progress in the knowledge of the pathophysiology of eczemas associated to ocular diseases could help to develop new immunobiological diagnostic methods and specific immunotherapy that could be used in AOD with skin involvement.

5. Conventional therapeutic intervention and new immunological treatments

Despite that AC is frequent, often is misdiagnosed and not adequately treated. Patients with these conditions may present to a variety of professionals-pharmacists, general practitioners, allergists/immunologists, otolaryngologist, and dermatologists; unfortunately, there is a lack of consensus in the multidisciplinary assessment for better treatment selection.
Treatments for allergic conjunctivitis have been continuously evolving since the early nineties, and several levels of therapeutic intervention have been described. Primary intervention is related to avoid offending antigens without pharmacological measures; secondary intervention is directed to control local effector functions of mast cells/eosinophils/basophils with H1- and H2-receptor antagonists, Disodium cromoglycate, Nedocromil sodium, anti-inflammatory drugs (non-steroids or steroids) (Bielory et al., 2005) and in severe cases, tertiary intervention with immune suppressor therapy, such as ciclosporin or tacrolimus has been used (Daniell et al., 2006; Vichyanond et al., 2004).

5.1 Other therapies

Autologous Serum (AS) has been used to treat dry eye syndrome for many years. It contains several growth factors, vitamins, fibronectin, albumin, lisozime and other components that have been considered important for corneal and conjunctival integrity (Kojima et al., 2008). To date few studies about AS use in AOD have been reported, improvement of signs and symptoms is not a constant in all patients (Goto et al., 2001; Gaytán-Melicoff et al., 2005). It would be interesting to replicate these studies isolating total or specific IgE from serum before application of autologus serum eye drops in ocular surface, because is a possibility that absence of improvement could be related with activation of local and migrating cells by FcεR, due to AS could contain high IgE concentrations in atopic patients.

5.2 Immune-based therapeutic approaches

All therapeutic interventions mentioned above are focused on topical agents in an effort to control "the effector side of the coin", than "the sensitization side of the coin". Research in immune-based therapeutic approaches is needed to perform deeply immunological changes that induce a better clinical outcome in AC patients; some of these therapeutic approaches are specific desensitization/immunotherapy and dialyzable leukocyte extracts. It is very important to clarify that both of these innovative therapies are still in evaluation, and until now there are not enough scientific information to ensure its efficacy in the treatment of AOD.

5.3 Specific immunotherapy

First described by Noon and Freeman in 1911, immunotherapy is thought to be the most specific treatment for allergic diseases, particularly asthma and allergic rhinitis. It is defined as the administration of low and calculated doses of the biological extract allergen or allergens implicated specifically in the disease of each patient (that is determined by the SPT), increasing gradually until get the highest dose clinically adequate. These vaccines comprise a complex mixture of proteins and glycoproteins that require dedicated standardization procedures to ensure batch-to-batch consistency. The whole desensitization process takes about 3 to 5 years, but the improvement should be reported during the first 3 to 6 months of treatment. There have been reported many ways for its administration, but nowadays only two have provided efficacy and safety: subcutaneous and sublingual (Shakir et al., 2010).

Possible mechanisms of action of subcutaneous immunotherapy, includes the down regulation of cytokines, inhibition of activation and recruitment of effector cells, and modulation of Th1 and Th2 balance, with IFN-γ secretion. This particular aspect seems to be of major relevance and explains by itself many of the changes related to improvement of the allergic symptoms in asthma and rhinitis, and the long lasting efficacy after discontinuation (Frew, 2010). Subcutaneous immunotherapy has been reported effective in patients with SAC in wich IgE-mediated hypersensitivity has been demonstrated with a convincingly diagnostic procedure. (Kari & Saari, 2010)

In the case of sublingual immunotherapy (SLIT), it has been reported that allergen is captured within the oral mucosa by Langerhans dendritic cells expressing high-affinity IgE receptors, producing IL-10 and TGF-β, and upregulating indoleamine dioxygenase (IDO), suggesting that such cells are prone to induce tolerance by T regs (Scadding et al., 2010). In humans, SLIT is capable to reduce the proliferative response of T lymphocytes and the inflammatory phenomena (cellular infiltration and adhesion molecule expression on epithelia) in nose and conjunctiva of atopic subjects, decrease methacholine responsiveness and, even it does not affect IgE levels, there are an increase of IgG1 and IgG4 (Moingeon et al., 2006). SLIT has been used in treatment of rhinoconjunctivitis, it success has been reported moderately effective in reducing total and individual ocular symptom scores (Calderon et al., 2011). Unfortunately, not convincing specific data have been presented to demonstrate if SLIT is significant effective during treatment of AOD and more clinical studies are needed to recognize the relevance of this therapy.

5.4 Dialyzable leukocyte extracts (DLE)

DLE or Transfer Factors, were described by Lawrence in 1955, who proved that the extract obtained from a dialyzed of viable leukocytes from a health donor presenting a positive percutaneous tuberculin test was able to transfer to a healthy receptor the ability to respond to this test (Lawrence, 1955). DLE are constituted by a group of numerous molecules all of them with a molecular weight between 1-6 KDa. DLE have been widely used as adjuvant for treating patients with infectious diseases, and deficient cell-mediated immune response (Wilson et al., 1984; Berrón et al., 2007). Transfer factors bind to antigens in an immunologically specific manner. This reactivity probably explains the specificity of individual transfer factors; it appears the purified materials are immunologically active and antigen-specific. (Kirckpatrick, 1993).

The most consistent effects of transfer factors on the immune system are expression of delayed-type hypersensitivity (DTH) and production of cytokines. DLE are able to induce secretion of macrophage migration inhibitory factor (Kirckpatrick, 1993), to restore the expression of TNFα and iNOS in a mouse model of tuberculosis, provoking inhibition of bacterial proliferation and significant increase of DTH (Fabre et al., 2004), and to induce expression of mRNA and IFN-γ in peripheral blood mononuclear cells from animal models and during treatment of human diseases (Estrada-Parra et al., 1998; Pineda et al., 2005; Luna-Baca et al., 2007; Santacruz-Valdes et al., 2010). Immune modulation induced by DLE therapy increase IFN-γ+ cells promoting Th1 response and restoring a Th2 balance, thus treatment with DLE has also been used in allergic diseases, such as AD (Sosa et al., 2001; Flores-Sandoval et al., 2005) and asthma (Valdés-Sánchez et al., 1993), in both diseases with promissory results, particularly in moderate persistent allergic asthma, helping to reduce the use of inhaled glucocorticoids (Espinosa Padilla et al., 2009). AOD treatment with DLE has not been enough studied yet; nonetheless, preliminary reports suggest that DLE improves clinical outcome in patients with negative skin reactivity to allergens, suggesting that DLE therapy could be used as therapeutic tool in such patients. (Jiménez-Martínez et al., 2010). However, more research is required to better understand exact indications of DLE in all types of AOD.

6. Biomarkers research and its applications in allergic ocular diseases

Biomarkers are common molecules, such as lipids, glycans or proteins, located in tissues, cells and secretions. Changes in concentration of these molecules, indicates a biological status from "normal" to "pathological" range. Biomarkers can be used as prognostic or diagnostic tools or as a target to new therapies (Hoffmann-Sommergruber et al., 2011). In this context proteomics, immunomics and bioinformatics could aid to explore and to know antigens recognized by immune system during allergic response.

Immunome is defined as the proteome subset of an antigen, recognized by the immune receptors (TCR or BCR) and the tools that help us to study immunome are named immunomics (De Groot, 2006). Exists different ways to analyze immunome, searching in immunome epitope databases could give us newly identified epitope; however, most databases involved TCR epitopes exclusively (Sette et al., 2005). To generate a functional profile for allergic conjunctivitis patients we can select epitopes from the growing, verified database of B cell epitopes (Prechl et al., 2010) but in the case of allergies is needed to know a biomarker candidate, this is only possible if we know the frequency of allergens in our population. Once we have an exploratory biomarker (most frequent allergen recognized by patients IgE antibodies), it could be used as a potential precursor for probable useful biomarker. Protein sequencing, and other functional procedures to evaluate functional proteins (i.e. ELISA, flow cytometry, immune histologyc techniques), followed by analytical test system (bioinformatics) could lead to identification or prediction of protein structure. (Goodsaid & Frueh, 2006). The last step in biomarker research is related to practical validation of putative biomarkers. If the new biomarker is related to diagnostic, studies should support specificity and sensitivity of the exploratory biomarker (Wilkins et al., 2006). Finally cross-validation processes will include independent validation of new biomarker by several researchers, and if results are reproducible, the biomarker may be considered valid (Hardouin et al., 2006).

All this process is needed to know peptides recognized by IgE antibody in allergic disease. Knowledge could be used to develop diagnostic test i.e. determination of specific IgE in tears or to develop second generation immunotherapy. Recombinant DNA technology could be used to obtain highly purified allergens in their native conformation. The recombinant allergens could then formulated with *ad hoc* adjuvants and/or mucoadhesive excipients so that they specifically target oral Langerhans cells and induce allergen-specific regulatory T cells (Moingeon, 2006).

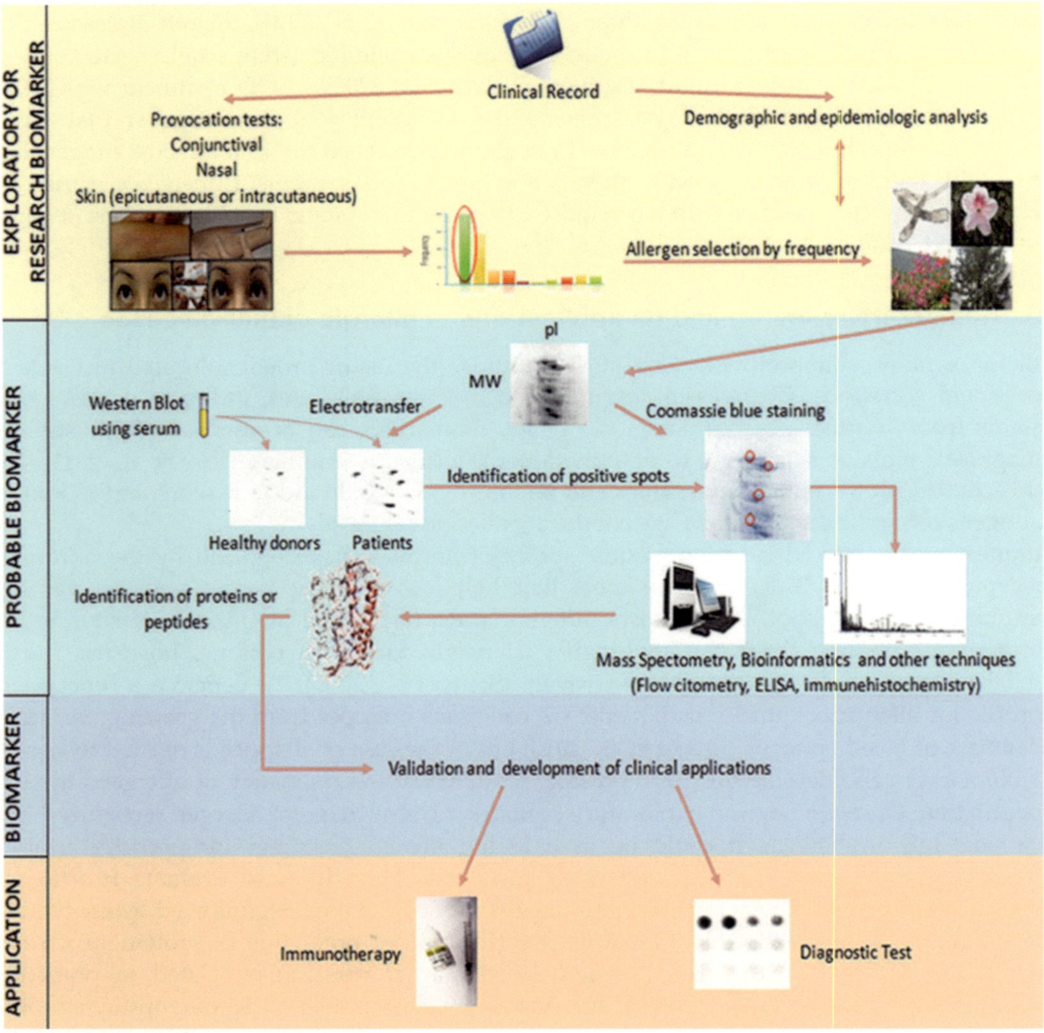

Fig. 3. Research flow in biomarkers related to allergic diseases.

7. Conclusions

Allergic ocular diseases have become a special concern for clinical and basic research. Their impact on quality of life among individuals, annually represent an important issue of investment to find better treatments, particularly to control the effects of chronic diseases which could threat vision and influence on daily life activities. Clinical diagnosis is still a challenger due to a wide range of overlapping entities which might respond differently to conventional treatments; such heterogeneity is important to be considered not only to focus on the ocular problem, but to approach the problem with an interdisciplinary medical group, including allergist/immunologist, ENT specialists, and dermatologist; all working together to improve ocular and systemic health of the allergic patient. Despite that important discoveries about immune pathophysiological mechanisms has brought light into the problem, there is not enough. Research efforts need to be also directed to the discovery of biomarkers and immune therapeutic management to control both, sensitization and effector phases of AOD. Knowledge about the molecular mechanisms involved, together with an interdisciplinary treatment group will support better results in allergic conjunctivitis patients.

8. Aknowledgments

ICYTDF PIFUT-P08124, Fundacion Conde de Valenciana, and Transfer Factor Project. Robles-Contreras A and Santacruz C must be considered as first authors indistinctly. The authors declare that they have no financial and personal relationships with other people or organizations that could inappropriately influence this work.

9. References

Abelson, MB., Chambers, WA., Smith LM. (1990). Conjunctival Allergen Challenge A Clinical Approach to Studying Allergic Conjunctivitis. Arch Ophthalmol. pp.84-88.

Abelson, MB., Smith L., & Chapin M. (2003). Ocular allergic disease: mechanisms, disease sub-types, treatment. Ocul Surf. pp. 127-149.

Abu El-Asrar, AM., Fatani, RA., Missotten, L. & Geboes, K. (2001). Expression of CD23/CD21 and CD40/CD40 ligand in vernal keratoconjunctivitis. Eye (Lond). pp. 217-224.

Aguilar-Velázquez, G, Santacruz-Valdés, C, Robles-Contreras, A, Ayala-Balboa, J, Bautista-de-Lucio, V, et al. (2009). Tear TNF as a Potential Link in the Pathogenesis of Allergic Conjunctivitis. Correlation between Tear IFNg/IL-5 and Clinical Data. Prodeedings of Allergy. Medimond. Argentina, pp.13-17.

Akdis, M., Verhagen, J., Taylor, A., Karamloo, F., Karagiannidis, C. et al. (2004). Immune responses in healthy and allergic individuals are characterized by a fine balance between allergen-specific T regulatory 1 and T helper 2 cells. J Exp Med. pp. 1567-1575.

Allansmith, MR., Hahn, GS., & Simon, MA. (1976). Tissue, tear, and serum IgE concentrations in vernal conjunctivitis. Am J Ophthalmol. pp. 506-511.

Al-Rawi, MM., Edelstein, DR. & Erlandson, RA. (1998). Changes in nasal epithelium in patients with severe chronic sinusitis: A clinicopathologic and electron microscopic study. Laryngoscope. pp. 1816-1823.

Anderson, DF., MacLeod, JD., Baddeley, SM., Bacon, AS., McGill, JI., et al. (1997). Seasonal allergic conjunctivitis is accompanied by increased mast cell numbers in the absence of leucocyte infiltration. Clin Exp Allergy. pp. 1060-1066.

Anderson, DF., Zhang, S., Bradding, P., McGill, JI., Holgate, ST., et al. (2001). The relative contribution of mast cell subsets to conjunctival TH2-like cytokines. Invest Ophthalmol Vis Sci. pp. 995-1001.

Annamalai, S., Kumar, NA., Madkour, MB., Sivakumar, S. & Kubba, H. (2003). An association between acquired epiphora and the signs and symptoms of chronic rhinosinusitis: a prospective case-control study. Am J Rhinol. pp. 111-114.

Bauer, S., Hangel, D. & Yu, P. (2007). Immunobiology of toll-like receptors in allergic disease. Immunobiology. pp. 521-533.

Berrón-Pérez, R., Chávez-Sánchez, R., Estrada-García, I., Espinosa-Padilla, S., Cortez-Gómez, R. et al. (2007). Indications, usage, and dosage of the transfer factor. Rev Alerg Mex. pp. 134-139.

Bielory, LJ. (2000). Allergic and immunologic disorders of the eye. Part I: immunology of the eye. Allergy Clin Immunol. pp. 805-816.

Bielory, L., Lien, KW. & Bigelsen, S. (2005). Efficacy and tolerability of newer antihistamines in the treatment of allergic conjunctivitis. Drugs. pp. 215-228.

Bonini, S., Bonini, S., Lambiase, A., Marchi, S., Pasqualetti, P. et al. (2000). Vernal keratoconjunctivitis revisited: a case series of 195 patients with long-term followup. Ophthalmology. pp. 1157-1163.

Bonini, S., Sacchetti, M., Mantelli, F. & Cambiase, A. (2007). Clinical grading of vernal keratoconjunctivitis. Curr Opin Allergy Clin Immunol. pp. 436-441.

Calderon, MA., Penagos, M., Sheikh, A., Canonica, GW. & Durham, S. (2011). Sublingual immunotherapy for treating allergic conjunctivitis. Cochrane Database Syst Rev. pp. CD007685.

Calonge, M. (2000). Ocular Allergies. Association with Immune Dermatitis. Acta Ophthalmol Scand. pp. 69-75.

Calonge, M. & Herreras, JM. (2007). Clinical grading of atopic keratoconjunctivitis. Curr Opin Alergy Clin Immunol pp. 442-445.

Chang SW, Chang CJ. (2001). Delayed tear clearance in contact lens associated papillary conjunctivitis. Curr Eye Res. pp. 253-257.

Choi, SH. & Bielory, L. (2008). Late-phase reaction in ocular allergy. Curr Opin Allergy Clin Immunol. pp. 438-444.

Cook, EB., Stahl, JL., Miller, ST., Gern, JE., Sukow, KA., et al. (1998). Isolation of human conjunctival mast cells and epithelial cells: tumor necrosis factor-alpha from mast cells affects intercellular adhesion molecule 1 expression on epithelial cells. Invest Ophthalmol Vis Sci. pp. 336-43.

Daniell, M., Constantinou, M., Vu, HT. & Taylor, HR. (2006). Randomised controlled trial of topical ciclosporin A in steroid dependent allergic conjunctivitis. Br. J Ophthalmol. pp. 461-464.

Dart, JK., Buckley, RJ., Monnickendan, M., & Prasad, J. (1986). Perennial allergic conjunctivitis: definition, clinical characteristics and prevalence. A comparison with seasonal allergic conjunctivitis. Trans Ophthalmol Soc U K. pp. 513-520.

De Groot, AS. (2006). Immunomics: discovering new targets for vaccines and therapeutics. Drug Discov Today. pp. 203-209.

De Groot, H., Brand, PL., Fokkens, WF. & Berger, MY. (2007). Allergic rhinoconjunctivitis in children. BMJ. pp. 985-988.

Del Culvillo, A., Montoso, J., Bartra, J., Valero, A., Ferrer, M. et al. (2010). Validation of ARIA duration and severity classifications in Spanish allergic rhinitis patients. The ADRIAL cohort study. Rhinology. pp. 201-205.

Dykewicz, MS. & Fineman, S. (1998). Executive Summary of Joint Task Force Practice Parameters on Diagnosis and Management of Rhinitis. Ann Allergy Asthma Immunol. pp. 463-468.

Engel, JM., Molinari, A., Ostfeld, B., Deen, M. & Croxatto O. (2009). Actinic Conjunctivits in children: Clinical features, relation to sun exposure, and proposed staging and treatment. J AAPOS. pp. 161-165.

Espinosa Padilla, SE., Orozco, S., Plaza, A., Estrada Parra, S., Estrada Garcia, I. et al. (2009) Efecto del factor de transferencia en el tratamiento con glucocorticoides en un grupo de paciente pediátricos con asma alérgica moderada persistente. Rev Aler Mex pp. 67-71.

Estrada-Parra, S., Nagaya, A., Serrano, E., Rodriguez, O., Santamaria, V. et al. (1998). Comparative study of transfer factor and acyclovir in the treatment of herpes zoster. Int J Immunopharmacol. pp. 521-535.

Fabre, RA., Pérez, TM., Aguilar, LD., Rangel, MJ., Estrada-Garcìa, I., et al.(2004) Transfer factors as immunotherapy and supplement of chemotherapy in experimental pulmonary tuberculosis. Clin Exp Immunol. pp. 215-23.

Flores-Sandoval, G., Gómez-Vera, J., Orea-Solano, M., López-Tiro, J., Serrano, E. et al. (2005). Transfer factor as specific immunomodulator in the treatment of moderate-severe atopic dermatitis. Rev Alerg Mex. pp. 215-20.

Forte, R., Cennamo, G., Del Prete, S., Napolitano, N., Farese, E. et al. (2009). Allergic conjunctivitis and latent infections. Cornea. pp. 839-842.

Foster, CS. & Calonge, M. (1990). Atopic Keratoconjunctivitis. Ophthalmology. pp. 992-1000.

Frew, AJ. (2010). Allergen immunotherapy. J Allergy Clin Immunol. pp. S306-313.

Fukagawa, K., Okada, N., Fujishima, H., Nakajima, T., Tsubota, K., Takano, Y. et al. (2002). CC-chemokine receptor 3: a possible target in treatment of allergy-related corneal ulcer. Invest Ophthalmol Vis Sci. pp. 58-62.

Fukushima, A., Ozaki, A., Jian, Z., Ishida, W., Fukata, K., et al. (2005). Dissection of antigen-specific humoral and cellular immune responses for the development of experimental immune-mediated blepharoconjunctivitis in C57BL/6 mice. Curr Eye Res. pp. 241-248.

Fukushima, F., Sumi, T. & Fukuda, K. (2006). Analysis of the interaction between IFNγ and IFNγR in the effector phase of experimental murine allergic conjunctivitis. Immunol Lett. pp.119-124

Fukushima, A., Sumi, T., Ishida, W., Ojima, A., Kajisako, M., et al. (2008). Depletion of thymus-derived CD4+CD25+ T cells abrogates the suppressive effects of alpha-galactosylceramide treatment on experimental allergic conjunctivitis. Allergol Int. pp. 241-246.

Gaytán-Melicoff, JA., Baca-Lozada, O., Velasco-Ramos, R. & Viggiano-Austria, D. (2005). Comparación entre suero autólogo, clorhidrato de olopatadina y fumarato de ketotifeno, en el manejo de la conjunctivitis alérgica. Rev Mex Oftalmol. pp. 25-31.

Goodsaid, F. & Frueh, F. (2006). Process map proposal for the validation of genomic biomarkers. Pharmacogenomics. pp. 773-782.

Goto, E., Shimmura, S., Shimazaki, J. & Tsubota, K. (2001) Treatment of superior limbic keratoconjunctivitis by application of autologous serum. Cornea. pp. 807-810.

Guglielmettia, S., Darta, JKG. & Calderd, V. (2010). Atopic keratoconjunctivitis and atopic dermatitis. Current Opinion in Allergy and Clinical Immunology. pp. 478–485.

Hardouin, J., Duchateau, M., Joubert-Caron, R. & Caron, M. (2006). Usefulness of an integrated microfluidic device (HPLC-Chip-MS) to enhance confidence in protein identification by proteomics. Rapid Commun Mass Spectrom. pp. 3236-3244.

Heath, H., Qin, S., Rao, P., Wu, L., LaRosa, G., et al. (1997). Chemokine receptor usage by human eosinophils. The importance of CCR3 demonstrated using an antagonistic monoclonal antibody. J Clin Invest. pp. 178-84.

Hoffmann-Sommergruber, .K, Paschinger, K. & Wilson, IB. (2011). Glycomarkers in parasitic infections and allergy. Biochem Soc Trans. pp. 360-364.

Ishida, W., Fukuda, K., Kajisako, M., Takahashi, A., Sumi, T., et al. (2010). Conjunctival macrophages act as antigen-presenting cells in the conjunctiva during the development of experimental allergic conjunctivitis. Mol Vis. pp. 1280-1285.

Jimenez-Martinez, MC., Aguilar, G., Santacruz, C., Robles-Contreras, A., Ayala, J. et al. (2010). Sublingual Desensitization or Immune Modulation with Dialyzable Leukocyte Extracts Improves the Clinical Outcome in Allergic Conjunctivitis. Clin Immunol. FOCIS 2010. Boston, USA. pp. S103.

Johansson, SG., Bieber, T., Dahl, R., Friedmann, PS., Lanier, BQ., et al. (2004). Revised nomenclature for allergy for global use: Report of the Nomenclature Review Committee of the World Allergy Organization, October, 2003. J Allergy Clin Immunol. pp. 832-6.

Kari, O & Saari KM. (2010) Updates in the treatment of ocular allergies. J Asthma Allergy. pp.149-158.

Kasetsuwan, N., Chatchatee, P., & Reinprayoon, U. (2010) Efficacy of local conjunctival immunotherapy in allergic conjunctivitis. Asian Pac J Allergy Immunol. pp. 237-241

Kirkpatrick, CH. (1993) Structural nature and functions of transfer factors. Ann N Y Acad Sci. pp. 362-368.

Kojima, T., Higuchi, A., Goto, E., Masumoto, Y., Dogru, M. et al. (2008). Autologous serum eye drops for the treatment of dry eye diseases. Cornea. pp.S25-S30.

Lawrence, HS. (1955). The transfer in humans of delayed skin sensitivity to streptococcal M substance and to tuberculin with disrupted leucocytes. J Clin Invest. pp. 219-230.

Lee, CH., Jang, JH., Lee, HJ., Kim, IT., Chu, MJ. et al. (2008). Clinical characteristics of allergic rhinitis according to allergic rhinitis and its impact on asthma guidelines. Clin Exp Otorhinolaryngol. pp. 196-200.

Leonardi, A., Brun, P., Tavolato, M., Abatangelo, G., Plebani, M. et al. (2000). Growth factors and collagen distribution in vernal keratoconjunctivitis. Invest Ophthalmol Vis Sci. 4175-4181.

Leonardi, A., Curnow, SJ., Zhan, H. & Calder, VL. (2006). Multiple cytokines in human tear specimens in seasonal and chronic allergic eye disease and in conjunctival fibroblast cultures. Clin Exp Allergy. pp. 777-784.

Leonardi, A., Fregona, IA. & Plebani, M. (2006). Th1- and Th2-type cytokines in chronic ocular allergy. Graefe's Arch Clin Exp Ophthalmol pp. 1240–1245.

Leonardi, A., De Dominicis, C. & Motterle, L. (2007). Immunopathogenesis of ocular allergy: a schematic approach to different clinical entities. Curr Opin Allergy Clin Immunol. pp. 429-435.

Lewkowich, IP., Herman, NS., Schleifer, KW., Dance, MP., Chen, BL., et al. (2005). CD4+CD25+ T cells protect against experimentally induced asthma and alter pulmonary dendritic cell phenotype and function. J Exp Med. pp. 1549-1561.

Litvyakova, LI. & Baraniuk, JN. (2001). Nasal provocation testing: a review. Ann Allergy Asthma Immunol. pp :355-364

Lobefalo, L., D'Antonio, E., Colangelo, L., Della Loggia, G., Di Gioacchino, M. et al. (1999). Dry eye in allergic conjunctivitis: role of inflammatory infiltrate. Int J Immunopathol Pharmacol. pp. 133-137.

Luna-Baca, GA., Linares, M., Santacruz-Valdes, C., Aguilar-Velazquez, G., Chavez, R. et al. (2007). Immunological study of patients with herpetic stromal keratitis treated with Dialyzable Leukocyte Extracts. Proceedings Immunology. pp. 67-71.

Matsuda, A., Okayama, Y., Ebihara, N., Yokoi, N., Hamuro, J., et al. (2009) Hyperexpression of the high-affinity IgE receptor-beta chain in chronic allergic keratoconjunctivitis. Invest Ophthalmol Vis Sci. pp. 2871-2877.

Matsuba-Kitamura, S., Yoshimoto, T., Yasuda, K., Futatsugi-Yumikura, S., Taki, Y., et al. (2010). Contribution of IL-33 to induction and augmentation of experimental allergic conjunctivitis. Int Immunol. pp. 479-489.

Moingeon, P. (2006). Sublingual immunotherapy: from biological extracts to recombinant allergens. Allergy. pp.15-19.

Moingeon, P., Batard, T., Fadel, R., Frati, F., Sieber, J. et al. (2006). Immune mechanisms of allergen-specific sublingual immunotherapy. Allergy. pp. 151-165.

Morgan, SJ., Williams, JH., Walls, AF., Holgate, ST. (1991) Mast cell hyperplasia in atopic keratoconjunctivitis. An immunohistochemical study. Eye (Lond) pp. 729-735.

Mortemousque, B. (2007). Les tests de provocation conjuntivaux. J Fr Ophtalmol pp. 300-305.

Moubayed, SP., Vu, TT., Quach, C. & Daniel, SJ. (2011). Periorbital cellulitis in the pediatric population: clinical features and management of 117 cases. J Otolaryngol Head Neck Surg. pp. 266-270.

Naclerio, RM., Bachert, C., Baraniuk, JN.(2010). Pathophysiology of nasal congestion. Int J Gen Med. pp. 47-57.

Nosbaum, A., Hennino, A., Berard, F. & Nicolas, JF. (2010). Patch testing in atopic dermatitis patients. Eur J Dermatol pp. 563-566.

Onguchi, T., Dogru, M., Okada, N., Kato, NA., Tanaka, M. et al. (2006). The impact of the onset time of atopic keratoconjunctivitis on the tear function and ocular surface findings. Am J Ophthalmol. pp. 569-571.

Ono, SJ. & Abelson, MB. (2005). Allergic conjunctivitis: update on pathophysiology and prospects for future treatment. J Allergy Clin Immunol. pp. 118-122.

Ownby, DR. (2001). Skin tests in comparison with other diagnostic methods. Immunol Aller Clin North Am pp. 355-367.

Pelikan, Z & Pelikan-Filipek M. (1989). Cytologic changes in the nasal secretions during the late nasal response. J Allergy Clin Immunol. pp. 1068-1079.

Pelikan, Z. (2009). Audiometric changes in chronic secretory otitis media due to nasal allergy. Otol Neurotol. pp. 868-875.

Pelikan, Z. (2009). The possible involvement of nasal allergy in allergic kertoconjunctivitis. Eye. pp.1653-1660.

Pelikan, Z. (2010). Allergic conjunctivitis and nasal allergy. Curr Allergy Asthma Rep. pp.295-302.

Pelikan Z. (2011) Delayed asthmatic response: a new phenotype of bronchial response to allergen challenge and soluble adhesion molecules in the serum. Ann Allergy Asthma Immunol. pp. 119-130

Pineda, B., Estrada-Parra, S., Pedraza-Medina, B., Rodriguez-Ropon, A., Pérez, R. et al. (2005). Interstitial transfer factor as adjuvant immunotherapy for experimental glioma. J Exp Clin Cancer Res. pp. 575-583.

Prechl, J., Papp, K. & Erdei, A. (2010). Antigen microarrays: descriptive chemistry or functional immunomics? Trends Immunol. pp. 133-137.

Reyes, NJ., Mayhew, E., Chen, PW., Niederkorn, JY. (2011) γδ T cells are required for maximal expression of allergic conjunctivitis. Invest Ophthalmol Vis Sci. pp. 2211-2216.

Rich, LF. & Hanifin, JM. (1985). Ocular complications of atopic dermatitis and other eczemas. Int Ophthalmol Clin. pp. 61-76.

Ryan, MW. & Brooks, EG. (2010). Rhinosinusitis and comorbidities. Curr Allergy Asthma Rep. pp. 188-193.

Sangwan, VS., Murthy, SI., Vemuganti, GK., Bansal, AK., Gangopadhyay, N. et al. (2005). Cultivated corneal epithelial transplantation for severe ocular surface disease in vernal keratoconjunctivitis. Cornea. pp. 426-430.

Santacruz-Valdes, C., Aguilar, G., Perez-Tapia, M., Estrada-Parra, S., Jimenez-Martinez, MC. (2010). Dialyzable Leukocyte extracts (Transfer factor) as adjuvant therapy for fungal keratitis. Am J Case Rep 2010 pp. 97-101.

Scadding, GW., Shamji, MH., Jacobson, MR., Lee, DI., Wilson, D. et al. (2010). Sublingual grass pollen immunotherapy is associated with increases in sublingual Foxp3-expressing cells and elevated allergen-specific immunoglobulin G4, immunoglobulin A and serum inhibitory activity for immunoglobulin E-facilitated allergen binding to B cells. Clin Exp Allergy. pp. 598-606.

Sette, A., Fleri, W., Peters, B., Sathiamurthy, M., Bui, HH. et al. (2005). A roadmap for the immunomics of category A-C pathogens. Immunity. pp. 155-61.

Shakir, EM., Cheung, DS. & Grayson, MH. (2010). Mechanisms of immunotherapy: a historical perspective. Ann Allergy Asthma Immunol. pp. 340-347.

Sosa, M., Flores, G., Estrada, S., Orea, M. & Gómez-Vera, J. (2001). Comparative treatment between thalidomide and transfer factor in severe atopic dermatitis. Rev Alerg Mex. pp. 56-64.

Spergel, JM. & Paller, AS. (2003). Atopic dermatitis and the atopic march. J Allergy Clin Immunol. pp. S118-27.

Stern, ME., Siemasko, K. & Gao, J. (2005).Role of Interferon-gamma in a mouse model of allergic conjunctivitis. Invest Ophthalmol Vis Sci pp. 3239–3246

Suzuki, S., Goto, E., Dogru, M., Asano-Kato, N., Matsumoto, Y., et al. (2006). Tear film lipid layer alterations in allergic conjunctivitis. Cornea. pp. 277-280.

Takhar, P., Smurthwaite, L., Coker, HA., Fear, DJ., Banfield, GK. et al. (2005). Allergen drives class switching to IgE in the nasal mucosa in allergic rhinitis. J Immunol. pp. 5024-5032.

Takhar, .P, Corrigan, CJ., Smurthwaite, L., O'Connor, BJ., Durham, SR., et al. (2007). Class switch recombination to IgE in the bronchial mucosa of atopic and nonatopic patients with asthma. J Allergy Clin Immunol. pp. 213-218.

Tanaka, M., Dogru, M., Takano, Y., Miyake-Kashima, M., Asano-Kato, N. et al. (2004). The relation of conjunctival and cornea findings in severe ocular allergies. Cornea. pp. 464-467.

Tuft, SJ., Kemeny, DM., Dart, JK. & Buckley, RJ. (1991). Clinical features of atopic keratoconjunctivitis. Ophthalmology pp. 150–158.

Uchio, E., Kimura, R., Migita, H., Kozawa, M.& Kadonosono, K. (2008) Demographic aspects of allergic ocular diseases and evaluation of new criteria for clinical assessment of ocular allergy. Graefes Arch Clin Exp Ophthalmol. pp. 291-296

Valdés-Sánchez, AF., Martín-Rodríguez, OL. & Lastra-Alfonso, G. (1993). Treatment of extrinsic bronchial asthma with transfer factor Rev Alerg Mex. pp. 124-131.

Vichyanond, P., Tantimongkolsuk, C., Dumrongkigchaipom, P., Jirapongsananuruk, O., Visitsunthorn, N. et al. (2004) Result of a novel therapy with 0.1% topical ophthalmic FK-506 ointment. J Allergy Clin Immunol. pp. 355-358.

Wilkins, MR., Appel, RD., Van-Eyk, JE., Chung, MC., Görg, A. et al. (2006). Guidelines for the next 10 years of proteomics. Proteomics. pp. 4-8.

Wilson, GB., Fudenberg, HH. & Keller, RH. (1984). Guidelines for immunotherapy of antigen-specific defects with transfer factor. J Clin Lab Immunol. pp. 51-58.

Wormald, R., Smeeth, L. & Henshaw, K. (2004). Evidence-based ophthalmology, BMJ publishing group.

Yuta, A., Ali, M., Sabol, M., Gaumond, E. & Baraniuk, JN. (1997). Mucoglycoprotein hypersecretion in allergic rhinitis and cystic fibrosis. Am J Physiol. pp. L1203-1207.

Zribi, H., Descamps, V., Hoang-Xuan, T., Crickx, B. & Doan, S. (2009). Dramatic improvement of atopic keratoconjunctivitis after topical treatment with tacrolimus ointment restricted to the eyelids. J Eur Acad Dermatol Venereol. pp. 489–490.

4

Mediators and Some Cytokines in Tears During the Late Conjunctival Response Induced by Primary Allergic Reaction in the Nasal Mucosa

Zdenek Pelikan
Allergy Research Foundation, Breda
The Netherlands

1. Introduction

The allergic conjunctivitis (AC) consists of five clinical types, a seasonal allergic conjunctivitis (SAC), perennial allergic conjunctivitis (PAC), vernal keratoconjunctivitis (VKC), atopic keratoconjunctivitis (AKC) and giant papillary conjunctivitis (GPC), having a common causal background, namely the involvement of allergic component, but different clinical features. [1-5] The five clinical types of AC can occur in 2 basic forms, a primary and a secondary form, with respect to the locality of the initial antigen-antibody/sensitized Th1 cells interaction with following steps, called initial allergic reaction. [6-12] In the primary AC forms, the initial allergic reaction with all subsequent steps, due to the direct exposure of conjunctivae by an external allergen, is localized in the conjunctival tissue. In these, classical, AC forms, the conjunctival tissue is the primary site of allergic reaction and together the primary target tissue affected directly by the allergic reaction and displaying the characteristic clinical symptoms. In the secondary AC forms, the initial allergic reaction taking place in the nasal mucosa, due to exposure to an external allergen, induces subsequently the secondary form of AC through various possible mechanisms and pathways. In this case, the conjunctival tissue is affected by factors released and generated by allergic reaction in the nasal mucosa and the conjunctival response displaying characteristic clinical symptoms may be considered as a consequence of the primary allergic reaction in the nose. [6-12]

In both the basic forms of AC as well as all five clinical types, various hypersensitivity mechanisms, such as immediate type (IgE-mediated Type I), late (Type III) or delayed (cell-mediated Type IV), may be involved.[1, 2, 5, 9-19] The involvement of various hypersensitivity types in AC results then in development of various types of conjunctival response (CR) to allergen exposure (challenge), an immediate (ICR), a late (LCR), a dual late (DLCR, being a combination of an immediate and a late type), a delayed (DYCR) and a dual delayed (DDYCR, being a combination of an immediate and a delayed type). [1-3, 5-14, 20] The primary forms of AC can be demonstrated by direct conjunctival provocation tests with allergens (CPTs), whereas the secondarily induced AC forms can only be confirmed by nasal provocation tests with allergens (NPTs) in combination with registration of the conjunctival signs and subjective symptoms.

Nevertheless, there is a great dearth of data concerning both the clinical and the immunologic features of the secondary CR and the mechanism(s) through which the allergic reaction initiated in the nasal mucosa induces the secondary CR types. [1-3, 5-42] The purpose of this study was to investigate: (1) the appearance and possible concentration changes of some important mediators, such as histamine, tryptase, eosinophil cationic protein (ECP), leukotrienes, myeloperoxidase (MPO) and cytokines, such as, interferon-γ (IFN-γ), IL-2, IL-4 and IL-5 in tears during the secondary late CR; (2) the possible significance of these mediators in tears for the mechanism(s) underlying the secondary late CR.

2. Material and methods

2.1 Patients

Thirty-one patients suffering from allergic conjunctivitis (SAC, n=13 and PAC, n=18) for more than 3 years, showing insufficient therapeutic compliance to the standard topical ophthalmologic treatment, having been referred to our Department of Allergology & Immunology (Institute of Medical Sciences "De Klokkenberg", Breda, The Netherlands), for more extensive diagnostic analysis of their AC complaints, and developing the secondary late conjunctival response(SLCR) to nasal provocation tests with allergens (NPTs),were randomly selected and volunteered to participate in this study.

These patients, 12 males and 19 females, 18-47 years of age (Table 1), have previously been treated with various topical and oral H1-receptor-antagonists, ophthalmic cromolyn formulation, topical ocular glucocorticosteroids, decongestant, topical vasoconstrictors and incidentally with NSAID drugs, without significant therapeutic effects. None of these patients suffered from other ocular disorders, infection, systemic diseases or immunodeffociency or had previously been treated with nasal cromolyn, nasal or systemic glucocorticosteroids, immunosuppressive drugs or immunotherapy. All of them demonstrated normal intraocular pressure. In 14 of these patients 19 conjunctival provocation tests (CPT) with inhalant allergen, performed previously, were negative.

The patients underwent a routine diagnostic procedure consisting of: a detailed disease history, general physical examination, basic laboratory tests, bacteriological screening of tears, nasal secretions, sputum and blood, roentgenogram of chest and paranasal sinuses in Water's projection, nasoscopy and cytologic examination of nasal secretions, skin tests with basic and supplementary inhalant and food allergens, determination of serum immunoglobulins, and ophthalmologic examination including ophthalmoscopy, slit-lamp evaluation, vital staining with fluorescein and cytologic examination of the tears. The routine diagnostic procedure performed in these 31 patients revealed positive or suspect history for nasal allergy (93%), positive skin (intracutaneous) tests with various inhalant allergens (100%), hyperaemic /livid and edematic nasal mucosa (97%), increased eosinophil and neutrophil counts in nasal secretions (87%), conjunctival hyperaemia and tearing to a slight degree (100%), appearance of incidental eosinophils and conjunctival epithelial cells in the tear specimens (84%), increased blood eosinophil counts (23%), positive specific IgE in the serum (ImmunoCAP) for some inhalant allergens (19%) and non-increased nasal responsiveness to histamine determined by means of nasal challenge with histamine (93%) (Table 1). No other abnormalities were found in these patients.

In these 31 patients, 54 nasal provocation tests (NPTs) with various inhalant allergens (Table 2)and 31 control challenges with PBS (phosphate-buffered saline)were performed using rhinomanometry in combination with simultaneous recording of the ocular signs and subjective symptoms (Tables 1, 2). The ocular signs and relevant subjective symptoms were evaluated by means of the Pelikan's scoring (grading) system (Table 3). [7, 9-12] The patients were investigated in a period without acute ocular and/or nasal complaints, without symptoms of an acute infection, outside the allergen-relevant period (season) and during. hospitalization. The long-acting H1-receptor antagonists, topical cromolyn and glucocorticosteroids were withdrawn 4 weeks, topical and oral short-acting H1 receptor antagonists, topical decongestants and other treatments were withdrawn 48 hours before each of the NPTs.

	Patients		Control subjects n=14
	SAC (n=13)	PAC (n=18)	
Age (years)	25 ± 7	31 ± 12	29 ± 9
Sex (M/F)	5/8	7/11	6/8
Disease history (years)	3.9±1.5	4.6±0.7	5.2 ± 1.1
Blood leukocyte count (x 10^9 /L) °	8.3±0.6	9.1±1.4	7.9±0.8
-increased	0	0	0
Blood eosinophil count (x 10^6 /L) °°	263±21	285±13	255±29
-increased	2	5	4
Increased total IgE in the serum ▫	0	0	0
Positive specific IgE in the serum ▫▫	1	5	2
Positive skin response •			
-Immediate type	4	7	8
-Late type	9	10	5
-Delayed type	0	1	1
Nasal provocation tests			
-positive	13	18	21
-negative	10	13	15

SAC= seasonal allergic conjunctivitis; PAC= perennial allergic conjunctivitis; ° = normal value 4.0-10.0 x 10^9/L; °° = normal value < 300 x 10^6/L; ▫ = normal value <500 IU/mL; ▫▫ = normal value <0.70 U/mL; • = positive skin response to the relevant allergen (=allergen producing positive nasal and conjunctival or nasal response only)

Table 1. Characteristics of the patients

The 31 positive NPTs producing the secondary late conjunctival response (SCLR) in these patients and 31 PBS control challenges were repeated 2-3 weeks later. The repeated NPTs and PBS control challenges were supplemented with a collection of the tears for the mediator determination (Table 4). A 4-day interval was always inserted between the end of the preceding test and the begin of the following test to prevent the carry-over effects and to allow the patient recovery. The study protocol was approved by the local ethical committee and informed consent was obtained from all study participants.

Allergen	Concentration	Nasal responses positive (n=31)	Conjunctival responses (n=31)		Nasal responses negative (n=23)
			SAC (n=13)	PAC (n=18)	
Dermatophagoides pteron	1000 BU/mL	5		5	3
Dermatophagoides farinae	1000 BU/mL	1		1	1
Animal danders					
-dog	3000 BU/mL	3		3	2
-horse	2000 BU/mL	2		2	0
-cat	2000 BU/mL	2		2	3
-guinea pig	2000 BU/mL	1		1	0
Feathers					
-parrot	3000 BU/mL	1		1	0
-parakeet	3000 BU/mL	1		1	1
Aspergillus fumigatus	1000 BU/mL	2		2	1
Pollen					
-grass mix I	1000 BU/mL	4	4		2
-grass mix II	1000 BU/mL	2	2		1
-flower mix	5000 BU/mL	1	1		2
-tree mix	3000 BU/mL	2	2		3
-weed mix	1000 BU/mL	1	1		2
-poplar	2000 BU/mL	1	1		0
-ragweed short	1000 BU/mL	1	1		1
-ragweed giant	1000 BU/mL	1	1		1

SAC = seasonal allergic conjunctivitis; PAC = perennial allergic conjunctivitis; BU/mL = biologic units per mL

Grasspollen mix I = *Dactylis glomerata, Lolium perenne, Phleum pratensis, Poa pratensis;*
Grasspollen mix II = *Festuca pratensis, Holcus lanatus, Agrostis alba, Anthoxanthum odoratum*
Flower pollen mix = *Dahlia variabilis, Solidago virgaurea, Primula variabilis, Forsythia suspensa*
Tree pollen mix = *Betula pendula, Corylus avellana, Juniperus communis, Salix alba*
Weed pollen mix = *Artemisia vulgaris,Plantago lanceolata, Rumex acetosa, Taraxacum officinale*

Table 2. Survey of the allergens used for nasal challenge

2.2 Allergens

Dialyzed and lyophilized allergen extracts (Allergopharma, Reinbek, Germany) were diluted in phosphate-buffered saline (PBS) and used for skin tests in concentrations of 100-500 BU/mL and for NPTs in concentrations of 1000-5000 BU/mL (Table 2), as recommended by the manufacturer. If indicated, higher dilutions of the allergen extracts were used both for the skin tests and for the NPTs.

2.3 Skin tests

Scratch tests with allergenic extracts in concentrations of 500 BU/mL were performed and the results evaluated after 20 minutes. If the results were negative, then intracutaneous tests in concentrations of 100 BU/mL and 500 BU/mL were carried out and evaluated 20 minutes and 6, 12, 24, 36, 48, 56, 72 and 96 hours after the intradermal injection. A skin wheal (>7.0 mm in diameter) occurring after 20 minutes was qualified as a positive immediate skin response, the skin infiltration appearing between 6 and 12 hours as a late skin response, and the skin induration recorded later than 48 hours as a delayed skin response.[8-13, 42-46]

2.4 Nasal provocation tests (NPTs)

Nasal challenges with allergens were performed using rhinomanometry, already described in our previous studies. [6-13, 23, 43-47] The nasal obstruction due to the edema of the nasal mucosa was evaluated by means of nasopharynx-nostril pressure gradient (NPG) parameters, which are the pressure differences (ΔP) between the nasopharyngeal cavity and the outside air, expressed in cm H_2O. NPTs were performed using the following schedule: (1) baseline values recorded at 0, 5 and 10 minutes before the challenge; (2) PBS control values recorded at 0, 5 and 10 minutes after a 3-minute application of PBS to the nasal mucosa of the non-intubated nasal cavity by means of a saturated wad of cotton wool on a nasal probe inserted under the middle turbinate; (3) post-challenge values recorded after a 3-minute challenge with allergen, carried out in the same manner as the challenge with PBS, at 0, 5, 10, 20, 30, 45, 60, 90 and 120 minutes, then every hour up to the 12th hour, and every second hour during the time-periods between the 24th-38th and 48th - 56th (60th) hour.[9-13] The allergens used for the NPTs were chosen with respect of the disease history and positive skin tests (Tables 1, 2). The nasal response (NR) was assessed to be positive when the post-challenge mean NPG values increased by at least 2.0 cm H_2O (1.2 ± 0.3, mean± SE) with respect to the mean baseline values, recorded at least at three consecutive time intervals[14, 23-26]. The NPG changes recorded within 60-120 minutes after the allergen challenge were considered to be an immediate NR (INR), those recorded within 4-12 hours to be a late NR (LNR), and the changes measured later than 24 hours to be a delayed NR (DYNR) [9-13, 43-45]

2.5 Control tests with phosphate-buffered saline (PBS)

The control nasal challenge with PBS was performed in each patient studied by the same schedule as that used for the NPTs with allergen, however 3 days later.

2.6 Conjunctival response

The objective conjunctival signs and relevant subjective symptoms were registered before and during all NPTs with allergens and PBS at the same time-points as the nasal NPG values. The features of the conjunctiva were assessed by ophthalmoscopy including a slit lamp. The conjunctival signs, hyperaemia (injection), chemosis, hyperlacrimation, and palpebral edema, and the subjective symptoms, such as itching (burning), blurred vision and photophobia, were registered and evaluated by means of the scale suggested by Abelson, however, modified by us (Pelikan's scale). [10-12] The evaluation criteria of the individual signs and symptoms were as follows: 0=absent, 1=mild (present to a slight degree), 2=moderate, 3= pronounced (moderately severe), 4=severe (Table 3). The differences in total sign score of 4 points or more (3 ± 1, mean ± SE), recorded at least at three consecutive time-intervals, were found to be statistically significant ($p<0.05$).

	Abelson I*	Abelson II**	Pelikan
I. OBJECTIVE SIGNS			
-Hyperemia (injection, redness)	0 - 4	0 - 3	0 - 4
-Chemosis		0 - 3	0 - 4
-Hyperlacrimation (tearing)		0 - 3	0 - 4
-Palpebral edema			0 - 4
II. SUBJECTIVE SYMPTOMS			
-Itching (burning)	0 - 4	0 - 4	0 - 4
-Photophobia			0 - 4
-Blurred vision			0 - 4

* = References 27, 28, 29; ** = References 21, 30
Abelson's grading scale: 0=None; 1=Mild (intermittent); 2=Moderate; 3=Severe; 4= extremely severe (or "incapacitating "itching); [Significant threshold: ≥+2]
Pelikan's grading scale: 0=Absent; 1=Mild (present to a slight degree or intermittent); 2=Moderate; 3= Pronounced (moderately severe); 4=Severe; [Significant difference: ≥4 points ($p<0.05$), with respect to the pre-challenge value, recorded at least at 3 consecutive time-points].

Table 3. Survey of Abelson's and our "modified" conjunctivitis grading scale and symptom score ("Pelikan's modified grading scale")

2.7 Collection and processing of tears

The tear specimens were collected from each of eyes separately by means of a micropipette from the inferior conjunctival fornix and/or lacus lacrimalis, before, 30 and 60 minutes, every second hour up to 12 hours and 24 hours after the allergen challenge. If necessary, a gentle pressure on the lacrimal sac from outside was applied. The tear samples (1-4 mL) were stored at -8°C and processed within 1 hours. The concentrations of appropriate factors in tears were measured by using commercially available kits, following the manufacturer's recommendations. The measurements of the factors were performed separately in tear samples from each of the eyes on each occasion, and the results were then calculated as the mean of both the eyes.

All measurements were performed in duplicate by a double-blind schedule. The intra-assay as well as the inter-assay coefficients of variations for all the assay kits employed were less than 10 %.

a. *Histamine* Histamine concentrations, so-called "blanks", were measured by the Siraganian's fluorometric method [48] Detection limits (DL): 1.0 ng/mL
b. *Tryptase* -ImmunoCAP (Pharmacia, Uppsala, Sweden). DL: 1.0 µg/L
c. *Eosinophil cationic protein (ECP)*-ImmunoCAP (Pharmacia Diagnostics, Uppsala, Sweden). DL: 2µg/L

d. *Leukotrienes B4, C4, E4* -EIA kits (Cayman Chemical Company, Ann Arbor/MI, USA). Detection limits (DL): LTB_4 = 4.8 pg/mL; LTC_4 = 2 pg/mL; LTE_4 = 3.7 pg/
e. *Myeloperoxidase (MPO)* - ELISA kit (Oxis International Inc, Portland /OR, USA). DL: 25 ng/mL
f. *Interferon-gamma (IFN-γ)* - ELISA kit (Bender MedSystems, Wien, Austria). DL: 1.0 pg/mL
g. *Interleukin 2 (IL-2)* - ELISA kit (R & D System (Minneapolis/MN, USA). DL: < 3.0 pg/mL
h. *Interleukin 4 (IL-4)* - ELISA kit (Bender MedSystems , Wien, Austria).DL: 0.6 pg/mL
i. *Interleukin 5 (IL-5)* - ELISA kit (R & D System (Minneapolis/MN, USA). DL: 3.0 pg/mL

2.8 Control group

Fourteen adults suffering from allergic rhinitis, confirmed by positive history, skin tests and positive NPTs with inhalant allergens, but without history of any ocular disease and with normal ophthalmologic findings, volunteered to participate as control subjects. In these patients 14 positive late nasal responses (LNR)with inhalant allergens were repeated and supplemented with registration of the conjunctival features and subjective symptoms and estimation of the above mentioned mediators in tears.

2.9 Statistical analysis

1. Nasal and conjunctival responses (mean total scores of conjunctival signs and subjective symptoms) to the allergen challenge as well as to the PBS control challenge in individual patients were statistically analyzed by Wilcoxon matched-pair signed rank test, comparing the post-challenge values at each of the time-points with the mean pre-challenge (baseline) values.
2. The mean NPG values and the mean total conjunctival score values were compared with corresponding PBS control values at each of the time-points and analyzed by the Mann-Whitney *U* test.
3. The post-challenge mediator values measured at each of the time points during the repeated SLCRs and PBS control in individual patients were compared with their pre-challenge values and statistically analyzed by Wilcoxon matched-pair signed rank test.
4. The mean post-challenge mediator values during the repeated SLCRs were compared with corresponding PBS values and statistically evaluated by Mann-Whitney *U* test. Statistical evaluation of the CR was performed separately for each of the eyes and then the mean from both the eyes was calculated. A P value < 0.05 was considered to be statistically significant.

3. Results

3.1 Nasal responses (NRs)

In the 31 patients 54 nasal provocation tests (NPTs) with various inhalant allergens (Tables 1, 2) and 31 PBS control challenges were performed. The 31 patients developed 31 late nasal responses (LNRs; $p<0.01$) and 23 negative nasal responses (NNRs; $p>0.1$)(Table 2). The LNR

began between 4-6 hours, reached its maximum between 6-8 hours and resolved within 12 hours after the nasal challenge with allergen.
The 31 PBS control tests were all negative ($p>0.1$). No significant differences were found in the appearance of the LNRs with respect to the individual allergens ($p>0.1$). The LNRs were associated with significant changes ($p<0.05$) in the counts (mostly temporary increase) of the neutrophils, eosinophils, epithelial and goblet cells, and to a lesser degree of the lymphocytes, in the nasal secretions. The counts of basophils, mast cells, monocytes and plasma cells were relatively low and without significant changes.
The repeated NPTs resulted in the development of similar and statistically significant LNRs as comparing the post-challenge with the pre-challenge (baseline) values ($p<0.001$) and with the PBS control values ($p<0.001$) (Fig. 1C). No statistical significant differences were found between the initial and the repeated LNRs ($p>0.2$).

3.2 Conjunctival responses (CRs)

The 31 positive LNRs, recorded in 31 patients, were associated with significantly positive secondary conjunctival responses of the late type (SLCR; $p<0.01$)(Table 2). The positive SLCR began between 5-6 hours, reached its maximum between 8-10 hours and resolved usually within 12, sometimes within 24 hours after the allergen challenge. The SLCR was represented by significant changes of the objective conjunctival signs ($p<0.01$) as well as subjective symptoms ($p<0.05$). No significant corneal signs were recorded in any SLCR. No conjunctival changes were recorded during the 23 negative nasal responses ($p>0.05$) or during the 31 PBS control challenges ($p>0.1$). The 31 repeated NPTs , have induced similar and statistically significant SLCRs , both as comparing the post-challenge with the pre-challenge (baseline) values ($p<0.01$) and as comparing with the PBS control challenge ($p<0.01$). (Fig. 1B). No statictically significant difference were found between the initial and the repeated SLCRs ($p>0.2$). No significant differences in the conjunctival changes recorded both during the initial and during the repeated SLCRs were observed between the right and left eye ($p>0.1$).

3.3 Changes of mediators and other factor in the tears during the SLCRs

The SLCRS were associated with significant changes in the concentrations ($p<0.05$) of histamine, EPC, LTC_4 , LTB_4 , MPO, IL-4 and IL-5 in the tears (Table 4; Fig. 1A). The pre-challenge concentrations of most of these factors were either very low or under the detection limit, whereas their post-challenge concentrations usually increased to various degrees at various time-points, followed by their decrease and disappearance from the tears within 24 hours after the allergen challenge (Table 4 ; Fig.1A). The concentrations of tryptase in tears was very low, sometimes under the detection limit and without significant changes ($p>0.05$). The INF-γ and IL-2 were recorded in the tears during the SLCRs irregularly and without any significant changes ($p>0.05$ and $p>0.05$, respectively). The LTE_4 was not detected in the tears during the positive SLCRs. No significant concentration changes of the investigated factors were recorded in tears during the 31 PBS control challenges and 23 negative CRs. Moreover, the concentrations of most of these factors were under the detection limits (Table 4). No significant differences in the concentrations of particular factors and their changes in tears have been found between the right and left eye, both during the SLCRs and during the PBS controls ($p>0.1$ and $p>0.2$, respectively).

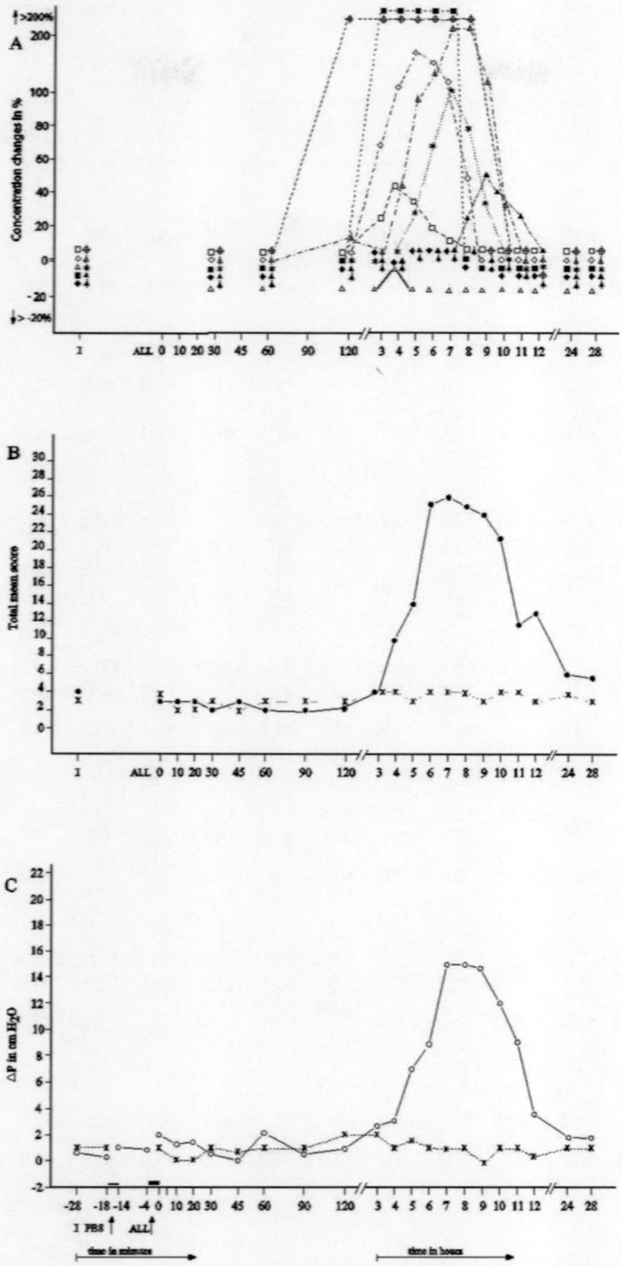

Fig. 1. The secondary late conjunctival responses (SLCRs; n=31) accompanying the isolated late nasal responses (ILNRs; n=31). **A.** The mean score of particular factors during the SLCR: □ = histamine, Δ = tryptase, ⌖ = EPC, ▲ = LTB_4, ◇ = LTC_4, ✶ = MPO, ■ = IL-4, ▲ = IL-5, ◆ = IFN-γ, ▲ = IL-2. **B.** The total mean score of conjunctival signs and symptoms during the SLCR (•) and PBS (**x**). **C.** The mean rhinomanometric values (NPG) recorded during ILNR (○) and PBS (x), I = Initial (baseline) values; PBS = Phosphate buffered saline; ALL = Allergen challenge

	Before the challenge	After the challenge (hours)														
		½	1	2	3	4	5	6	7	8	9	10	11	12	24	28
Histamine *ng/mL*																
- *SLCR*	< 1.0	< 1.0	< 1.0	< 1.0	2.6 ± 0.3*	4.7 ± 0.5*	3.4 ± 0.7*	1.9 ± 0.6+	1.2 ± 0.1	<1.0	<1.0	<1.0	<1.0	<1.0	<1.0	1.3 ± 0.2
- *PBS*	< 1.0	< 1.0	< 1.0	< 1.0	<1.0	<1.0	1.1 ± 0.1	<1.0	<1.0	<1.0	<1.0	<1.0	<1.0	<1.0	<1.0	<1.0
Tryptase *µg/L*																
- *SLCR*	1.3±0.3	<1.0	<1.0	1.1 ± 0.1	<1.0	1.3 ± 0.2	<1.0	<1.0	<1.0	<1.0	<1.0	<1.0	<1.0	<1.0	<1.0	<1.0
- *PBS*	< 1.0	<1.0	<1.0	<1.0	1.2 ± 0.2	<1.0	<1.0	<1.0	<1.0	<1.0	<1.0	<1.0	<1.0	<1.0	<1.0	<1.0
EPC µg/L																
- *SLCR*	2.3±0.2	2.5 ± 0.4	2.2 ± 0.1	4.5 ± 0.7+	5.3 ± 1.1+	9.5 ± 2.3*	13.8 ± 3.2**	15.6 ± 2.0**	7.3 ± 1.8*	6.0 ± 1.4*	2.4 ± 0.2	<2.0	<2.0	<2.0	<2.0	<2.0
- PBS	2.7±0.6	<2.0	<2.0	2.4 ± 0.4	2.5 ± 0.3	<2.0	<2.0	2.8 ± 0.5	2.3 ± 0.3	2.5 ± 0.2	2.1 ± 0.1	2.2 ± 0.1	<2.	2.4 ± 0.3	<2.	<2.
LTB4 pg/mL																
- *SLCR*	<4.8	<4.8	<4.8	5.5 ± 0.6	4.9 ± 0.1	6.8 ± 1.0+	9.3 ± 2.1*	11.2 ± 3.1*	23.0 ± 2.6**	28.5 ± 1.4**	10.7 ± 1.9*	6.6 ± 0.5+	5.1 ± 0.4	5.0 ± 0.2	<4.8	<4.8
- PBS	<4.8	<4.8	<4.8	5.1 ± 0.2	<4.8	<4.8	<4.8	<4.8	5.0±0.2	<4.8	<4.8	<4.8	<4.8	<4.8	<4.8	<4.8
LTC4 pg/mL																
- *SLCR*	2.2±0.1	<2.0	<2.0	2.3 ± 0.3	3.8 ± 0.7+	5.2 ± 0.5*	6.1 ± 0.4*	5.8 ± 0.3*	4.9 ± 0.8*	3.3 ± 0.2	2.3 ± 0.2	<2.0	<2.0	<2.0	<2.0	<2.0
- *PBS*	<2.0	<2.0	<2.0	<2.0	<2.0	<2.0	<2.0	<2.0	<2.0	2.2 ± 0.2	2.1 ± 0.1	<2.0	<2.0	<2.0	<2.0	<2.0
MPO *ng/mL*																
- *SLCR*	<25.0	<25.0	<25.0	<25.0	<25.0	<25.0	31.9 ± 5.5+	43.8 ± 3.6*	51.5 ± 4.0**	45.1 ± 2.8*	34.2 ± 1.7*	26.3 ± 1.0	<25.0	<25.0	<25.0	<25.0
- PBS	<25.0	<25.0	<25.0	<25.0	<25.0	<25.0	28.6 ± 2.7	<25.0	<25.0	<25.0	<25.0	<25.0	<25.0	<25.0	<25.0	<25.0
IFN-γ *pg/mL*																
- *SLCR*	<1.0	<1.0	<1.0	<1.0	<1.0	<1.0	<1.0	<1.0	<1.0	<1.0	<1.0	<1.0	1.2 ± 0.1	1.2 ± 0.2	<1.0	<1.0
- PBS	<1.0	<1.0	<1.0	<1.0	<1.0	<1.0	<1.0	<1.0	<1.0	<1.0	<1.0	<1.0	<1.0	<1.0	<1.0	<1.0
IL-2 pg/mL																
- *SLCR*	< 3.0	< 3.0	3.2 ± 0.2	<3.0	<3.0	<3.0	<3.0	<3.0	<3.0	3.3 ± 0.3	<3.0	<3.0	<3.0	3.2 ± 0.1	<3.0	<3.0
- PBS	< 3.0	< 3.0	< 3.0	< 3.0	< 3.0	3.1 ± 0.1	< 3.0	< 3.0	< 3.0	< 3.0	< 3.0	< 3.0	< 3.0	< 3.0	< 3.0	< 3.0
IL-4 *pg/mL*																
- *SLCR*	<0.6	<0.6	<0.6	<0.6	2.4 ± 1.0+	5.7 ± 0.8*	7.9 ± 1.5**	4.0 ± 0.6*	1.8 ± 0.5	<0.6	<0.6	<0.6	<0.6	<0.6	<0.6	<0.6
- PBS	<0.6	<0.6	<0.6	<0.6	<0.6	<0.6	<0.6	<0.6	<0.6	<0.6	<0.6	<0.6	1.3 ± 0.4	<0.6	<0.6	<0.6

	Before the challenge	After the challenge (hours)														
		½	1	2	3	4	5	6	7	8	9	10	11	12	24	28
IL-5 *pg/mL*																
- *SLCR*	<3.0	<3.0	<3.0	<3.0	<3.0	<3.0	<3.0	<3.0	<3.0	3.7 ± 0.6	4.6 ± 0.4*	4.3 ± 0.7*	3.8 ± 0.2	<3.0	<3.0	<3.0
- PBS	<3.0	<3.0	<3.0	<3.0	<3.0	<3.0	<3.0	<3.0	<3.0	<3.0	<3.0	<3.0	<3.0	<3.0	3.1 ± 0.1	<3.0

SLCR = Secondary late conjunctival response; PBS = Phosphate-buffered saline; Significance of mean post-challenge values with respect to the mean pre-challenge (baseline) value:
+ = $p \leq 0.05$; * = $p < 0.05$; ** = $p < 0.01$

Table 4. Concentration of particular factors in tears during the secondary late conjunctival response (SLCR)

3.4 Control patients

The 14 control patients developed an isolated late nasal response (ILNR) during the initial as well as the repeated NPTs ($p < 0.001$ and $p < 0.001$ respectively). No significant conjunctival signs or subjective symptoms were recorded during the 14 repeated LNRs ($p > 0.2$). No significant changes in concentrations of the investigated factors were recorded in tears during the repeated LNRs in these control patients.

4. Discussion

The relationship between the conjunctivae and the nose includes both the anatomical and the functional aspect. [1, 10-12] The conjunctiva is connected with the nasal cavity not only by means of the naso-lacrimal duct, being a part of lacrimal ways, through which opening the tear drainage into the nasal cavity is facilitated, but also by means of the blood vessel network, lymphatic tissue system and neurogenic network. All of them express a number of mutual links and share various common properties.[1, 10-12] Allergic reactions taking place primarily in the nasal mucosa due to the intranasal exposure to inhalant allergen may affect the conjunctiva and subsequently also other ocular tissues, such as the cornea, in various ways and upon involvement of various mechanisms.[9-12, 33, 49-58] These mechanisms may include: (1) Various cell types participating in the allergic reaction occurring in the nasal mucosa, such as mucosal mast cells, eosinophils, basophils, neutrophils, B-lymphocytes/plasma cells, particular subsets of T-lymphocytes (Th`1, Th2, Th 17, T-regulatory cells, natural killer cells), dendritic cells, monocytes thrombocytes, macrophages, epithelial and endothelial cells, and mucosal goblet cells, can migrate into the bloodstream and/or lymphatic system, and under extreme conditions also into lacrimal ways, and thereby attain the conjunctiva; (2) The various cell types, activated and/or inhibited during the allergic reaction in the nasal mucosa, generate and release a number of factors (classical mediators, eicosanoids, cytokines, chemokines, adhesion molecules, chemotactic and other factors), which could then reach conjunctiva either directly by the retrograde penetration through the naso- lacrimal duct and lacrimal ways or indirectly through the related blood and/or lymphatic vessel system; (3) The allergic reaction could also activate the local neurogenic system (sensory nerves, sympathetic and parasympathetic fibres) releasing then the neuropeptides which can reach the conjunctiva either along or through the related nerves, such as nervus trigemini, nervus nasociliaris and ganglion pterygopalatinum; (4) The allergic reaction or its particular stages and parts can also stimulate the local nasal mucosal lymphatic system called "nose-associated lymphatic tissue" (NALT), being a part of the"mucosa- associated lymphatic system" (MALT). The MALT system facilitates a multiple and mutual communication among the particular lymphatic organ-related sub-systems, in this case between the NALT on one hand and the "eye-associated lymphatic tissue "(EALT), "conjunctiva- associated lymphatic tissue"(CALT), "tear-associated lymphatic tissue "(TALT) and "lacrimal drainage-associated lymphatic tissue"(LDALT) on the other hand. The abundance of the relationship and communication among the individual parts of lymphatic system allow not only a multiple transmission of various signals (e.g. cell-cell, cell-receptor, receptor-receptor), but also a reciprocal (both- directional) traffic of various types of circulating cells, such as B-lymphocytes/plasma cells producing immunoglobulins of individual classes and sub-classes, particular sub-sets of T-lymphocytes (Th1- and Th2-cells, cytotoxic, regulatory and natural killer cells), antigen-presenting cells (APC), other cell types, or finally, under certain circumstances, of some cells resident in the mucosal membrane.

The cell traffic can be effectuated not only through various attraction mechanisms governed by chemotactic factors, cytokines, chemokines and adhesion molecules, but also through a special, so-called, "homing mechanism" of B- and T-lymphocytes, controlled by a number of homing factors.[10-12, 55, 56]

The disturbed homing mechanism leads to migration of particular cell types (e.g. B- or T-lymphocytes) to locations different from the predetermined destinations. By this way, the particular sub-sets of lymphocytes having been initially activated in a certain tissue (mucosal locality), after migrating into the bloodstream and/or lymphatic network to finish their maturation process, do not return to this original tissue, but due to the disturbed homing factors they terminate their route by entering into another tissue, different from the original one. This process is called "wrong homing". [10-12, 45-56]

The occurrence and possible role of various mediators, cytokines, chemokines and adhesion molecules in tears has already been extensively studied in patients suffering from various forms of allergic conjunctivitis. [14-16, 18, 20, 26, 32-35, 37-42, 57-83]

The mediators having been most frequently studied in tears included histamine,[20, 37, 40, 41,59-62, 64, 66] tryptase,[14, 26, 35, 37, 62, 66, 67] ECP,[14, 26, 32, 63, 66, 68, 69] LTB_4,[20, 64, 70-74] LTC_4,[20, 37, 41, 73, 74] LTD_4,[73] MPO,[63, 66] Prostaglandins (PGD_2, PGE_2) [41, 60, 62, 72] and various cytokines [1, 3, 5, 12, 16-18, 26, 36, 62, 63, 66, 76-83]

In most of these studies a single determination of the mediators in tears of patients suffering from primary forms of allergic conjunctivitis (SAC, PAC) or keratoconjunctivitis (VKC, AKC) has been performed. The papers addressing the determination of the mediators during the conjunctival provocation tests with allergens (CPTs) are not numerous.[14, 20, 26, 32, 35, 37, 38, 40, 60, 66, 83] Studies following the concentration changes of the above mentioned mediators in tears for a longer period of time as a serial determination during the particular types of conjunctival response (immediate/ early and/or late) due to the conjunctival challenge with allergen are relatively rare.[14, 20, 32, 37, 61-63, 83] The primary immediate/early conjunctival response (ICR) to conjunctival challenge with allergen (CPT) has been reported to be accompanied by concentration changes (mostly increase) of histamine, [14, 20, 26, 37, 38, 40, 41,

[60-62, 66, 83] tryptase,[14, 35, 37, 62] ECP,[63] LTB_4,[20, 73] LTC_4,[20, 37, 41, 73] MPO,[63] PGD_2,[41, 60, 83] kinin,[41, 60] TAME-esterase[41, 60] and various cytokines[62, 63] in tears. The primary late conjunctival response (LCR) to conjunctival challenge with allergen (CPT) has been reported to be associated with increased concentrations of histamine,[14, 20, 61, 83] ECP,[14, 32, 63] LTB_4,[20] LTC_4[20] and some cytokines [16, 62] in tears. Our results demonstrating increased concentrations of histamine, EPC, LTB_4, LTC_4, MPO in tears during the secondary late conjunctival response (SLCR) would indicate their active role in the development of this type of CR. However, they were most probably released by the eosinophils, neutrophils and mast cells or basophils in the nasal mucosa, the place of the primary allergic reaction due to the initial allergen exposure. This fact may be supported by results of our other studies,[7, 9, 84] demonstrating only limited numbers of these cell types in tears during the later stages of SLCR. Moreover, these cells were in a non-activated condition, which means their cytoplasmic granules were not degranulated. In contrast, the primary LCR due to the direct conjunctival challenge with allergen is usually accompanied by the abundant appearance of eosinophils and neutrophils and sporadical mast cells, all of them having been exhausted and demonstrating empty cytoplasmic granules (=degranulation) (our not yet published data).

Another interesting result was evidence of slightly increased concentrations of cytokines IL-4 and IL-5 in the tears, whereas IFN-γ and IL-2 appeared in the tears only irregularly and without any concentration changes. This finding may suggest an involvement of Th_2 -lymphocytes in the mechanism leading to the SLCR, however, during the initial phase of this mechanism taking place in the nasal mucosa.

An interesting, but also somewhat conflicting, result was the absence of specific allergen-IgE antibody in serum of most the patients developing the SLCR. Moreover, in another supplementary pilot study, which results are not shown, we did not record any allergen-specific IgE antibody in the nasal secretions or even in the tears during the SLCR. This finding is then partly in contrast to the increased histamine concentrations in the tears during this CR type. The absence of specific IgE antibody in the serum as well as in the nasal secretions and tears of the patients developing the SLCR would suggest either that the concentration of IgE both in the serum and in the nasal secretions and tears were under the detection limits, or a possible involvement of topical IgE being limited to the nasal mucosa only and without any migration outside the nasal mucosa, or finally involvement of non-IgE mechanism in the SLCR. Unfortunately, at this moment we have no acceptable explanation for these phenomena. Further investigation, such as biopsy and immunohistochemical methods of the conjunctival and adjacent tissues will be necessary to provide more clarity on this field.

The results of this study would also stress the importance of provocation tests with allergens. The conjunctival provocation tests with allergens (CPTs), performed directly on the conjunctiva, confirm the role of allergic reaction taking place in the conjunctiva due to a direct exposure of conjucntival tissue to an inhalant allergen. The CPTs result in the manifestation of various types of primary conjunctival response, such as immediate, late or delayed, characterized by various conjunctival signs and subjective symptoms. The CPTs are therefore suitable for demonstrating and confirming the primary types of CR. Nevertheless, the secondary or secondarily induced CR types can only be demonstrated and confirmed by means of nasal provocation tests with allergens (NPTs) combined with simultaneous registration of the conjunctival signs and subjective symptoms. An important requirement for both the CPTs and NPTs is registration of the particular representative parameters before and repeatedly after the allergen challenge, thus for a sufficiently long period of time, allowing measurement of the particular response type in its whole and dynamic course.

5. References

[1] Barney NP, Graziano FM, Cook EB, Stahl JL. Allergic and immunologic diseases of the eye. In: Adkinson NF, Bochner BS, JW, Busse WW, Holgate ST, Lemanske RF, Simons FE, eds. Middleton's Allergy, principles & practice (7th Ed). Philadelphia: Mosby -Elsevier Inc 2009: 1117-1137

[2] McGill JI, Holgate ST, Church MK, Anderson DF, Bacon A. Allergic eye disease mechanisms. Br J Ophthalmol 1998; 82: 1203-1214

[3] Bielory L. Allergic and immunologic disorders of the eye; Part I: Immunology of the eye; Part II: Ocular allergy. J Allergy Clin Immunol 2000; 106: 805-816, 1019-1032

[4] Dart JK, Buckley RJ, Monnickendan M, Prasad J. Perennial allergic conjunctivitis: definition, clinical characteristics and prevalence. A comparison with seasonal allergic conjunctivitis. Trans Ophthalmol Sci UK 1986; 105: 513-520

[5] Bielory L, Friedlaender MH. Allergic conjunctivitis. Immunol Allergy Clin N Am 2008; 28: 43-57

[6] Pelikan Z. Allergic conjunctivitis: primary and secondary role of the allergy reaction in the nose. Dutch J Med (Ned Tijdschr Geneesk) 1988; 132: 561-563

[7] Pelikan Z. The causal role of the nasal allergy in some patients with allergic conjunctivitis. Allergy 2002: 57 (Suppl 73): 230

[8] Pelikan Z. Late nasal response-its clinical characteristics, features, and possible mechanisms. In: Dorsch W (Ed). Late Phase Allergic Reactions. Boca Raton, Ann Arbor, Boston (USA): CRC Press 1990: 111-155

[9] Pelikan Z. The late nasal response. Thesis. Amsterdam: The Free University of Amsterdam 1996

[10] Pelikan Z. Seasonal and perennial allergic conjunctivitis: the possible role of nasal allergy. Clin Exp Ophthalmol 2009; 37:448-457

[11] Pelikan Z. The possible involvement of nasal allergy in allergic keratoconjunctivitis. Eye 2009; 23: 1653-1660

[12] Pelikan Z. Allergic conjunctivitis and nasal allergy. Curr Allergy Asthma Rep 2010; 10: 295-302

[13] Melillo G, Bonini S, Cocco G, Davies RJ, De Monchy JGR, Frølund L, Pelikan Z. Provocation tests with allergens. Allergy 1997; 52 (Suppl 35): 5-36

[14] Bacon AS, Ahluwalia P, Irani AM, Schwartz LB, Holgate ST, Church MK, McGill JI. Tear and conjunctival changes during the allergen-induced early- and late-phase responses. J Allergy Clin Immunol 2000; 106: 948-954

[15] Calder VL. Cellular mechanisms of chronic cell-mediated allergic conjunctivitis. Clin Exp Allergy 2002; 32: 814-817

[16] Leonardi A, Fregona IA, Plebani M, Secchi AG, Calder VL. Th1- and Th2-type cytokines in chronic ocular allergy. Graefe's Arch Clin Exp Ophthalmol 2006; 244: 1240-1245

[17] Stahl JL, Barney NP. Ocular allergic disease. Curr Opin Allergy Clin Immunol 2004; 4 455-459

[18] Leonardi A, Curnow SJ, Zhan H, Calder VL. Multiple cytokines in human tear specimens in seasonal and chronic allergic eye disease and in conjunctival fibroblast cultures. Clin Exp Allergy 2006; 36: 777-784

[19] Metz DP, Hingorani M, Calder VL, Buckley RJ, Lightman SL. T-cell cytokines in chronic allergic eye disease. J Allergy Clin Immunol 1997; 100: 817-824

[20] Bonini S, Bonini S, Berruto A, Tomassini M, Carlesimo S, Bucci MG, Balsano F. Conjunctival provocation test as a model for the study of allergy and inflammation in humans. Int Arch Allergy Appl Immunol 1989; 88: 144-148

[21] Abelson MB, Chambers WA, Smith LM. Conjunctival allergen challenge. A clinical approach to studying allergic conjunctivitis. Arch Ophthalmol 1990; 108: 84-88

[22] Friedlaender MH. Conjunctival provocation testing: Overview of recent clinical trials in ocular allergy. Int Ophthalmol Clin 2003; 43: 95-104

[23] Pelikan M, Pelikan Z. The role of the nasal mucosa in some cases of allergic conjunctivitis and the effects of Disodium Cromoglycate (DSCG). J Allergy Clin Immunol 1985; 75 (Suppl to No 1): 186

[24] Abelson MB, Loeffler O. Conjunctival allergen challenge:models in the investigation of ocular allergy. Curr Allergy Asthma Rep 2003; 3: 363-368

[25] Anderson DF. The conjunctival late-phase reaction and allergen provocation in the eye. Clin Exp Allergy 1996;26:1105- 1107

[26] Leonardi A. In-vivo diagnostic measurements of ocular inflammation. Curr Opin Allergy Clin Immunol 2005; 5: 464-472

[27] Abelson M, Howes J, George M. The conjunctival provocation test model of ocular allergy: Utility for assessment of an ocular corticosteroid, Loteprednol etabonate. J Ocular Pharmacol & Therap 1998; 14: 533-542

[28] Abelson MB, Spitalny L. Combined analysis of two studies using the conjunctival allergen challenge model to evaluate Olopatadine hydrochloride, a new ophthalmic antiallergic agent with dual activity. Am J Ophthalmol 1998;125:797-804

[29] Abelson MB. Evaluation of Olopatadine, a new ophthalmic antiallergic agent with dual activity, using the conjunctival allergen challenge model. Ann Allergy Asthma Immunol 1998; 81: 211-218

[30] Abelson MB, George MA, Schaefer K, Smith LM. Evaluation of the new ophthalmic antihistamine, 0.05% levocabastine in the clinical allergen challenge model of allergic conjunctivitis. J Allergy Clin Immunol 1994; 94: 458-464

[31] Kari O. Atopic conjunctivitis, a cytologic examination. Acta Ophthalmol (Copenh) 1988; 66: 381-386

[32] Montan PG, Hage-Hamsteren van M, Zetterström O. Sustained eosinophil cationic protein release into tears after a single high-dose conjunctival allergen challenge. Clin Exp Allergy 1996; 26: 1125-1130

[33] Sacchetti M, Micera A, Lambiase A, Speranza S, Mantelli F, Petrachi G, Bonini S, Bonini S. Tear levels of neuropeptides increase after specific allergen challenge in allergic conjunctivitis. Mol Vis 2011;17:47-52

[34] Bonini S, Bonini S, Vecchione A, Naim DM, Allansmith MR, Balsano F. Inflammatory changes in conjunctival scrapings after allergen provocation in humans. J Allergy Clin Immunol 1988; 82: 462-469

[35] Leonardi A, Busato F, Fregona I, Plebani M, Secchi AG. Anti-inflammatory and antiallergic effects of ketorolac tromethamine in the conjunctival provocation model. Br J Ophthalmol 2000; 84: 1228-1232
[36] Choi SH, Bielory L. Late-phase reaction in ocular allergy. Curr Opin Allergy Clin Immunol 2008; 8: 438-444
[37] Mita H, Sakuma Y, Shida T, Akiyama K. Release of chemical mediators in the conjunctival lavage fluids after eye provocation with allergen or compound 48/80. Arerugi 1994; 43: 800-808
[38] Callebaut I, Spielberg L, Hox V, Bobic S, Jorissen M, Stalmans I, Scadding G, Ceuppens JL, Hellings PW. Conjunctival effects of a selective nasal pollen provocation. Allergy 2010; 65: 1173-1181
[39] Leonardi A, De Dominics C, Motterle L. Immunopathogenesis of ocular allergy: a schematic approach to different clinical entities. Curr Opin Allergy Clin Immunol 2007; 7: 429-435
[40] Kari O, Salo OP, Halmepuro L, Suvilehto K. Tear histamine during allergic conjunctivitis challenge. Graefe's Arch Clin Exp Ophthalmol 1985; 223: 60-62
[41] Friedlaender MH. Conjunctival provocative tests: A model of human ocular allergy. Tr Am Ophthalmol Soc 1989; 87:577-597
[42] Helintö M, Renkonen R, Tervo T, Vesaluoma M, Saaren-Seppälä, Haahtela T, Kirveskari J. Direct in vivo monitoring of acute allergic reactions in human conjunctiva. J Immunol 2004; 172:3235-3242
[43] Pelikan Z. Late and delayed response of the nasal mucosa to allergen challenge. Ann Allergy 1978; 41: 37-47
[44] Pelikan Z, Pelikan-Filipek M. Cytologic changes in the nasal secretions during the late nasal response. J Allergy Clin Immunol 1989; 83: 1068-1079
[45] Pelikan Z, Pelikan-Filipek M. Cytologic changes in the nasal secretions during the immediate nasal response. J Allergy Clin Immunol 1988; 82: 1103-1112
[46] Pelikan Z, Pelikan-Filipek M. Intracellular changes in some cell types in nasal secretions (NS) during the late nasal response(LNR) to allergen challenge (NPT). Clin Exp Allergy 1990; 20 (Suppl to No 1): 60 (Abstr P 131)
[47] Pelikan Z, Feenstra L, Barree GOF. Response of the nasal mucosa to allergen challenge measured by two different methods of rhinomanometry. Ann Allergy 1977; 38: 263-267
[48] Siraganian RP. Histamine release and assay methods for the study of human allergy. In: Rose NR, Friedman H, Fahey JL, Eds. Manual of clinical laboratory immunology. 3rd Ed. Washington (DC): American Society of Microbiology 1986;675-684
[49] Dua HS, Gomes JA, Donoso LA, Laibson PR. The ocular surface as part of the mucosal immune system: conjunctival mucosa-specific lymphocytes in ocular surface pathology. Eye 1995; 9: 261-267
[50] Paulsen F. The human nasolacrimal ducts. Adv Anat Embryol Cell Biol 2003; 170: 1-106
[51] Sirigu P, Maxia C, Puxeddu R, Zucca I, Piras F, Perra MT. The presence of a local immune system in the upper blind and lower part of the human nasolacrimal dust. Arch Histol Cytol 2000; 63: 431-439
[52] Knop E, Knop N. Lacrimal drainage-associated lymphoid tissue (LDALT): a part of the human mucosal immune system. Invest Ophthalmol Vis Sci 2001; 42: 566-74

[53] Knop N, Knop E. Conjunctiva-associated lymphoid tissue in the human eye. Invest Ophthalmol Vis Sci 2000;41:1270-1279
[54] Paulsen FP, Schaudig U, Thale AB. Drainage of tears: impact on the ocular surface and lacrimal system. Ocul Surf 2003; 1: 180-191
[55] O'Sullivan NL, Montgomery PC, Sullivan DA. Ocular mucosal immunity. In: Mestecky J, Binnenstock J, Lamm M, Strober W, McGhee J, Mayer L (eds). Mucosal immunology (3rd Ed). Burlington (MA,USA), San Diego (CA,USA), London: Elsevier- Academic Press 2005: 1477-1496
[56] Youngman KR, Lazarus NH, Butcher EC. Lymphocyte homing: Chemokines and adhesion molecules in T cell and IgA plasma cell localization in the mucosal immune system. In: Mestecky J, Binnenstock J, Lamm M, Strober W, McGhee J, Mayer L (eds). Mucosal immunology (3rd). Burlington (MA,USA), San Diego (CA,USA), London: Elsevier-Academic Press 2005: 667-680
[57] Motterle L, Diebold Y, De Salamanca AE, Saez V, Garcia-Vazquez C, Stern ME, Calonge M, Leonardi A. Altered expression of neurotransmitter receptors and neuromediators in vernal keratocinjunctivitis. Arch Ophthalmol 2006; 124: 462-468
[58] Zoukhri D. Effect of inflammation on lacrimal gland function. Exp Eye Res 2006; 82: 885-898
[59] Leonardi A. Role of histamine in allergic conjunctivitis. Acta Ophthalmol Scand 2000; 78: 18-21
[60] Proud D, Sweet J, Stein P, Settipane RA, Kagey-Sobotka A, Friedlaender MH, Lichtenstein LM. Inflammatory mediator release on conjunctival provocation of allergic subjects with allergen. J Allergy Clin Immunol 1990; 85: 896-905
[61] Leonardi A, Smith LM, Fregona IA, Salmaso M, Secchi AG. Tear histamine and histaminase during the earlt (EPR) and late (LPR) phases of the allergic reaction and the effects of lodoxamide. Eur J Ophthalmol 1996; 6: 106112
[62] Leonardi A, Motterle L, Bortolotti M. Allergy and the eye. Clin Exp Immunol 2008; 153 (Suppl 1):17-21
[63] Leonardi A, Borghesan F, Faggian D, DePaoli M, Secchi AG, Plebani M. Tear and serum soluble leukocyte activation markers in conjunctival allergic diseases. Am J Ophthalmol 2000; 129:151-158
[64] Uchio E, Miyakawa K, Ikezawa Z, Ohno S. Systemic and local immunological features of atopic dermatitis patients with ocular complications. Br J Ophthalmol 1998; 82: 82-87
[65] Margrini L, Bonini S, Centofanti M, Schiavone M, Bonini S. Tear tryptase levels and allergic conjunctivitis. Allergy 1996; 51: 577-581
[66] Leonardi A. Vernal keratoconjunctivitis: pathogenesis and treatment. Progr Retinal Eye Res 2002; 21: 319-339
[67] Tabbara KF. Tear tryptase in vernal keratoconjunctivitis. Arch Ophthalmol 2001; 119: 338-342
[68] Leonardi A, Borghesan F, Faggian D, Secchi A, Plebani M. Eosinophil cationic protein in tears of normal subjects and patients affected by vernal keratoconjunctivitis. Allergy 1995; 50: 610-613
[69] Oh JE, Shin JC, Jang SJ, Lee HB. Expression of ICAM-1 on conjunctival epithelium and ECP in tears and serum of children with allergic conjunctivitis. Ann Allergy Asthma Immunol 1999; 82: 579-585

[70] Lambiase A, Bonini S, Rasi G, Coassin M, Bruscoloni A, Bonini S. Montelukast, a leukotriene receptor antagonist, in vernal keratoconjunctivitis associated with asthma. Arch Ophthalmol 2003; 121: 615-620

[71] Thakur A, Willcox MD. Cytokine and lipid inflammatory mediator profile of human tears during contact lens associated inflammatory diseases. Exp Eye Res 1998; 67: 9-19

[72] Nathan H, Naveh N, Meyer E. Levels of prostaglandin E2 and leukotriene B4 in tears of vernal conjunctivitis patients during a therapeutical trial with indomethacin. Doc Ophthalmol 1994; 85: 247-257

[73] Bisgaard H, Ford-Hutchinson AW, Charleson S, Taudorf E. Production of leukotrienes in human skin and conjunctival mucosa after specific allergen challenge. Allergy 1985; 40: 417-423

[74] Akman A, Irkec M, Orhan M, Erdener U. Effect of lodoxamide on tear leukotriene levels in giant papillary conjunctivitis associated with ocularprothesis. Ocul Immunol Inflamm 1998; 6: 179-184

[75] Wakamatsu TH, Okada N, Kojima T, Matsumoto Y, Ibrahim OMA, Dogru M, Adan ES, Fukagawa K, Katakami C, Tsubota K, Shimazaki J, Fujishima H. Evaluation of conjunctival inflammatory status by confocal scanning laser microscopy and conjunctival brush cytology in patients with atopic keratoconjunctivitis. Mol Vis 2009;15:1611-1619

[76] Leonardi A, Sathe S, Bartolotti M, Beaton A, Sack R. Cytokines, matrix metalloproteases, angiogenic and growth factors in tears of normal subjects and vernal keratoconjunctivitis patients. Allergy 2009; 64: 710-717

[77] Uchio E, Ono SY, Ikezawa Z, Ohno S. Tear levels of interferon-gamma, interleukin (IL)-2, IL-4 and IL-5 in patients with vernal keratoconjunctivitis, atopic keratoconjunctivitis and allergic conjunctivitis. Clin Exp Allergy 2000;30: 103-109

[78] Sack RA, Conradi L, Krumholz D, Beaton A, Sathe S, Morris C. Membrane array characterization of 80 chemokines, cytokines, and growth factors in open- and closed-eye tears: angiogenin and other defense system constituents. Invest Ophthalmol Vis Sci 2005; 45: 1228-1238

[79] Uchino E, Sonoda S, Kinukawa N, Sakamoto T. Alteration pattern of tear cytokines during the course of day: Diurnal rhythm analyzed by multicytokine assay. Cytokine 2006; 33: 36-40

[80] Bonini S, Lambiase A, Sachhetti M, Bonini S. Cytokines in ocular allergy. Int Ophthalmol Clin 2003; 43: 27-32

[81] Cook EB. Tear cytokines in acute and chronic ocular allergic inflammation. Curr Opin Allergy Clin Immunol 2004; 4: 441-445

[82] Calder VL, Jolly G, Hingorani M, Adamson P, Leonardi A, Secchi AG, Buckley RJ, Lighman S. Cytokine production and mRNA expression by conjuctival T-cell lines in chronic allergic eye disease. Clin Exp Allergy 1999;29: 1214-1222

[83] Ahluwalia P, Anderson DF, Wilson SJ, McGill JI, Church MK. Nedocromil sodium and levocabastine reduce the symptoms of conjunctival allergen challenge by different mechanisms. J Allergy Clin Immunol 2001;108:449-454

[84] Pelikan Z. Cytologic changes in tears during the late type of secondary conjunctival response induced by nasal allergy. In: Conjunctivitis-Monography. Intech; 2011

5

Cytologic Changes in Tears During the Late Type of Secondary Conjunctival Response Induced by Nasal Allergy

Zdenek Pelikan
Allergy Research Foundation, Breda
The Netherlands

1. Introduction

Allergic conjunctivitis (AC),a disorder of the conjunctiva in which an allergic component plays a key role, affects approximately 15-25% of the adult and pediatric population [1-8]. Estimates in the literature indicate that the seasonal allergic conjunctivitis (SAC) occurs most frequently, followed by atopic keratoconjunctivitis (AKC), vernal keratoconjunctivitis (VKC), perennial allergic conjunctivitis (PAC), whereas giant papillary conjunctivitis (GPC) occurs only sporadically [1-9]. However, according to our clinical experience, the PAC occurs most frequently, followed by SAC, AKC and VKC, whereas the GPC represents only 0.5- 1% of all AC cases [10-17].

The allergic conjunctivitis (AC) can be divided into two basic forms with respect to the localization of the antigen-antibody or antigen-sensitized Th1 cell interaction with subsequent steps (allergic reaction) [10-16] In the primary form of AC, the allergic reaction due to the direct exposure of conjunctiva to an external allergen takes place primarily in the conjunctiva,. In this case, the conjunctiva is the primary site of the allergic reaction which results in the development of the primary (or classical) AC form. The secondary form of AC is induced by the allergic reaction occurring primarily in the nasal mucosa due to the exposure of nasal mucosa to an external allergen via various possible mechanisms which are described in the discussion. Moreover, the initial allergic reaction in the nasal mucosa usually can, but does not necessarily, cause also the concomitant nasal response characterized by nasal mucosal edema resulting in nasal obstruction, hypersecretion and sneezing [10, 12].

Various hypersensitivity types, such as immediate type (type I, IgE-mediated), late type (type III) or delayed type (type IV, cell-mediated) can participate both in the primary and in the secondary form of AC.[1, 3, 5, 6, 10-36] The involvement of various hypersensitivity mechanisms in AC may result in development of three basic types of conjunctival response (CR), an immediate (ICR), a late (LCR) or a delayed (DYCR) type, and two supplementary types of CR, such as dual late (DLCR), being a combination of an immediate and a late CR, and a dual delayed (DDYCR), a combination of an immediate and a delayed CR.[1, 6, 8, 9, 10-16, 19, 20, 24, 25, 28, 36- 40] Additionally, the non-specific hyperreactivity resulting from direct stimulation of mucosal, glandular, or neurogenic receptors/elements in the nasal mucosa and/or conjunctival tissue by non-specific agents might also participate in the conjunctivitis complaints/response, however, usually to a lesser degree.[3, 12, 41]

There is a dearth of information concerning both the role of an allergic reaction occurring initially in the nasal mucosa in the conjunctiva and possible induction of the secondary conjunctival and corneal response [10-16]. Moreover, no data are available to illustrate the appearance of the individual cell types and the cytologic changes in the tears accompanying the particular types of secondary CR [12, 13].

The purpose of this study, which is a continuation of our earlier work,[10-16] was to: (1) investigate the appearance of particular cell types and the changes in their counts in the tears during the secondary late conjunctival response, (2) to evaluate the possible significance of the individual cell types and their count changes in the tears for the diagnostic approach as well as for the clarification of the mmunologic mechanism(s) underlying this CR.

2. Material and methods

2.1 Patients

One hundred sixty–nine patients suffering from allergic conjunctivitis for more than 3 years and responding insufficiently to the topical ophthalmologic treatment, had been referred to our Department of Allergology & Immunology (Institute of Medical Sciences "De Klokkenberg", Breda, The Netherlands) for more extensive diagnostic and therapeutical analysis Thirty-five of 169 patients, developing the secondary late conjunctival response (SLCR) to the nasal provocation tests with allergen (NPT) performed as a part of the routine diagnostic procedure, volunteered to participate in this study.

These patients, 15 males and 20 females, 19-43 years of age, suffering from SAC (n=16) or PAC (n=19) showed subjective symptoms and objective signs of conjunctivitis and positive skin tests to various inhalant allergens. In 6 of these patients also positive specific IgE in the serum (RAST) to Dermatophagoides pteronyssinus or farinae and/or grasspollen was recorded. All these patients had normal intraocular pressure. None of them suffered from other ocular disorders, infections, systemic disease or immunodeficiency. Twelve patients had previously undergone 17 conjunctival provocation tests CPT) with various inhalant allergens, which were negative. They had previously been treated with topical and systemic H1-receptor antagonists, topical ocular cromolyn, topical ocular glucocorticosteroids, decongestants, topical vasoconstrictors and some of them also with NSAID drugs, however, without any substantial improvement of their conjunctival complaints.

Patients underwent a routine diagnostic procedure consisting of: a detailed disease history, general examination to exclude systemic or other disorders, basic laboratory tests, bacteriological screening of the tears and nasal secretions, basic and supplementary skin tests with inhalant and food allergens, X-ray of the paranasal sinuses in Water's projection, nasoscopy and cytologic examination of the nasal secretions, and ophthalmologic examination including ophthalmoscopy, slit-lamp evaluation, vital staining with fluorescein and cytologic examination of the tears.

The diagnostic procedure revealed a positive history for nasal allergy, positive skin tests with various inhalant allergens,, hyperaemic and edematous nasal mucosa, increased eosinophil and neutrophil counts in the nasal secretions, conjunctival hyperaemia and tearing to a slight degree, appearance of incidental eosinophil and/or conjunctival epithelial cell in the tear specimens and non-increased nasal responsiveness to histamine. In 4 patients a significant blood eosinophilia was also recorded. No other abnormalities were detected.

In these 35 patients, 47 nasal provocation tests (NPT) with various inhalant allergens (Table 1), with respect to the positive skin tests and/or suspect disease history and 35 PBS

(phosphate-buffered saline) control tests were performed by means of rhinomanometry [10-16, 42-47] combined with recording of the ocular signs and symptoms. [10-14] The patients were investigated in a period without acute ocular and nasal complaints, without symptoms of an acute infection, outside the allergen-relevant season and during hospitalization.
Long-acting H1-receptor antagonists and topical (nasal) glucocorticosteroids were withdrawn 6 weeks, topical and oral short- acting H1-receptor antagonists, topical decongestants and other treatments were withdrawn 48 hours before each of the NPTs. In these 35 patients, 35 NPTs with the same allergens producing the secondary late CR and 35 PBS control challenges (Table 1) were repeated 2 weeks later. The repeated SLCR and PBS controls (Fig. 1C) were supplemented with collection of the tears for the cytologic examination. A 4-day interval was always inserted between the end of the preceding test and the begin of the following test to prevent the carry-over effects and to allow for patient recovery. The study protocol was approved by the local ethical committee and informed consent was obtained from all study participants.

Allergen	Concentration	Nasal responses positive (n=35)	Conjunctival responses (n=35)	
			SAC (n=16)	PAC (n=19)
Dermatophagoides pteron	1000 BU/mL	6		6
Animal danders				
-dog	3000 BU/mL	3		3
-cat	2000 BU/mL	4		4
-hamster	2000 BU/mL	2		2
Feathers				
-canary	3000 BU/mL	1		1
-parrot	3000 BU/mL	2		2
Aspergillus fumigatus	1000 BU/mL	1		1
Pollen				
-grass mix I	1000 BU/mL	5	5	
-grass mix II	1000 BU/mL	2	2	
-flower mix	5000 BU/mL	3	3	
-tree mix	3000 BU/mL	1	1	
-weed mix	1000 BU/mL	1	1	
-birch	1000 BU/mL	4	4	

Grasspollen mix I= *Dactylis glomerata, Lolium perenne, Phleum pratensis, Poa pratensis;*
Grasspollen mix II=*Festuca pratensis, Holcus lanatus, Agrostis alba, Anthoxanthum odoratum*
Flower pollen mix=*Dahlia variabilis, Solidago virgaurea, Primula variabilis, Forsythia suspensa*
Tree pollen mix= *Betula pendula, Corylus avellana, Juniperus communis, Salix alba*
Weed pollen mix=*Artemisia vulgaris,Plantago lanceolata, Rumex acetosa, Taraxacum officinale*

Table 1. Survey of the allergens used for nasal challenge

2.2 Allergens

Dialyzed and lyophilized allergen extracts (Allergopharma, Reinbek, Germany) were diluted in phosphate-buffered saline (PBS) and used for skin tests in concentrations of 100-500 BU/mL and for NPTs in concentrations of 1000-5000 BU/mL (Table 1), as recommended by the manufacturer. If indicated, higher dilutions of the allergen extracts were used both for the skin tests and for the NPTs.

2.3 Skin tests

Scratch tests with allergenic extracts in concentrations of 500 BU/mL were performed and the results evaluated after 20 minutes. If the results were negative, then intracutaneous tests in concentrations of 100 BU/mL and 500 BU/mL were performed and evaluated 20 minutes and 6, 12, 24, 36, 48, 56, 72 and 96 hours after the intradermal injection. A skin wheal (>7.0 mm in diameter) occurring 20 minutes after the intracutaneous injection was qualified as a positive immediate skin response, the skin infiltration appearing between 6 and 12 hours as a late skin response, and the skin induration recorded later than 48 hours as a delayed skin response.[10-17, 42-47]

2.4 Nasal provocation tests (NPTs)

Nasal challenges with allergens were performed by means of rhinomanometry, already described in our previous studies.[10-16, 42-47] The nasal mucosa response (nasal obstruction due to the nasal mucosa edema) was evaluated by means of nasopharynx- nostril pressure gradient (NPG) parameters, which are the pressure differences (ΔP) between the nasopharyngeal cavity and the outside air, expressed in cm H_2O. NPTs were performed by the following schedule: (1) baseline values recorded at 0, 5 and 10 minutes before the challenge; (2) PBS control values recorded at 0, 5 and 10 minutes after a 3-minute application of PBS to the nasal mucosa of the non-intubated nasal cavity by means of a saturated wad of cotton wool on a nasal probe inserted under the concha media; (3) post-challenge values recorded after a 3-minute challenge with allergen, carried out in the same manner as the challenge with PBS, at 0, 5, 10, 20, 30, 45, 60, 90 and 120 minutes, and subsequently every hour up to the 12th hour, and then every second hour during the time-periods between the 24th-38th and 48th – 56th (60th) hour [12, 42-47]. The allergens used for the NPTs were chosen with respect of the disease history and positive skin tests (Table 1). The nasal response (NR) was assessed to be positive when the post-challenge mean NPG values increased by at least 2.0 cm H_2O (1.2 ± 0.3, mean± SE) with respect to the mean baseline values, recorded at least at three consecutive time intervals[12, 42-47]. The NPG changes recorded within 60-120 minutes after the allergen challenge were considered to be an immediate nasal response (INR), those recorded within 4-12 hours to be a late nasal response (LNR), and the changes measured later than 24 hours to be a delayed nasal response (DYNR) [10-15, 42-47].

2.5 Control tests with phosphate-buffered saline (PBS)

The control nasal challenge with PBS was performed in each patient studied following the same schedule as that used for the NPTs with allergen, however, 3 days later.

2.6 Conjunctival response

The objective conjunctival signs and relevant subjective symptoms were registered before and during all NPTs with allergens and PBS at the same time-points as the nasal NPG values. The features of the conjunctiva were assessed by ophthalmoscopy including a slit lamp. The conjunctival signs, such as hyperaemia (injection), chemosis, hyperlacrimation, and palpebral edema, and the subjective symptoms, such as itching (burning), blurred vision and photophobia, were registered and evaluated by means of the scale suggested previously by Abelson [48-51], but modified by us (Pelikan's scale). [10, 11, 13, 14] The evaluation criteria of the individual signs and symptoms were as follows: 0=absent, 1=mild (present to a slight degree), 2=moderate, 3= pronounced (moderately severe), 4=severe (Table 2). Differences in total sign score of 4 points or more (3 ± 1, mean ± SE), recorded at least at three consecutive time-intervals, were found to be statistically significant (p<0.05).[13, 14]

	Abelson I*	Abelson II**	Our score
I. OBJECTIVE SIGNS			
-Hyperemia (injection, redness)	0 - 4	0 - 3	0 - 4
-Chemosis		0 - 3	0 - 4
-Hyperlacrimation (tearing)		0 - 3	0 - 4
-Palpebral edema			0 - 4
II. SUBJECTIVE SYMPTOMS			
-Itching (burning)	0 - 4	0 - 4	0 - 4
-Photophobia			0 - 4
-Blurred vision			0 - 4

* = References 48-50; ** = References 51

Abelson's grading scale: 0=None; 1=Mild (intermittent); 2=Moderate; 3=Severe; 4=extremely severe or "incapacitating "itching; [Significant threshold: ≥+2]

Our evaluation scale: 0=Absent; 1=Mild (present to a slight degree or intermittent); 2=Moderate; 3= Pronounced (moderately severe); 4=Severe; [Significant difference: ≥4 points (p<0.05), with respect to the pre-challenge value, recorded at least at 3 consecutive time-points].

Table 2. Survey of Abelson's and our "modified" conjunctivitis grading scale and symptom score

2.7 Collection and processing of tears

The tear specimens were collected from each of eyes separately by means of micropipette from the fornix (corner) before, then after 30 and 60 minutes and every second hour up to 12 hours and 24 hours after the allergen challenge. The specimens were divided into 3 portion transferred to the microscopic slides and spread out on the slide surface using a glass probe. The first series of the air-dried specimens was fixed by polyethylene glycol and stained by Hansel's method modified by us.[12, 42- 44] The second air-dried series was stained by May-Grünwald-Giemsa, modified by us.[12, 42- 44] The third series fixed by methanol was stained by toluidine blue method.[12, 42-44] Specimens were dehydrated by methyl alcohol, mounted in Canada balsam and scanned microscopically.[12, 42-44]The absolute numbers of the individual cell types have been counted per microscopic field at magnification x250 and means were calculated from 20 fields, per each eye separately. The mean values from both the eyes were finally calculated.

Doubtful cells were re-examined under oil immersion at magnification x1200. The appearance of particular cell types was evaluated by the following scale: - = no appearance; ± = sporadical; + =slight; +± =moderate; ++ =pronounced; ++± =distinct; +++ = large; ++++ = very large appearance. The statistically significant magnitude of changes in the count of particular cell types in tears between two consecutive count degrees (mean ±SD) for secondary CRs was as follows: eosinophils 4 (4.15±0.38); neutrophils 5(4.61±0.72); basophils 1 (0.58±0.30); mast cells 1 (0.65±0.41); lymphocytes 2 (1.83±0.26); monocytes 1(0.53±0.39); epithelial cells 5 (4.97±0.51). The lowest statistically significant magnitude of the cell count is expressed as + (slight).

2.8 Control group

Eleven young adults suffering from allergic rhinitis, confirmed by positive history, skin tests and NPTs with inhalant allergens, but without history of any ocular disease and with normal ophthalmologic findings, volunteered to participate as control subjects. In these patients 11 positive late nasal responses (LNR) to inhalant allergens were repeated and supplemented with registration of the conjunctival features, subjective symptoms and cytologic examination of the tears.

2.9 Statistical analysis

The dynamic course of the nasal as well as the conjunctival responses were statistically evaluated by means of generalized multivariate analysis of variance model (MANOVA)[52]. The polynomials were fitted to the mean curves over time(8 time points within 120 minutes, 18 time points between 2 and 12 hours and 8 time points between 24 an 52 hours after the allergen challenge), and the appropriate hypotheses were tested by the modified MANOVA computerized system. [52]

1. The mean NPG values and the mean total conjunctival score values of the same type of response were compared with corresponding PBS control values at each of the time-points and analyzed by the Mann-Whitney *U* test.
2. The changes in the count of particular cell types in tears during the NPTs as well as the PBS control challenges were analyzed by the Wilcoxon matched-pair signed rank test, comparing the post-challenge values with the mean pre-challenge (baseline) values at each of the time-points. Statistical evaluation of the CR was performed separately for each of the eyes and then the mean from both the eyes was always calculated. A *p* value <0.05 was considered to be statistically significant.

3. Results

3.1 Nasal responses (NRs)

In the 35 patients 47 nasal provocation tests (NPTs) with various inhalant allergens (Table 1) and 35 PBS control challenges were performed. The 35 patients developed 35 late nasal responses (LNRs; p<0.001) and 12 negative nasal responses (NNRs; p>0.1). The LNR began between 4-6 hours, reached its maximum between 6-8 hours and resolved within 12 hours after the nasal challenge with allergen.

The 35 PBS control tests were all negative (p>0.2) No significant differences were found in the appearance of the LNRs with respect to the individual allergens (p>0.1). In 6 patients positive IgE in the serum to various inhalant allergens and in 4 patients increased blood eosinopil count were found. The LNRs were associated with significant changes ($p<0.05$) in the counts (mostly temporary increase) of the neutrophils, eosinophils, epithelial and goblet cells, and to a lesser degree of the lymphocytes, in the nasal secretions. The counts of basophils, mast cells, monocytes and plasma cells were relatively low and mostly without significant changes.

The repeated NPTs resulted in the development of a similar and statistically significant LNRs comparing the post-challenge with the pre-challenge (baseline) values ($p<0.01$) as well as with the PBS control values ($p<0.001$) (Fig. 1C). No statistical significant differences were found between the initial and the repeated LNRs ($p>0.1$).

3.2 Conjunctival responses (CRs)

The 35 positive LNRs, recorded in 35 patients, were associated with significantly positive secondary conjunctival responses of the late type (SLCR; $p<0.01$). The positive SLCR began between 5-6 hours, reached its maximum between 8-10 hours and resolved usually within 12, sometimes within 24 hours after the allergen challenge. The SLCR was represented by significant changes in the objective conjunctival signs ($p<0.01$) well as subjective symptoms ($p<0.05$) (Table 3). No SLCR has been accompanied by significant corneal signs. No significant conjunctival changes were recorded during the 12 negative nasal responses ($p>0.05$) or during the 35 PBS control challenges ($p>0.1$). No significant differences in the conjunctival changes were observed between the right and left eye ($p>0.1$).

The repeated NPTs have induced similar and statistically significant SLCRs, both comparing the post-challenge with the pre-challenge (baseline) values ($p<0.01$) and comparing with the PBS control challenge ($p<0.01$) (Fig. 1B). No statistically significant difference were found between the initial and the repeated SLCRs ($p>0.2$).

	SLCR Total ocular symptom score (TOSS)											
	minutes			hours								
	0	30	60	2	3	4	6	8	10	12	24	28
ILNR	-	-	-	-	-	*	***	***	***	*	-	-

SLCR= Secondary late conjunctival response (total mean conjunctival score values);
ILNR=Isolated late NR (NPG values);
- = $p>0.05$; * = $p<0.05$; **= $p<0.01$; ***= $p<0.001$

Table 3. Significance of the correlation between positive SLCR and positive ILNR

3.3 Cytologic changes in the tears during SLCRs

The repeated SLCRs were accompanied with low cellular counts in tears as compared with counts observed in tears during the primary types of allergic conjunctivitis.[11] The SLCRS were associated with significant changes in the count of eosinophils and neutrophils, but not of other cell types (Fig. 1A, Table 4). Before the NPTs the eosinophils as well as the neutrophils appeared in tears only sporadically. The counts of eosinophils increased between 6 and 8 hours ($p<0.05$), then they decreased and disappeared from the tears at 10 hours after the allergen challenge. The counts of neutrophils increased significantly (p<0.05) between 8 and 10 hours, decreased at 12 hours and persisted to a slight, non-significant, degree up to 24 hours after the allergen challenge. The counts of epithelial cells increased slightly between 10 and 12 hours after the allergen challenge, but they did not reach a significant degree (p>0.05). The other cell types, such as basophils, mast cells, lymphocytes and monocytes, appeared in tears during the SLCRs only sporadically. The cells appearing in tears were intact and they did not demonstrate any changes of their cytoplasmic granules. During the 35 PBS control tests as well as during the 12 negative nasal responses (NNRs) only sporadic epithelial cells and no other cell types were observed. No significant differences in results were found between both the eyes.

	Before the challenge	After the challenge (hours)														
		½	1	2	3	4	5	6	7	8	9	10	11	12	24	28
Eosinophils																
- *SLCR*	1	0	2	1	2	0	3	2	5*	6*	7*	5*	3	2	0	0
- *PBS*	1	1	1	0	0	1	0	0	1	1	0	1	0	0	1	0
Neutrophils																
- *SLCR*	0	1	0	0	0	2	1	1	3	7*	8*	8*	9*	4	1	0
- *PBS*	0	0	1	2	2	0	0	0	1	0	0	3	0	1	0	0
Mast cells																
- *SLCR*	0	0	0	0	0	0	0	0	0	0	0	0	0	0	0	0
- PBS	0	0	0	0	0	0	0	0	0	0	0	0	0	0	0	0
Basophils																
- *SLCR*	0	0	0	0	0	0	0	0	0	0	1^{+}	0	0	0	0	0
- PBS	0	0	0	0	0	0	0	0	0	0	0	0	0	0	0	0
Lymphocytes																
- *SLCR*	0	0	0	0	1	1	3^{+}	3^{+}	0	1	0	3^{+}	2	1	0	0
- *PBS*	0	0	1	0	0	1	1	0	2	0	1	1	0	0	0	0
Monocytes																
- *SLCR*	0	0	0	0	0	0	0	0	0	1^{+}	1^{+}	0	0	0	0	0
- PBS	0	0	0	0	0	0	0	0	0	0	0	0	0	0	0	0
Goblet cells																
- *SLCR*	0	0	0	0	0	0	0	0	0	0	0	0	0	0	0	0
- PBS	0	0	0	0	0	0	0	0	0	0	0	0	0	0	0	0
Epithelial cells																
- *SLCR*	1	1	2	1	3	2	4	0	2	2	3	6*	6*	7*	3	1
- PBS	1	0	0	2	0	1	0	2	0	0	1	1	1	0	1	1

SLCR = Secondary late conjunctival response; PBS = Phosphate-buffered saline; Significance with respect to the baseline (before the challenge): $^{+}$ = *p<±0.05*; * = *p<0.05*;

Table 4. Mean numbers of particular cell types in tears during the positive SLCR and PBS control challenge

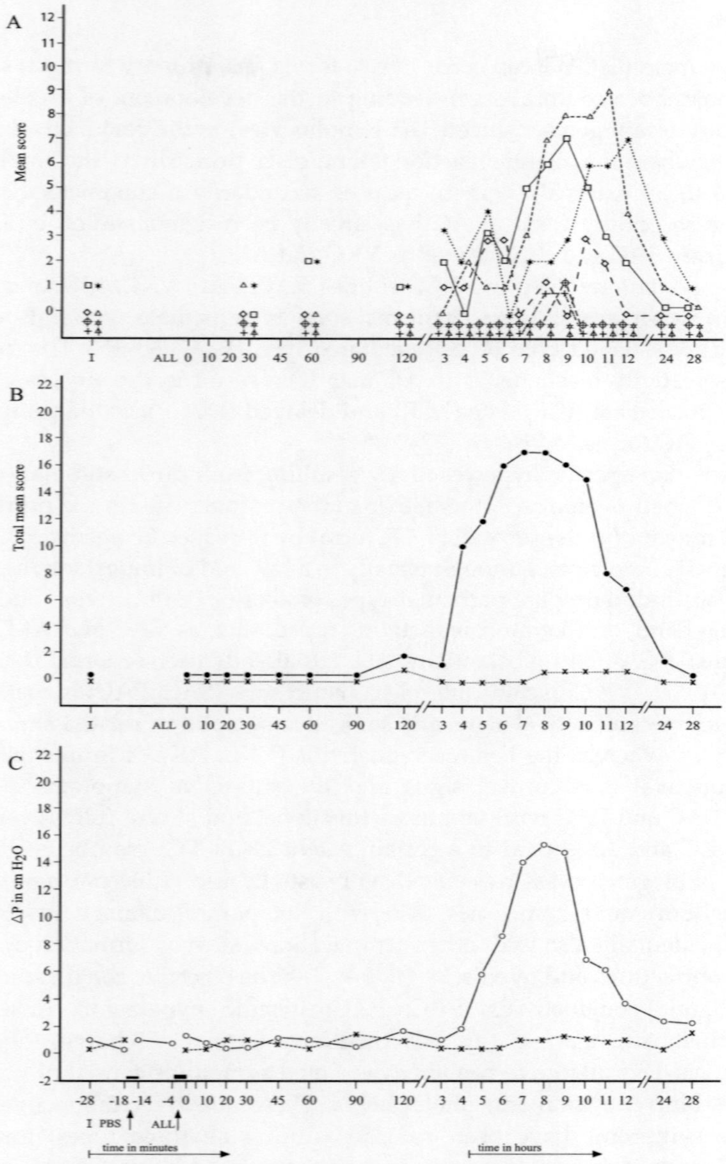

Fig. 1. The secondary late conjunctival responses (SLCRs; n=35) accompanying the isolated late nasal responses (ILNR; n= 35). **A.** The mean score of particular cell counts during the SLCR : □ = Eosinophils, Δ = Neutrophils; ⌖ = Basophils, ⍋ = Mast cells, ◇ = Lymphocytes, + = Monocytes, ✵ = Goblet cells, ✶ = Conjunctival epithelial cells. **B.** The mean total score of conjunctival signs and symptoms during the SLCR (●) and PBS (**x**). **C.** The mean rhinomanometric values (NPG) recorded during ILNR (○) and PBS (x). I = Initial (baseline) values, PBS = Phosphate buffered saline; ALL = Allergen challenge

4. Discussion

The allergic conjunctivitis (AC) can occur in two forms, in a primary form caused by a direct exposure of conjunctiva to an allergen leading to the development of an allergic reaction (antigen-antibody or antigen-sensitized Th1 lymphocytes) in the conjunctival tissue, or in a secondary form, where the allergic reaction taking place primarily in the nasal mucosa, due to its exposure to an external allergen, induces secondarily a conjunctival response. The existence of the secondary form of AC has already been demonstrated by us in patients suffering both from SAC and PAC as well as VKC and AKC. [10-16]

The allergic component involved in all AC entities, SAC, PAC, VKC, AKC and GPC, may be due to different hypersensitivity mechanisms, such as immediate type (IgE-mediated type I), late (type III) or delayed type (C cell-mediated type IV).[1, 3, 5, 6, 10-36] The involvement of various hypersensitivity mechanisms in AC may then result in three types of conjunctival response (CR), immediate (ICR), late (LCR) and delayed (DYCR), of the primary as well as of the secondary AC forms.[1, 6, 8-16, 19, 20, 25, 28, 36-40, 53-55]

Additionally, the non-specific hyperreactivity resulting from direct stimulation of mucosal, glandular and/or neurogenic receptors either in the conjunctivae (in the primary CR form) or in the nasal mucosa (in the secondary CR form) by non-specific agents might participate in the conjunctival complaints, although usually to a low and unimportant degree.[3, 12, 41]

The pathogenesis underlying the particular types of allergic conjunctivitis, such as SAC and PAC on the one hand, and keratoconjunctivitis types, such as VKC and AKC on the other hand and finally GPC, differs substantially, as it has already been reported in the literature.[1-16, 18, 22, 24, 26, 27, 33, 35, 39, 53, 54] Clinically, allergic conjunctivitis (SAC, PAC) is characterized by a number of objective conjunctival signs and subjective symptoms, related almost exclusively to the conjunctiva, whereas the keratoconjunctivitis (VKC, AKC) features include both the objective conjunctival and corneal signs and the subjective symptoms. [1-15, 26, 33, 35, 55] Generally, the SAC and PAC represent more functional and almost fully reversible process, whereas the VKC and AKC (and to a certain extent also GPC) may be characterized as a functional-morphologic process associated with usually reversible damage of the corneal surface (epithelium), and sometimes also with temporary damage of limbus and/or papillae, and incidentally also with other complications, such as formation of corneal scars, lacrimal way contractures and uveitis. [1, 6, 8, 9, 18, 26, 33- 35] The objective conjunctiva-related signs typical for allergic conjunctivitis (SAC, PAC) include hyperaemia (injection) of the conjunctiva, chemosis, tearing (hyperlacrimation, watery discharge) and sometimes palpebral oedema. The subjective conjunctiva-related symptoms consist of itching, burning and sometimes blurred vision and photophobia. These objective conjunctiva-related signs and subjective symptoms have been recorded during all three types (immediate, late, delayed) of CR, both in their primary and in their secondary form.[10-16, 19, 20, 26, 33, 36, 39, 48-51, 53-55] However, the appearance and participation of individual objective signs and subjective symptoms in the clinical picture exhibited some differences with respect to the particular CR types (immediate, late, delayed), to the individual CR forms (primary vs. secondary) and to the particular clinical AC entities, such as SAC, PAC, VKC, AKC and GPC. [10-17, 19, 20, 26, 28, 29, 33, 36, 39, 51, 53-55]

The objective signs and subjective symptoms of AC and their appearance during the conjunctival provocation tests (CPTs) as well as during the nasal provocation tests (NPTs) can be evaluated by a scoring (grading) system. Various scoring systems have been proposed in the literature up to date.[1, 3-9, 19, 33, 37, 53-56] One of the widely used scoring system has been suggested by Abelson et al.[48-52] However, the proposed scoring systems differ with respect to the parameters registered and the numbers of the grading points. Moreover, in the proposed scoring systems, including that suggested by Abelson et al, not all conjunctival and corneal signs and subjective symptoms typical for AC forms are included. Therefore, we have developed an improved and modified scoring (grading) system (Pelikan's scoring system)[10, 11, 13- 15], including additionally conjunctival chemosis, palpebral edema, burning, blurred vision and photophobia (Table 2).

In our system, predominantly the relative values, which means the difference between the post-challenge mean signs and symptoms and their pre-challenge values, as well as their dynamic course have been considered to be basic parameters for the assessment of the CSs. Using our model, the statistically significant differences in the total signs and symptoms have been calculated to be at least 4 points ($p<0.05$; Fig.1B). We belief that evaluation of the CRs by means of repeated comparison of the relative values of particular clinical parameters (conjunctival signs and symptoms) in their time-course may increase the credibility of the results.

The relationship between the conjunctivae and lacrimal ways on one hand and the nasal mucosa on the other hand is effectuated both on the anatomic and on the functional level.[1, 3, 5-31, 33-36, 55-66] Both the levels include connection of the conjunctiva with the nasal cavity through the naso-lacrimal duct, facilitating the tear drainage into the nasal cavity, but allowing also retrograde migration of factors from the nasal cavity into the conjunctivae, and connection of both the organs through the blood vessels, lymphatic tissue and the neurogenic network, all showing some links and sharing some common properties.

An allergic reaction occurring initially in the nasal mucosa can affect the conjunctiva in different manners upon involving of different mechanisms: (1) This reaction leads to release of a number of mediators, immunoglobulins, cytokines, adhesion molecules, chemotactic and other factors, which can then reach the conjunctiva via a retrograde penetration through the naso-lacrimal duct and system; [5, 6, 15, 18-31, 35, 55, 63, 64] (2) The released mediators and factors can be transported by the bloodstream through the local blood vessel system, e.g. *arteria maxillaries-pars pterygopalatina, vena facialis and plexus pterygoideus;*[5, 6, 12-15, 19, 35, 65] (3) This reaction can stimulate the local neurogenic network (sensory nerves, sympathetic and parasympathetic fibers) and released neuropeptides may reach conjunctiva along and/or through the particular nerves, such as *nervus trigeminus, nervus nasociliaris and ganglion pterygopalatinum;* [63, 64] (4) Various cell types participating in the allergic reaction occurring in the nasal mucosa, such as mast cells, basophils, eosinophils, neutrophils, plasma cells, monocytes , thrombocytes, B- and particular sub-sets of T-lymphocytes (Th1, Th2, Th 17, T-regulatory and natural killer cells), dendritic cells and macrophages can migrate through the bloodstream and/or the lymphatic stream into the ocular tissue;[11-14, 33, 61] (5) The allergic reaction occurring in the nasal mucosa and released factors can stimulate the local nasal mucosal lymphatic system *"nose-associated lymphatic tissue"* [NALT], expressing manifold mutual communication with the lymphatic network both of the lacrimal system, such as *" tear duct-associated lymphatic tissue"*[TALT], *"lacrimal drainage-associated lymphoid tissue"* [LDALT], and that of conjunctiva, called *"conjunctiva-associated lymphatic tissue"* [CALT]and *"eye-associated lymphatic tissue"* [EALT].[12-16, 57-62, 65, 66] In this way not only the transmission of certain intercellular and cellular-tissue receptor signals but also cellular traffic of various cell types , e.g. of T-lymphocytes (Th1, Th2),antigen-presenting cells (APC) and B-cells (plasma cells) can be realized.[10, 12-15, 19, 29, 30, 35, 39, 62, 65, 66] An additional mechanism playing also a role in the cellular traffic among the particular organ-associated lymphatic tissues , under certain circumstances, is the defective "homing mechanism" of the B- and T-lymphocytes, controlled by a number of homing factors.[10, 12-15, 29, 61, 62, 65, 66]

The allergy reaction in the conjunctival tissue, similarly to the nasal mucosa, is a dynamic process caused by a certain external allergen in which various types of cells are involved in various steps of this process.[1-16, 18-40, 42-44, 54-56, 61, 62, 65-67] This is also an exfoliative process leading to release and migration of various cell types, usually after finishing of their active involvement, into the particular fluids(media), such as nasal secretions or tears.[1-19, 24-26, 28, 29, 32-35, 38-40, 42-44, 53-56, 58-62, 65, 67, 68] These fluids may therefore be considered not only as a conditioning means of the particular organ, but also as waste media serving for drainage and removal of the exhausted and no longer active cells migrating from the mucosal membrane or being eliminated by the mucosal tissues after finishing their active participation in the allergic reaction. [8, 9, 12, 19, 24, 35, 42-44, 61, 67]

The numbers as well as the stage and condition of the eliminated cells can also indicate the qualitative as well as quantitative aspects of the running and/or passing allergic reaction in the particular mucosal membrane, in this case conjunctival tissue and/or nasal mucosa. [11, 12, 14] However, the current or passing involvement of the individual cell types in the allergic reaction can only be characterized by comparing their counts and conditions before and repeatedly after a well-defined intervention, which is a challenge with a certain allergen in a certain dose during a certain interval of time.[10-16, 19, 33, 37, 39, 42-49, 51, 56, 68] The cytologic examination of tears, as with the nasal secretions, is a relatively easy and valuable technique for evaluation of changes in the particular cell types appearing in tears during the allergic reaction. [19, 22, 34, 35, 57, 59] However, this method is limited only to tears and does not allow full evaluation of the cellular changes in the mucosal membrane itself. This may only be derived from a biopsy of the mucosal (conjunctival) tissue only.[19, 29, 31, 38, 68]

The cytologic examination of the conjunctiva can be performed by means of various techniques, such as brush, impression and scraping technique and classical biopsy technique.[4, 19, 24, 28, 31, 35, 37-39, 46, 54, 55, 65, 67-74] The brush and impression techniques may be considered to be in fact already semi-invasive methods, whereas scraping and biopsy are typical invasive methods. Each of these methods has its advantages and disadvantages. The major disadvantage of these techniques, except the brush method, is the use of anesthetics. Certain traumatizing effects of the conjunctival (ocular) tissue, stimulation/irritation of the tissue and blood capillary neurogenic receptors causing some of the undesirable reflexes and their unsuitability for the serial application, may also be qualified as a disadvantage. These techniques cannot be performed repeatedly on the same conjunctival location owing to traumatizing effects and tissue repair and *vice versa* the results attained from different localities are not fully comparable. Recently, a new promising technique, the confocal laser scanning microscopy, has been introduced. [71] On the other hand, the cytologic examination of the tears, collected by means of aspiration with a micropipette, is a very simple and easy method, which can be repeated almost endlessly, requires no anesthesia, does not traumatize the ocular tissue and is most similar to the natural clearance of the eye and drainage of tears. [19-23, 27, 30-34, 37, 39, 54, 64] The tear specimens can be processed and stained applying various methods and techniques, such as Hansel's stain, Wright's stain, May-Grünwald-Giemsa, Leishman stain, Winkler-Schultze method, Kardoz-Gemisch technique, Romanowski stain, Shorr's stain, Alcian blue-Safranin method, Astra blue, Azure A stain, Toluidine blue, Papanicolaou stain or

Carnoy's fixation-Periodic-Acid-Schiff (PAS).[4, 37, 39, 54, 55, 67, 69, 72-74] We have employed May-Grünwald-Giemsa staining as a basic method, and the Hansel's and toluidine blue staining as a supplementary technique, analogically to the staining technique a of the nasal secretions. [11, 12, 42-44]

Studies concerning the cytologic examination of tears in patients with allergic conjunctivitis, especially the appearance of particular cell types in tears and their changes, are not numerous. [39, 69, 73, 75, 76] The appearance of particular cell types has been investigated by means of a single tear cytogram , revealing increased numbers of eosinophils, mast cells, epithelial cells and sometimes neutrophils in tears.

The data gathered by brush, impressive or scrapping methods as well as by conjunctival biopsy performed in AC patients demonstrated some variations in presence of particular cell types as well as their numbers both in the epithelial and sub- epithelial layers of the conjunctiva. Mostly eosinophils and neutrophils, sporadically mast cells and lymphocytes were found in conjunctival epithelium and subepithelial layers. [19, 20, 31, 37, 55, 67- 69, 73, 76] However, since these methods are not fully suitable to be performed repeatedly on the same location, the course of cellular changes remain to be unknown.

Nevertheless, there is a dearth of data documenting dynamic course of the changes of individual cell types in tears during particular types of the primary conjunctival response to the allergen challenge using conjunctival provocation tests (CPTs).[19, 37, 55, 68, 73, 76] Moreover, no information has been found by us in the literature concerning the cytologic changes in the tears during the secondarily induced conjunctival responses by the primary nasal response to allergen challenge. Our results cannot be therefore compared with other data.

Our findings of relatively low counts of all cell types in tears during the SLCRs and only slightly increased eosinophil and neutrophil counts at the peak of the SLCRs , 8-10 hours after the nasal allergen challenge, may suggest the following hypotheses:

1. The primary allergic reaction occurring in the nasal mucosa induces the secondary conjunctival response of the late type;
2. The cells, especially the eosinophils and neutrophils, appearing in the tears during the SLCR did not probably participate directly in the allergic reaction either in the conjunctival tissue or in the nasal mucosa. These cell did not originate primarily from either conjunctival tissue or from nasal mucosa during the early stages of allergic reaction, but they probably migrated from the dilated conjunctival capillaries during the later stages of conjunctival response as a consequence of effects of the mediators and other factors released during the primary allergic reaction in the nasal mucosa and subsequently penetrating into the conjunctival tissue. This hypothesis may be supported by the intact condition of these cells, which cytoplasmic granules were not degranulated;
3. The discrepancy between the low counts of eosinophils and neutrophils in the tears during the SLCR and their relatively high counts in the nasal secretions during the primary late nasal response, would oppose the possible migration of these cells from the nose into the conjunctival tissue;
4. The SLCR may probably be induced by mediators released primarily in the nasal mucosa and subsequently penetrating into the conjunctivae.

Nevertheless, the exact manner and route by which these factors penetrate and achieve the conjunctivae is not yet clarified and will need more concurrent studies comparing levels of particular mediators in the nasal secretions, lacrimal ways and tears.

5. References

[1] Bielory L, Friedlaender MH. Allergic conjunctivitis. Immunol Allergy Clin N Am 2008; 28: 43-57

[2] Uchio E, Kimura R, Migita H, Kozawa M, Kadonosono K. Demographic aspects of allergic ocular diseases and evaluation of new criteria for clinical assessment of ocular allergy. Graefe's Arch Clin Exp Ophthalmol 2008; 246: 291-296

[3] Bielory L. Ocular allergy overview. Immunol Allergy Clin N Am 2008; 28: 1-23

[4] Dart JK, Buckley RJ, Monnickendan M, Prasad J. Perennial allergic conjunctivitis: definition, clinical characteristics and prevalence. A comparison with seasonal allergic conjunctivitis. Trans Ophthalmol Sci UK 1986; 105: 513-520

[5] McGill JI, Holgate ST, Church MK, Anderson DF, Bacon A. Allergic eye disease mechanisms. Br J Ophthalmol 1998; 82: 1203-1214

[6] Bielory L. Allergic and immunologic disorders of the eye; Part II: Ocular allergy. J Allergy Clin Immunol 2000; 106: 1019-1032

[7] Ziskin A. Allergic conjunctivitis. Current Allergy & Clin Immunol 2006; 19: 56-59

[8] Barney NP, Graziano FM, Cook EB, Stahl JL. Allergic and immunologic diseases of the eye. In: Adkinson NF, Bochner BS, Busse WW, Holgate ST, Lemanske RF, Simons FE, eds. Middleton's Allergy, principles & practice. 7th Ed. Philadelphia: Mosby-Elsevier Inc 2009; 1117-1137

[9] Hingorani M, Lightman S. Ocular allergy. In: Kay AB, ed. Allergy and Allergic Diseases. Oxford: Blackwell Sci 1997: 1645-1670

[10] Pelikan Z. Allergic conjunctivitis: primary and secondary role of the allergy reaction in the nose. Dutch J Med (Ned Tijdschr Geneesk) 1988; 132: 561-563

[11] Pelikan Z. The causal role of the nasal allergy in some patients with allergic conjunctivitis. Allergy 2002: 57 (Suppl 73): 230

[12] Pelikan Z. The late nasal response. Thesis. Amsterdam: The Free University of Amsterdam 1996

[13] Pelikan Z. Seasonal and perennial allergic conjunctivitis: the possible role of nasal allergy. Clin Exp Ophthalmol 2009; 37: 448-457

[14] Pelikan Z. The possible involvement of nasal allergy in allergic keratoconjunctivitis. Eye 2009; 23: 1653-1660

[15] Pelikan Z. Allergic conjunctivitis and nasal allergy. Curr Allergy Asthma Rep 2010; 10: 295-302

[16] Pelikan M, Pelikan Z. The role of the nasal mucosa in some cases of allergic conjunctivitis and the effects of Disodium Cromoglycate (DSCG). J Allergy Clin Immunol 1985; 75 (Suppl to No 1): 186

[17] Pelikan Z. Late nasal response-its clinical characteristics, features, and possible mechanisms. In: Dorsch W (Ed). Late Phase Allergic Reactions. Boca Raton, Ann Arbor, Boston (USA): CRC Press 1990: 111-155

[18] Ono SA, Abelson MB. Allergic conjunctivitis: Update on pathophysiology and prospects for future treatment. J Allergy Clin Immunol 2005; 115: 118-122

[19] Bacon AS, Ahluwalia P, Irani AM, Schwartz LB, Holgate ST, Church MK, McGill JI. Tear and conjunctival changes during the allergen-induced early- and late-phase responses. J Allergy Clin Immunol 2000; 106: 948-954

[20] Anderson DF. The conjunctival late-phase reaction and allergen provocation in the eye. Clin Exp Allergy 1996;26:1105-1107

[21] Bonini S, Lambiase A, Sacchetti M, Bonini S. Cytokines in ocular allergy. Int Ophthalmol Cli 2003; 43: 27-32
[22] Cook EB. Tear cytokines in acute and chronic ocular allergic inflammation. Curr Opin Allergy Clin Immunol 2004; 4: 441-445
[23] Calder VL, Jolly G, Hingorani M, Adamson P, Leonardi A, Secchi AG, Buckley RJ, Lighman S. Cytokine production and mRNA expression by conjuctival T-cell lines in chronic allergic eye disease. Clin Exp Allergy 1999;29: 1214-1222
[24] Calder VL. Cellular mechanisms of chronic cell-mediated allergic conjunctivitis. Clin Exp Allergy 2002; 32: 814-817
[25] Leonardi A, Fregona IA, Plebani M, Secchi AG, Calder VL. Th1- and Th2-type cytokines in chronic ocular allergy. Graefe's Arch Clin Exp Ophthalmol 2006; 244: 1240-1245
[26] Stahl JL, Barney NP. Ocular allergic disease. Curr Opin Allergy Clin Immunol 2004; 4: 455-459
[27] Leonardi A, Curnow SJ, Zhan H, Calder VL. Multiple cytokines in human tear specimens in seasonal and chronic allergic eye disease and in conjunctival fibroblast cultures. Clin Exp Allergy 2006; 36: 777-784
[28] Magone MT, Whitcup SM, Fukushima A, Chan CC, Silver PB, Rizzo LV. The role of IL-12 in the induction of late-phase cellular infiltration in a murine model of allergic conjunctivitis. J Allergy Clin Immunol 2000; 105: 299-308
[29] Metz DP, Hingorani M, Calder VL, Buckley RJ, Lightman SL. T-cell cytokines in chronic allergic eye disease. J Allergy Clin Immunol 1997; 100: 817-824
[30] Baudouin Ch, Liang H, Bremond-Gignac D, Hamard P, Hreiche R, Creuzot-Garcher C, Warnet JM, Brignole-Baudouin F. CCR4 and CCR5 expression in conjunctival specimens as differential markers of T_{H1}/T_{H2} in ocular surface disorders. J Allergy Clin Immunol 2005; 116: 614-619
[31] Metz DP, Bacon AS, Holgate ST, Lightman SL. Phenotypic characterization of T cells infiltrating the conjunctiva in chronic allergic eye disease. J Allergy Clin Immunol 1996; 98: 686-696
[32] Stern ME, Siemasko KF, Niederkorn JY. The Th1/Th2 paradigm in ocular allergy. Curr Opin Allergy Clin Immunol 2005; 5: 446-450
[33] Friedlaender MH. Conjunctival provocation testing: Overview of recent clinical trials in ocular allergy. Int Ophthalmol Clin 2003; 43: 95-104
[34] Uchio E, Ono SY, Ikezawa Z, Ohno S. Tear levels of interferon-gamma, interleukin (IL)-2, IL-4 and IL-5 in patients with vernal keratoconjunctivitis, atopic keratoconjunctivitis and allergic conjunctivitis. Clin Exp Allergy 2000;30: 103-109
[35] Leonardi A, De Dominics C, Motterle L. Immunopathogenesis of ocular allergy: a schematic approach to different clinical entities. Curr Opin Allergy Clin Immunol 2007; 7: 429-435
[36] Choi SH, Bielory L. Late-phase reaction in ocular allergy. Curr Opin Allergy Clin Immunol 2008; 8: 438-444 [cytol]
[37] Callebaut I, Spielberg L, Hox V, Bobic S, Jorissen M, Stalmans I, Scadding G, Ceuppens JL, Hellings PW. Conjunctival effects of a selective nasal pollen provocation. Allergy 2010; 65: 1173-1181
[38] Anderson DF, MacLeod JDA, Baddeley SM, Bacon AS, McGill JL, Holgate ST, Roche WR. Seasonal allergic conjunctivitis is accompanied by increased mast cell numbers in the absence of leukocyte infiltration. Clin Exp Allergy 1997; 27: 1060-1066

[39] Bonini S, Bonini S, Berruto A, Tomassini M, Carlesimo S, Bucci MG, Balsano F. Conjunctival provocation test as a model for the study of allergy and inflammation in humans. Int Arch Allergy Appl Immunol 1989; 88: 144-148
[40] Lambiase A, Normando EM, Vitiello L, Micera A, Sacchetti M, Perrella E, Racioppi L, Bonini S, Bonini S. Natural killer cells in vernal keratoconjunctivitis. Mol Vis 2007;13:777-784
[41] Sacchetti M, Lambiase A, Aronni S,Griggi T, Ribatti V, Bonini S, Bonini S. Hyperosmolar conjunctival provocation for the evaluation of nonspecific hyperreactivity in healthy patients and patients with allergy. J Allergy Clin Immunol 2006; 118: 872-877
[42] Pelikan Z, Pelikan-Filipek M. Cytologic changes in the nasal secretions during the late nasal response. J Allergy Clin Immunol 1989; 83: 1068-1079
[43] Pelikan Z, Pelikan-Filipek M. Cytologic changes in the nasal secretions during the immediate nasal response. J Allergy Clin Immunol 1988; 82: 1103-1112
[44] Pelikan Z, Pelikan-Filipek M. Intracellular changes in some cell types in nasal secretions (NS) during the late nasal response (LNR) to allergen challenge (NPT). Clin Exp Allergy 1990; 20 (Suppl to No 1): 60 (Abstr P 131)
[45] Pelikan Z, Feenstra L, Barree GOF. Response of the nasal mucosa to allergen challenge measured by two different methods of rhinomanometry. Ann Allergy 1977; 38: 263-267
[46] Melillo G, Bonini S, Cocco G, Davies RJ, De Monchy JGR, Frølund L, Pelikan Z. Provocation tests with allergens. Allergy 1997; 52 (Suppl 35): 5-36
[47] Pelikan Z. Late and delayed response of the nasal mucosa to allergen challenge. Ann Allergy 1978; 41: 37-47
[48] Abelson M, Howes J, George M. The conjunctival provocation test model of ocular allergy: Utility for assessment of an ocular corticosteroid, Loteprednol etabonate. J Ocular Pharmacol & Therap 1998; 14: 533-542
[49] Abelson MB, Spitalny L. Combined analysis of two studies using the conjunctival allergen challenge model to evaluate Olopatadine hydrochloride, a new ophthalmic antiallergic agent with dual activity. Am J Ophthalmol 1998;125:797-804
[50] Abelson MB. Evaluation of Olopatadine, a new ophthalmic antiallergic agent with dual activity, using the conjunctival allergen challenge model. Ann Allergy Asthma Immunol 1998; 81: 211-218
[51] Abelson MB, Chambers WA, Smith LM. Conjunctival allergen challenge. A clinical approach to studying allergic conjunctivitis. Arch Ophthalmol 1990; 108: 84-88
[52] Tabachnick BG, Fidell LS. Using multivariate statistics. New York: Harper Collins College Publishers 1996
[53] Helintö M, Renkonen R, Tervo T, Vesaluoma M, Saaren-Seppälä, Haahtela T, Kirveskari J. Direct in vivo monitoring of acute allergic reactions in human conjunctiva. J Immunol 2004; 172:3235-3242
[54] Leonardi A. In-vivo diagnostic measurements of ocular inflammation. Curr Opin Allergy Clin Immunol 2005; 5: 464-472
[55] Friedlaender MH. Conjunctival provocative tests: A model of human ocular allergy. Tr Am Ophthalmol Soc 1989; 87: 577-597

[56] Montan PG, Hage-Hamsteren van M, Zetterström O. Sustained eosinophil cationic protein release into tears after a single high-dose conjunctival allergen challenge. Clin Exp Allergy 1996; 26: 1125-1130
[57] Paulsen F. The human nasolacrimal ducts. Adv Anat Embryol Cell Biol 2003; 170: 1-106
[58] Sirigu P, Maxia C, Puxeddu R, Zucca I, Piras F, Perra MT. The presence of a local immune system in the upper blind and lower part of the human nasolacrimal dust. Arch Histol Cytol 2000; 63: 431-439
[59] Knop E, Knop N. Lacrimal drainage-associated lymphoid tissue (LDALT): a part of the human mucosal immune system. Invest Ophthalmol Vis Sci 2001; 42: 566-74
[60] Paulsen FP, Paulsen JL, Thale AB, Schaudig U, Tillmann BN. Organized mucosa-associated lymphoid tissue in human nasolacrimal ducts. Adv Exp Med Biol 2002; 506: 873-876
[61] Paulsen FP, Schaudig U, Thale AB. Drainage of tears: impact on the ocular surface and lacrimal system. Ocul Surf 2003; 1: 180-191
[62] O'Sullivan NL, Montgomery PC, Sullivan DA. Ocular mucosal immunity. In: Mestecky J, Binnenstock J, Lamm M, Strober W, McGhee J, Mayer L (eds). Mucosal immunology (3rd Ed). Burlington (MA,USA), San Diego (CA,USA), London: Elsevier- Academic Press 2005: 1477-1496
[63] Youngman KR, Lazarus NH, Butcher EC. Lymphocyte homing: Chemokines and adhesion molecules in T cell and IgA plasma cell localization in the mucosal immune system. In: Mestecky J, Binnenstock J, Lamm M, Strober W, McGhee J, Mayer L (eds). Mucosal immunology (3rd). Burlington (MA,USA), San Diego (CA,USA), London : Elsevier-Academic Press 2005: 667-680
[64] Calonge M, De Salamanca AE, Siemasko KF, Diebold Y, Gao J, Juárez-Campo M, Stern ME. Variation in the expression of inflammatory markers and neuroreceptors in human conjunctival epithelial cells. Ocul Surf 2005; 3 (4 Suppl): 145-148
[65] Sacchetti M, Micera A, Lambiase A, Speranza S, Mantelli F, Petrachi G, Bonini S, Bonini S. Tear levels of neuropeptides increase after specific allergen challenge in allergic conjunctivitis. Mol Vis 2011;17:47-52
[66] Dua HS, Gomes JA, Donoso LA, Laibson PR. The ocular surface as part of the mucosal immune system: conjunctival mucosa-specific lymphocytes in ocular surface pathology. Eye 1995; 9: 261-267
[67] Takano Y, Fukagawa K, Dogru M, Asano-Kato N, Tsubota K, Fujishima H. Inflammatory cells in brush cytology samples correlate with severiry of corneal lesions in atopic keratoconjunctivitis. Br J Ophthalmol 2004; 88: 1504-1505
[68] Bonini S, Bonini S, Vecchione A, Naim DM, Allansmith MR, Balsano F. Inflammatory changes in conjunctival scrapings after allergen provocation in humans. J Allergy Clin Immunol 1988; 82: 462-469
[69] Leonardi A. Vernal keratoconjunctivitis: pathogenesis and treatment. Progr Retinal Eye Res 2002; 21: 319-339
[70] Trocme SD, Leiferman KM, George T, Bonini S, Foster CS, Smit EE, Sra SK, Grabowski LR, Dohlman CH. Neutrophil and eosinophil participation in atopic and vernal keratoconjunctivitis. Curr Eye Res 2003; 26: 319-325
[71] Wakamatsu TH, Okada N, Kojima T, Matsumoto Y, Ibrahim OMA, Dogru M, Adan ES, Fukagawa K, Katakami C, Tsubota K, Shimazaki J, Fujishima H. Evaluation of conjunctival inflammatory status by confocal scanning laser microscopy and

conjunctivsl brush cytology in patients with atopic keratoconjunctivitis. Mol Vis 2009;15:1611-1619

[72] Tsubota K, Takamura E, Hasegawa T, Kobayashi T. Detection by brush cytology of mast cells and eosinophils in allergic and vernal conjunctivitis. Cornea 1991; 10: 525-531

[73] Kari O. Atopic conjunctivitis, a cytologic examination. Acta Ophthalmol (Copenh) 1988; 66: 381-386

[74] Kari O, Haahtela T, Laine P, Turunen JP, Kari M, Sarna S, Laitinen T, Kovanen PT. Cellular characteristics of non-allergic eosinophilic conjunctivitis. Acta Ophthalmol 2010; 88: 245-250

[75] Leonardi A, Busato F, Fregona I, Plebani M, Secchi AG. Anti-inflammatory and antiallergic effects of ketorolac tromethamine in the conjunctival provocation model. Br J Ophthalmol 2000; 84: 1228-1232

[76] Bonini S, Bonini S, Berruto A, Tomassini M, Carlesimo S, Bucci MG, Balsano F. Conjunctival provocation test as a model for the study of allergy and inflammation in humans. Int Arch Allergy Appl Immunol 1989; 88: 144-148

Part 3

Treatment and Therapeutical Management of Conjunctivitis

6

Management of Conjunctivitis in General Practice

Soumendra Sahoo[1], Adnaan Haq[2],
Rashmirekha Sahoo[3] and Indramani Sahoo[4]
[1]*Melaka Manipal Medical College*
[2]*St George University of London*
[3]*Nilai University College*
[4]*Retired Professor Ophthalmology*
[1,3]*Malaysia*
[2]*UK*
[4]*India*

1. Introduction

This chapter will describe various treatment options for infective conjunctivitis, allergic conjunctivitis, conjunctivitis in immunological disorders and other varieties of conjunctivitis that can be effectively managed in general practice whilst also highlighting various RCTs and systematic reviews on treatment of conjunctivitis.

The conjunctiva is a vascularised mucus membrane that covers some anterior portion of the globe and the inner aspects of eye lids. Like all mucous membranes, it also consists of epithelial and stromal layers. The continuum of the epithelial cell layer occurs in one side with epidermis of the lids at the lid margin and with the corneal epithelium at the limbus. Because of this anatomical architecture we call this pouch as conjuctival cul-de sac. The conjunctiva has enormous potential for combating infections mainly because of a) high vascularity b) different types of cells present in conjunctiva initiating and participating in defence inflammatory reactions c) immunopotent cells present in conjunctiva d) enzymatic activity of conjunctiva neutralising many pathogens including viruses. However the conjunctival sac is rarely sterile and is prone to external insult as well as victim of immunological reactions. It has been found that the normal conjunctival flora shares organisms with the skin and respiratory tract. The major organisms found are *Staphylococcus, Diptheroids, Anaerobes, Streptococcus, Pneumococcus, Hemophilus, E.Coli* etc. However, as most of these potential pathogens are in their dormant stage, they rarely cause infection. Bacterial or infective conjunctivitis is mainly due to organisms of exogenous source. Though many forms of such infections are self-limiting because of barrier function of the conjunctival epithelium, there are exceptions for certain virulent organisms such as *N.gonorrhea, Listeria monocytogens ,Corynobacterium diptheriae* and the *Haemophilus* group. These bacteria possess proteolyitic enzymes which damage the parenchymal structure of the conjunctiva. Some conjunctival infections may signify an underlying disease something more sinister such as a systemic disease. In neonates, infective conjunctivitis poses a greater threat to the vision in comparison to adult varieties and therefore any visual problems must be assessed thoroughly.

1.1 Role of general practitioner in managing conjunctivitis

The majority of conjunctivitis cases report to their general practitioner for initial management. In a study in 1992, most general practitioners expressed confidence of managing conjunctivitis by themselves although many expressed that to refer the cases later if necessary. (Featherstone P I et al 1992)
The general practitioner needs to be well versed in diagnosing the type of conjunctivitis and rendering initial advices to the sufferer. Although conjunctivitis looks like a minor ailment, it can be frustrating and has social implications especially at work places.

1.2 Guidelines for GPs in achieving the following goals

- Identify patients at risk of developing conjunctivitis
- Accurately diagnose conjunctivitis of diverse origins
- Improve the quality of care rendered to patients with conjunctivitis
- Initiate appropriate treatment for conjunctivitis
- Reduce the potentially adverse effects of conjunctivitis
- Inform and educate patients and other health care providers about the diagnosis and management of conjunctivitis.

2. Management of conjunctivitis

It is essential to differentiate conjunctivitis from other vision threatening conditions that produce red eye such as in acute congestive glaucoma and uveitis. The GP should try to extract as much information from history taking. The second task with them is to find out the type of conjunctivitis. Cases with bacterial conjunctivitis will most likely present with white discharge, whilst watering of the eye has been associated with viral conjunctivitis. Itching is a prominent symptom in case of allergic conjunctivitis. Other forms of conjunctivitis such as in immunological disorders can be identified after finding some form of clinical clue during systemic examination. While managing cases of conjunctivitis, general practitioners must try to avoid contaminating themselves as well as clinic items.

2.1 Management of bacterial conjunctivitis

Although most cases of bacterial conjunctivitis run through benign course and self-healing, depending on the immune status of the patient, it might lead to severe lasting and with threat to vision too. As mentioned earlier, bacterial conjunctivitis usually presents with sticky eyes with white discharges. Unilateral conjunctivitis may be due to chemical, toxic, mechanical factors or may be due to the involvement of lacricamal gland or even a case of glaucoma, which the GP should be aware of while treating them.
Although there has been a tremendous decrease in incidence of most dangerous varieties of bacterial conjunctivitis such as caused by *Gonococcus* and *Diphtheria,* bacterial conjunctivitis still continues as commonest type of conjunctivitis in developing nations. The outbreak is usually during monsoon season. Conjunctival discharge (usually white) used to be the main diagnostic feature apart from red and gritty eye as major complains. Once a GP is certain of bacterial conjunctivitis, their first approach would be to clean the discharge with cotton

soaked with warm water, and to explain the same procedure to the patients, so they can do in home before applying medications. Generally most of the bacterial conjunctivitis cases are treated as outpatient cases but whenever any corneal involvement is suspected it would be ideal to treat the patient as an inpatient.

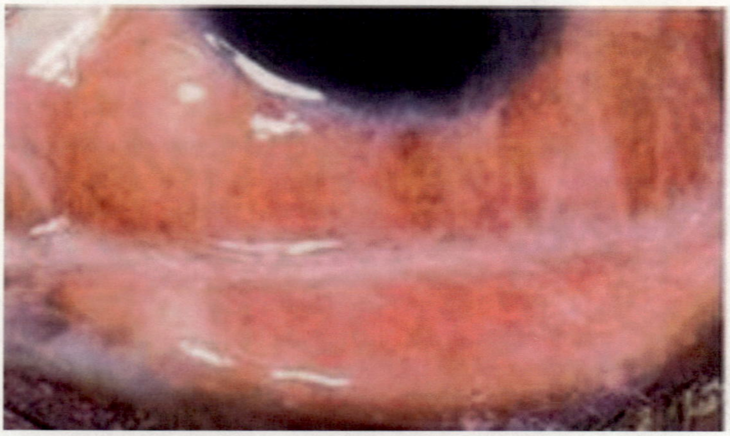

Fig. 1. Bacterial conjunctivitis (Look for the mucous discharge)

There are three categories of approaches of treating conjunctivitis in a GP setting; no use of antibiotic eye drops, delayed use of antibiotics and early use of antibiotics in conjunctivitis. (Everitt HA 2006).

The fundamental treatment of bacterial conjunctivitis is application of topical antibiotics. However, the pattern of antibiotics prescription varies in different practices. Most GPs prefer to start with broad spectrum antibiotics. The most commonly used broad-spectrum antibiotics are Ciloxan (ciprofloxacin) or Ocuflox (ofloxacin), Gatifloxacin ,which are commonly prescribed. Sulfacetamide is also acceptable though not commonly used now days. Although aminoglycosides like Gentamycin and Tobramycin are often used they sometimes retard epithelial healing process, and so they should be used with caution. Polytrim (trimethoprim/sulfamethoxazole) is a reasonable choice particularly in children. Chloramphenicol eye drop is also a preferred choice especially in developing countries where the common organisms responsible are gram positive bacteria. The usual practice is to instil drops every 2 hours, although there is also an ointment that can be used at night or every 4-6 hours throughout the day.

To give a better idea on effectiveness of various topical antibiotics used in bacterial conjunctivitis we are quoting few study reports below.

A) Study on fluoroquinolone group of topical antibiotics:

One randomized, multicenter, double-masked, vehicle-controlled study, with a total of 957 patients aged 1 year and older with bacterial conjunctivitis were randomized to treatment with besifloxacin ophthalmic suspension 0.6% or vehicle applied topically three times daily for 5 days. It has been found that:

Three hundred and ninety patients had culture-confirmed bacterial conjunctivitis. Clinical resolution and microbial eradication were significantly greater with besifloxacin ophthalmic suspension than with vehicle at Visit 2 (45.2% vs. 33.0%, $p = 0.0084$; and 91.5% vs.

59.7%, $p < 0.0001$, respectively) and Visit 3 (84.4% vs. 69.1%, $p = 0.0011$; and 88.4% vs. 71.7%, $p < 0.0001$, respectively). They had expressed that the results of secondary endpoints of individual clinical outcomes were consistent with primary endpoints. They also found that only few eyes receiving besifloxacin ophthalmic suspension experienced adverse events than those receiving vehicle (9.2% vs. 13.9%; $p = 0.0047$). They concluded by saying that the Besifloxacin ophthalmic suspension produced clinical resolution and microbial eradication rates significantly better than vehicle and was safe for the treatment of bacterial conjunctivitis. (Michael E T 2009)

In one recent comparative study on currently prescribed antibiotics in bacterial conjunctivitis, the authors evaluated the speed of clinical efficacy for two currently available topical antibiotics: polymyxin B sulfate/trimethoprim (polymyxin/trimethoprim) and 0.5% moxifloxacin ophthalmic solution. They had enrolled eighty-four eyes of 56 patients younger than 18 years with a clinical diagnosis of bacterial conjunctivitis in a multicenter study. Patients were randomly assigned to receive either 1 drop of polymyxin/ trimethoprim four times daily for 7 days or 1 drop of 0.5% moxifloxacin three times daily for 7 days. Ocular signs and symptoms were evaluated at baseline and 24 and 48 hours after the start of dosing. Microbiological cultures were collected at baseline and 48 hours. They had noted patients rated ocular symptoms and adverse events on day 7 via telephone interview. They had included primary efficacy assessment as relief of all signs and symptoms of bacterial conjunctivitis. According to their reports all patients bar one completed all visits. At the 48-hour visit, complete resolution of ocular signs and symptoms was observed in 81% of the patients treated with moxifloxacin and 44% of the patients treated with polymyxin/trimethoprim (P = .001). No adverse events were reported in both the groups. They concluded by saying that Moxifloxacin 0.5% administered three times daily was safe and could cure bacterial conjunctivitis more effectively and significantly faster than polymyxin/trimethoprim dosed four times daily. The majority of patients were cured and symptom-free by 48 hours. They commented that moxifloxacin is cost-effective and significantly more efficacious than polymyxin/trimethoprim in the speed by which it reduced the symptoms and disease transmission. (Granet DB 2008)

B) Study on aminoglycoside group of topical antibiotics:

Similarly, one more comparative study was done for Gentamycin and Merimycin topical preparations in bacterial conjunctivitis. That study compared the clinical and microbiologic value of topical netilmicin with that of gentamicin in the treatment of acute bacterial conjunctivitis. It was a double-blind, randomized, prospective, controlled study, which was performed in 209 patients. One to two drop(s) of either antibiotic was applied to the affected eye(s) four times a day for up to 10 days. They examined the cases at the time of diagnosis and after 3, 5, and 10 days. Clinical efficacy was measured as the cumulative sum score (CSS) of the key signs and symptoms of acute bacterial ocular infection. Sensitivity/resistance was evaluated using the disk diffusion method. The drug efficacy assessment was restricted only to patients with positive baseline culture results ($n = 121$) in that study. Of the isolated organisms, 96.9% were sensitive to netilmicin, whereas only 75.0% were sensitive to gentamicin ($p = 0.00001$). They also observed that Netilmicin provided a broad-spectrum coverage comparable with that of ciprofloxacin, ofloxacin, and norfloxacin. Netilmicin also was more effective than gentamicin in eradicating infections ($p = 0.001$ at day 5 and $p = 0.037$ at day 10) and in ameliorating the CSS ($p = 0.037$ at day 3, $p = 0.001$ at both day 5 and day 10). Only minor adverse events occurred in patients

treated with either netilmicin or gentamicin. They concluded by saying that netilmicin was a safe and effective antibiotic that could be used as first-line therapy for the treatment of acute bacterial conjunctivitis. (Papa V 2002)
A study in Canada done by Jackson WB compared 1% fucidic acid viscous drop with 0.3% tobramycin eye drop in treating acute bacterial conjunctivitis and came with the conclusion that the clinical and bacteriologic efficacy of fusidic acid viscous drops combined with the convenience of a twice-daily dosage regimen establishes this antibiotic as first-line treatment for suspected acute bacterial conjunctivitis and a favourable alternative to other broad-spectrum antibiotics.

C) Recent study reports on Azithromycin eye drop:

Of late, studies on the use of Azithromycin in bacterial conjunctivitis provide some positive responses. Azithromycin 1% showed successful therapeutic intervention because therapy could be completed with 7 drops administered over 5 days, whilst high bactericidal levels were sustained in the eye overnight. they believed that there was the potential for reduction in the development of resistance by effectively killing sensitive organisms. (Friedlaender MH 2007).
Similarly, another study in 2008 showed that the topical therapy with azithromycin 1.5% administered only twice daily for 3 days effectively eradicated most pathogenic bacteria associated with bacterial conjunctivitis. Those microbiologic results were in accordance with the observed clinical outcome. The study claimed that the new anti-infective product had the advantage of a short treatment course which could lead to an improvement in patient compliance. (Denis F 2008)
One more study highlighted the kinetics of Azithromycin in treating bacterial conjunctivitis. This study tested the hypothesis that azithromycin demonstrates a bactericidal, concentration-dependent antibiotic effect at concentrations corresponding to and exceeding published tear and conjunctival levels. The antibacterial activity of different concentrations of azithromycin 1% in DuraSite® (AzaSite®; Inspire Pharmaceuticals Inc, Durham, NC, USA) was evaluated in this study by using a kinetics-of-kill model. Recent conjunctivitis isolates of *Staphylococcus aureus, Streptococcus pneumoniae* or *Haemophilus influenzae* were exposed to four concentrations of azithromycin (100, 250, 500 and 750 μg/ml). Starting concentrations were similar to the maximum concentrations (Cmax) that have been demonstrated in conjunctiva (83 μg/g) and tears (288 μg/ml) following topical ocular administration. The percentage of surviving bacteria at 30 and 60 minutes following exposure to each concentration were determined. Azithromycin failed to demonstrate bactericidal activity (i.e. a 3-log reduction in surviving bacteria) against *S. aureus, S. pneumoniae* or *H. influenzae*. Furthermore, the rate and extent of antibacterial activity with azithromycin did not change with higher concentrations, even at the highest tested concentration of 750 μg/ml .They concluded by saying that azithromycin demonstrated bacteriostatic activity against common conjunctival pathogens up to the maximum tested concentration of 750 μg/ml (i.e. 2.6-times and 9-times published Cmax tear and conjunctival concentration, respectively). Azithromycin's bacteriostatic effects and prolonged elimination half-life would likely lead to a corresponding increase in the emergence of macrolide-resistant isolates. (Mark S 2008)
The advantages of Azithromycin eye drop in bacterial conjunctivitis is its shorter duration of effective treatment. In one comparative study the authors compared the three day treatment bacterial conjunuctivitis with 1.5% Azithromycin eye drop versus 7 days treatment with

Tobramycin eye drop. They compared the efficacy and safety of Azyter, azithromycin 1.5% eye drops, for 3 days with tobramycin 0.3% for 7 days to treat purulent bacterial conjunctivitis. That was a multicentre, randomised, investigator-masked study including 1043 children and adults with purulent bacterial conjunctivitis. Patients received either azithromycin 1.5% twice-daily for 3 days or tobramycin 0.3%, 1 drop every two hours for 2 days, then four times daily for 5 days. Clinical signs were evaluated and cultures obtained at D0, D3 and D9 (where D refers to "day"). Primary variable was the clinical cure at the Test-of-Cure (TOC)-visit (D9±1), for patients with D0-positive cultures. The cure was defined as: bulbar conjunctival injection and discharge scores of 0.They documented that among 471 patients with D0-positivity in the per protocol set, 87.8% of the azithromycin 1.5% group and 89.4% of the tobramycin group were clinically cured at the TOC-visit. Azithromycin was non-inferior to tobramycin for clinical and bacteriological cure. Clinical cure was significantly higher with azithromycin 1.5% at D3. The safety profile of azithromycin was satisfactory with a good patient and investigator's acceptability. They concluded by saying that Azithromycin 1.5% for 3 days was as effective and as safe as tobramycin for 7 days. Furthermore, more azithromycin than tobramycin patients presented an early clinical cure at Day 3. Due to its twice daily dosing regimen for 3 days, azithromycin represents a step forward in the management of purulent bacterial conjunctivitis, especially in children. (Isabelle C 2006)

To start or not start antibiotics, or a delayed start of antibiotics?

There has been debate on this question. We quote few study reports which did not find much difference in antibiotic treated group and those not given antibiotics.

In one of the Cochrane systematic reviews the meta analysis reveals that acute bacterial conjunctivitis is frequently a self-limiting condition, as clinical remission occurred by days 2 to 5 in 64% (95% confidence interval (CI) = 57-71) of those treated with placebo. But the treatment with antibiotics was, however, associated with significantly better rates of clinical remission (days 2 to 5: relative risk (RR) = 1.31, 95% CI = 1.11-1.55), with a suggestion that this benefit was maintained for late clinical remission (days 6 to 10: RR = 1.27, 95% CI = 1.00-1.61).They concluded by saying that the acute bacterial conjunctivitis is frequently a self-limiting condition but the use of antibiotics is associated with significantly improved rates of early clinical remission, and early and late microbiological remission. (A Sheikh and B Hurwitz).

Similarly, one randomised control trial involving 30 GP centres in UK, Everitt HA et al compared the three management strategies; no antibiotic, immediate antibiotic and delayed antibiotic and came to a conclusion that the delayed prescribing approach may be the best approach. Compared with no initial offer of antibiotics, delayed prescribing had the advantage of reduced antibiotic use (almost 50%), no evidence of hospitalisation, similar symptom control to immediate prescribing, and reduced re-attendance for eye infections.(Everitt HA 2006)

In view of antibiotic eye drops being costly in various parts of developing countries an alternate way of treating with povidone iodine, especially in children, can serve as alternative. This was documented in one of the studies, which was done to report the efficacy of povidone-iodine as a treatment for conjunctivitis in paediatric patients. It was a double-masked, controlled, prospective clinical trial. The study was done in a general hospital in Manila, Philippines, 459 children (mean (SD) age 6.6 (6.6) years; range, 7 months-21 years) with acute conjunctivitis were studied. Infected eyes were cultured for bacteria and underwent immunofluorescent testing for *Chlamydia trachomatis*. Viral conjunctivitis was diagnosed if bacterial cultures were negative and diagnostic criteria were met. Subjects were alternated to receive povidone-iodine 1.25% or neomycin-polymyxin-B-gramicidin ophthalmic solution, one drop 4 times daily in the affected eye. Ocular inflammation was evaluated daily by the family or patient and weekly by an ophthalmologist. The main outcome measures were days until cured and proportion cured after 1 and 2 weeks of treatment. It was found that despite adequate statistical power (power >80% for a 1-day difference and $P < .05$), there was no significant difference between treatment groups regarding the number of days to cure or proportion cured at 1 or 2 weeks whether caused by bacteria or virus ($P = .133–.824$ for the four comparisons). After 1 week of treatment, povidone-iodine cured marginally more chlamydial infections than the antibiotic ($P = .057$). By 2 weeks, fewer chlamydial infections were cured than those of viral or bacterial etiology ($P = .0001$). The younger the patient, the faster their conjunctivitis resolved (R = 0.13, $P = .013$).The authors concluded in saying that povidone-iodine 1.25% ophthalmic solution was as effective as neomycin-polymyxin B-gramicidin for treating bacterial conjunctivitis, somewhat more effective against chlamydia, and as ineffective against viral conjunctivitis. Povidone-iodine ophthalmic solution should be strongly considered as treatment for bacterial and chlamydial conjunctivitis, especially in developing countries where topical antibiotics are often unavailable or costly. (Sherwin JI 2002)

The overall idea of a successful treatment of bacterial conjunctivitis is to go for proper diagnosis and follow up. GPs should restrain themselves from early initiation of antibiotics; rather follow the case with maintenance of ocular hygiene. The choice of antibiotic should also measure cost effectiveness and availability. And worsening of symptoms and signs should prompt GPs in referring cases to the Consultants.

It is interesting to note that in one of the studies comparing treatment with different antibiotics, it did not demonstrate that any one antibiotic is superior. It said that the choice of antibiotic should be based on consideration of cost and bacterial resistance. The present practice of prescribing antibiotics in most cases is not necessary. (Rose P 2007)

Although the very severe form of conjunctivitis resulting from *gonococcal* infections are always referred and treated by consultants, GPs should have knowledge on treatment and preventative measures of *gonoccocal* conjunctivitis. Infection by *N gonorrhoeae* in the newborn also requires systemic treatment of the neonate, the mother, and at-risk contacts. In usual practice, general practitioners refer the cases for consultant's intervention. The neonate may be treated with intravenous aqueous penicillin G 100 units per kg per day in 4 divided doses for 1 week. The mother and at-risk contacts may be treated with a single dose of intramuscular ceftriaxone 125 mg followed by oral doxycycline 100 mg twice daily for 7 days. Common regime for prophylaxis for such occurrence is by instillation of 1% silver nitrate solution, 1% tetracycline ointment, or 0.5% erythromycin ointment just after birth. Patients with *gonococal* conjunctivitis should be seen daily until resolution of conjunctivitis at the same time each case should be simultaneously treated for Chlamydia trachomatis infection.

2.2 Management of viral conjunctivitis

Viral induced conjunctivitis is another form of conjunctivitis and although self limiting in many cases, they take longer duration for healing. The most common viral organisms responsible for this form of conjunctivitis are Herpes simplex virus (HSV), Varicella Zoster virus (VZV), pox virus, measles virus, immunodeficiency virus (HIV) etc. In all these forms of conjunctivitis, the common presentation is the development of conjunctival follicles, which arise due to hypertrophied lymphoid tissue caused by the inflammatory reaction from the viral presence.

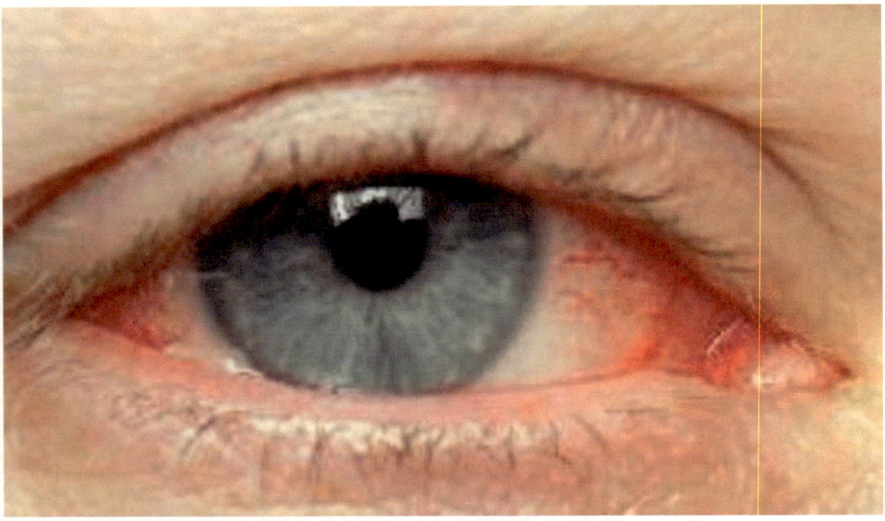

Fig. 2. Viral conjunctivitis (Look for pink eye without any discharge)

Herpes infection of the eye may be acquired as the patient's first exposure to the virus (primary infection) or as involvement of a new anatomical site (the eye) in a patient with previous HSV infection. In either case, patients with herpetic eye infection risk recurrent eye disease throughout their lives. The infective lesions of the corneal epithelium (dendritic and geographic ulcers) occasionally develop into non-infective indolent or trophic ulcers, particularly under the influence of cauterizing chemicals or corticosteroids. Inflammation of the corneal stroma may accompany herpetic epithelial lesions or occur independently. Stromal keratitis probably represents the host's immune response to viral antigens filtering down from epithelial lesions or from viral replication in stromal cells.

The choice of the optimal technique for diagnosing viral and chlamydial keratoconjunctivitis depends upon the efficiency, speed, and cost of the test. The performance of conventional laboratory procedures is relatively poor, and the interpretative difficulties documented with these tests are well recognised. Owing to their inherent sensitivity and high specificity, nucleic acid amplification procedures, in particular PCR, are recognised as the ultimate modern diagnostic tool for the identification of adenovirus, HSV, and *C trachomatis* in clinical eye swab samples. However, in laboratories without access to PCR, the conventional techniques of enzyme immunoassay, culture. (Elfath ME et al 1999)

Most cases of viral conjunctivitis, like that caused by adenovirus, need supportive treatment. No evidence exists that demonstrates efficacy of antiviral agents. Patients should be instructed to use cold compresses and lubricants, such as artificial tears, for comfort and symptom relief. For some susceptible individuals, a topical astringent or antibiotic may be used to prevent a bacterial super infection. Extreme caution should be taken when using corticosteroids, as they may worsen an underlying HSV infection. Recent reports suggest there is a beneficial effect of topical iodine povidone-iodine at a concentration of 1:10 (0.8%) in adenoviral conjunctivitis. Patients with acute conjunctivitis or those with corneal involvement, such as ulceration, herpetic keratitis, should be referred to an ophthalmologist without further delay.

General practitioners should not prescribe antibiotics in all cases of viral conjunctivitis, rather, they should offer supportive treatments such as cold compress, cleaning the discharges with sterile cotton and sometimes prescribing artificial tears. They may also encourage using darker glasses as this not only reduces the photophobia experienced but also masks the virulent look of a red and swollen eye.

2.2.1 Tips on precautions during treatment

Patient instruction during treatment of viral conjunctivitis:

- Warning patients on contagious nature. They need to wash hand frequently and to avoid direct contact with others
- They need to be isolated from office/work place and from school at least for couple of weeks
- They need to know that the condition may get worse and should consult doctor frequently

Professional precautions:

- Hand washing before and after examining such cases
- Try to avoid contact of instruments
- If instruments get contaminated try to clean or sterilise. Immersing the instrument with 1-2% solution of sodium hypochlorite or 3% hydrogen peroxide is ideal

2.3 Management of allergic conjunctivitis

Allergic conjunctivitis comprises a group of diseases affecting the ocular surface and is usually associated with type 1 hypersensitivity reactions. Two acute disorders, seasonal allergic conjunctivitis and perennial allergic conjunctivitis, exist, as do 3 chronic diseases, vernal keratoconjunctivitis, atopic keratoconjunctivitis, and giant papillary conjunctivitis.

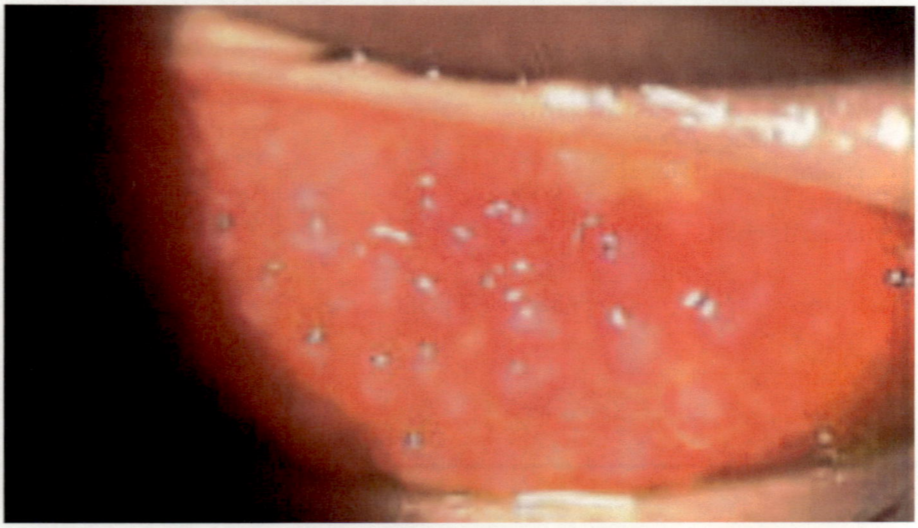

Fig. 3. Allergic conjunctivitis (Look for follicles and papillae)

The ocular surface inflammation (usually mast cell driven) results in itching, tearing, lid and conjunctival oedema-redness, and photophobia during the acute phase and can lead to a classic late-phase response (with associated eosinophilia and neutrophilia) in a subset of individuals. As is the case in other allergic diseases, a chronic disease can also develop, accompanied by remodelling of the ocular surface tissues. In severe cases, the patient experiences extreme discomfort and sustains damage to the ocular surface.

There are many varieties of both topical and systemic medications available for allergic conjunctivitis. It is often too confusing to select any one specifically for a purpose. Table 1 gives a broad idea on type of medication commonly available for treating allergic conjunctivitis with some examples and indications.

Group	*Generic name*	*Indications*
Systemic antihistamines	Cetrizine, Loratidine, Fexofenadine etc	Presence of systemic allergy along with conjunctivitis
Mast cell stabilisers	Cromolyn sodium, Lodoxamide, Nedocromil sodium	Effective in chronic conjunctivitis such as vernal conjunctivitis
Antihistamines with added property of mast cell stabilisation	Olopatadine, Ketotifen	Very good response in acute allergic conjunctivitis and in long run helps in stabilising mast cells too
Topical Steroids (Idealy the GPs should refrain from prescribing steroids; let this group used by Ophthalmologists only)	Fluorometholone, Loteprednol	Used for severe variety of allergic conjunctivitis but always look for toxicity in long term therapy
Vasoconstrictors	Naphazoline/Pheniramine	Any form of conjunctivitis as a support therapy but chronic use to be avoided
Topical NSAIDs	Keterolac	Symptomatic relief of itching in severe cases

Table 1. Summary of commonly available medications for allergic conjunctivitis

For such cases, there is no highly effective and safe treatment regimen. Topical administration of corticosteroids is used in severe cases but is associated with an increased risk for the development of cataracts and glaucoma. Thus, there is a worldwide search for new bio targets for the treatment of these diseases. Here, we provide a brief update of the clinical symptoms associated with these diseases, the rationale for disease classification, recent advances in our understanding of the pathogenesis of the diseases, and an update on both preclinical and clinical advances toward refined therapies for these diseases. (Santa JO et al 2005)

Another variety of conjunctivitis is produced because of the susceptibility of conjunctiva to allergens. They may be either exogenic or endogenic in nature. The conjunctival reaction is determined by the immune status of individuals. This variety of conjunctivitis is more challenging to treat than that resulted out of specific bacterial infections.

The primary aim of treating a conjunctivitis case is to relieve the common symptoms such as ocular itching, grittiness and discharge .Although many of the infective conjunctivitis have a self limiting course, patients often go to their General Practitioners or optometrists. General practitioners invariably prescribe antibiotics for a faster resolution of the symptoms whereas optometrists may offer a range of symptom relieving over the counter medication.

Mast cell stabilisers are another group which are used alone or in combination with steroid preparations. Commonly used are cromolyn sodium and lodoxamide (Alomide). Olopatadine (Patanol), nedocromil (Alocril), and ketotifen (Zaditor) . Nonsteroidal anti-inflammatory drugs (NSAIDs) which act on the cyclooxygenase metabolic pathway and inhibit production of prostaglandins and thromboxanes are found to be alternative to cortecostroids and can be a better option. It is usually safe to prescribe vasoconstrictors in general practice due to the relatively low dose and fewer side effects. Common vasoconstrictors include naphazoline, phenylephrine, oxymetazoline, and tetrahydrozoline.

As mono-therapy, oral antihistamines are an excellent choice when attempting to control multiple early-phase, and some late-phase, allergic symptoms in the eyes, nose and pharynx. Topical antihistaminic agents not only provide faster and superior relief than systemic antihistamines, but they may also possess a longer duration of action than other classes including vasoconstrictors, pure mast cell stabilisers, NSAIDs and corticosteroids. Unfortunately, despite their efficacy in relief of allergic symptoms, systemic antihistamines may result in unwanted adverse effects, such as drowsiness and dry mouth. Newer second-generation antihistamines (cetirizine, fexofenadine, loratadine and desloratadine) are preferred over first-generation antihistamines in order to avoid the sedative and anticholinergic effects that are associated with first-generation agents. Finally it can be said that when the allergic symptom or complaint, such as ocular pruritus, is isolated, focused therapy with topical (ophthalmic) antihistamines is often efficacious and clearly superior to systemic antihistamines, either as monotherapy or in conjunction with an oral or intranasal agent.

Topical cyclosporine A is an effective treatment in the management of severe allergic conjunctivitis refractory to other medications mentioned earlier. It has additional benefit as a steroid-sparing agent. (Ozcan et al 2007)

In spite of using all the verities of above mentioned topical preparations allergic conjunctivitis sometimes more challenging and frustrating in general practice. They often

prompted for using steroid eye drops. The use of corticosteroid should aim at relatively weak steroids, such as rimexolone, medrysone, and fluorometholone, that tend to have less potency with fewer ocular adverse effects but can be prescribed for a longer durations. Topical corticosteroids may be considered for severe seasonal ocular allergy symptoms, although long-term use should be avoided because of risks of ocular adverse effects, including glaucoma and cataract formation. (Leonard B et al 2005).So it is better advisable for GPs not to start steroid eye drops.
Having said this, although the treatment for allergic conjunctivitis has markedly expanded in recent years, providing opportunities for more focused therapy, it often leaves both physicians and patients confused over the variety of options. Therefore a proper assurance and frequent counselling to the sufferers holds the key to successful management of allergic conjunctivitis.

2.3.1 Atopic keratoconjunctivitis

AKC is a bilateral inflammation of conjunctiva and eyelids, which has a strong association with atopic dermatitis. It is also a type I hypersensitivity disorder with many similarities to VKC, yet AKC is distinct in a number of ways.
In 1953, Hogan first described the association between atopic dermatitis and conjunctival inflammation.1 He reported 5 cases of conjunctival inflammation in male patients with atopic dermatitis.1 Atopic dermatitis is a common hereditary disorder that usually has its onset in childhood; symptoms may regress with advancing age. Approximately 3% of the population is afflicted with atopic dermatitis, and, of these, approximately 25% have ocular involvement. General practitioners should try with antihistamines and if not responding should refer the cases to Ophthalmologists.

2.3.2 Giant papillary conjunctivitis (GPC)

GPC is an immune-mediated inflammatory disorder of superior tarsal conjunctiva. As the name implies, the primary finding is the presence of "giant" papillae, which are typically greater than 0.3 mm in diameter. It is believed that GPC represents an immunologic reaction to a variety of foreign bodies, which may cause prolonged mechanical irritation to the superior tarsal conjunctiva. Although contact lenses (hard and soft) are the most common irritant, ocular prostheses, extruded scleral buckles, and exposed sutures following previous surgical intervention may precipitate GPC. Topical mast cell stabilisers can be given to such cases.

2.3.3 Follow-up of allergic conjunctivitis cases

Follow up is an important strategy while treating allergic conjunctivitis because of the following purposes

- GPs need to diagnose steroid related complication or steroid dependence early so that idiosyncrasy is saved
- GPs should go for change of medication or to go for some combination therapy if the initial response found ineffective.
- GPs should provide health education during all visits so that avoidance of allergy sensitive factors become a habit of the individual
- GPs should provide assurance to the cases and their relatives on every follow up.

Type of Conjunctivitis	Clinical features	Treatment	Prevention
Bacterial Conjunctivitis	Red eye Photophobia Discharge	Cleanliness of eyes Symptomatic If Antibiotics : 1. Ciprofloxacin, Ofloxacin, Gatifloxacin, Moxyfloxacin, 2. Chloramphenicol 3. Gentamycin	Hand washing Avoid share of napkins Cleaning and disinfectiveness of instruments used Avoid contact lens
Viral Conjunctivitis	Red eye Watering of eye Mild itching Sometimes with subconjunctival haemorrhage Presence of follicles	Mostly symptomatic with the use of cold compress In longstanding cases might prescribe antibiotics for secondary infection. No substantial benefit of antivirals.	Personal hyegine:Washing hands Disinfect the instruments used
Allergic Conjunctivitis	Red eye Intense Itching Lacrimation Cobblrestone appearance Giant paoillae Tranta's spot Presence of mucus threads	Assurance 1. Steroid eye drops 2. Antihistamine eye drops 3. Disodium chromoglycate eye drops 4. Lodoxamide eye drop 5. Olapatadine eye drop	Avoidance of allergy Desensitisation in some cases
Conjunctivitis from Immunological	Red eye Dry eye Involvement of cornea and sclera Presence of systemic features depending on the case	Lubricant eye drops Corticosteroids in some cases Topical NSAIDs	Periodic Ophthalmic checkups in the presence of systemic immunological disorders
Other forms of conjunctivitis 1. Cicatrizing conjunctivitis 2. Superior limbic conjunctivitis	1.Dry eye,conjunctival scarring,corneal involvement 2.Foreign body sensation,photophobia,mucoid discharge & dry eye	1. Topical steroids,topical lubricating agents,surgical repair 2. Topical lubricants,Mast cell stabilisers	

Table 2. A quick guide to the diagnosis and treatment of various forms of conjunctivitis by general practitioners

2.4 Management of conjunctivitis from immunological reactions

Some examples of conjunctivitis resulted out of immunological reactions are cicatricial pemphigoid, conjunctivitis in erythema multiform, conjunctival reaction in Stevens Johnson syndrome etc..In most form of these immunological conjunctivitis there use to be great amount of scarring and cicatrisation of conjunctival tissue. The treatment of these conditions may require some surgical approach apart from medicinal therapy. Hence these are out of scope in treating at the hand of general practitioners. However, GPs should be aware of such conditions and it would not be a bad idea from their side to start topical antibiotic earliest to avoid secondary infections. They should know to start topical antibiotics along with steroid if happen to see a case of Stevens Johnson syndrome. They should also be able to counsel the cases on severity of such cases and inform the cases regarding possible surgical interventions like ocular surface reconstruction, keratoprosthesis etc.

3. Preventive aspects of various forms of conjunctivitis

Prevention of infective conjunctivitis relies primarily on good personal hygiene. The bacterial conjunctivitis is uncommon but can be spread by the hands or from upper respiratory tract infections. Gonnoccal infection is transmitted from the genital tract or urine to the eye by hands. This is a serious breach of normal hygiene. Ophthalmia neonatorum can be prevented by the use of povidone iodine drops, tetracycline eye ointment or other antiseptics or antibiotics at birth.

Viral conjunctivitis can sweep through a community or an institution such as a school very rapidly. This is highly infectious and needs to be controlled by the enforcement of strict hygiene standards. Contamination through possible articles like towels, face cloths and hands need to be avoided. Prevention of allergic conjunctivitis is not possible unless the patient is able to change his or her environment or job or identify the allergen causing the allergy and remove it, e.g., pollen, animal fur. Drugs such as atropine, neomycin can cause allergy and needs prompt withdrawal if detected.

4. Conclusion

Conjunctivitis is very frustrating and has social implications especially at work places if it is not treated comprehensively. General Practitioners must remain vigilant when suspecting conjunctivitis and have the ability to quickly determine whether it has been caused by bacteria, viruses or allergens. They should know that a past history of infectious conjunctivitis and complaints of itching invariably excludes the possibility of bacterial conjunctivitis, whereas complaints such as glued eye are indicative of bacterial conjunctivitis.

Another fact that general practitioners must take into consideration is that viral conjunctivitis is more prevalent and has a stronger tendency to recur than a bacterial conjunctivitis. Conjunctivitis with a dominant itch indicates an allergic cause. Failure to differentiate what the cause is may lead to wrong treatment and may, in some cases, prolong treatment. It must also be noted that General Practitioners should also remain aware of the differential diagnoses, such as uveitis, acute congestive glaucoma and instruct patients to seek follow-up care if the expected improvement does not occur or if vision becomes affected.

5. Acknowledgement

We would like to acknowledge the constant encouragement and support of the Chief Executive of MMMC, Malaysia and Pro-Vice Chancellor of Manipal University, India Prof Datuk Dr Razzak, Dean of Faculty of Medicine, MMMC Prof Jaspal, Deputy Dean Academic, Faculty of Medicine, MMMC Prof Adinegara in writing this chapter.

6. References

Denis F et al. Microbiological efficacy of 3-day treatment with azithromycin 1.5% eye-drops for purulent bacterial conjunctivitis. *Eur J Ophthalmol*. 2008 Nov-Dec , Vol.18,No.6, 858-68.

Elfath m elnifro & robert j cooper. Diagnosis of viral and chlamydial keratoconjunctivitis: which laboratory test?Br J Ophthalmol, 1999, Vol.83, 622-627.

Everitt HA et al. Randomised controlled trial of management strategies for acute infective conjunctivitis in general practice. *BMJ*, 2006, 333-321.

Featherstone PI et al. General practitioners' confidence in diagnosing and managing eye conditions: a survey in south Devon. *Br J Gen Pract*, 1992 January , Vol.42,No.354, 21–24.

Friedlaender MH and Protzko E. Clinical development of 1% azithromycin in DuraSite®, a topical azalide anti-infective for ocular surface therapy. *Clin Ophthalmol*, 2007 March, Vol.1,No.1, 3–10.

Granet DB et al. A Multicenter Comparison of Polymyxin B Sulfate/Trimethoprim Ophthalmic Solution and Moxifloxacin in the Speed of Clinical Efficacy for the Treatment of Bacterial Conjunctivitis. *J of Ped Oph and Stabismus*, 2008, Vol.45, No.6, 340-49.

Isabelle C et al. 3-day treatment with azithromycin 1.5% eye drops versus 7-day treatment with tobramycin 0.3% for purulent bacterial conjunctivitis: multicentre, randomised and controlled trial in adults and children. *Br J Ophthalmol*, 2007, Vol. 91, 465-469.

Jackson WB. Differentiating conjunctivitis of diverse origins. *Surv Ophthalmol.*, 1993 Jul-Aug, Vol.38, Suppl, 91-104.

Leonard Bielory; Kenneth W. Lien; Steve Bigelsen. Efficacy and Tolerability of Newer Antihistamines in the Treatment of Allergic Conjunctivitis. *Drugs*, 2005 , Vol. 65, No. 2, 215-228.

Michael ET et al. Phase III efficacy and safety study of besifloxacin ophthalmic suspension 0.6% in the treatment of bacterial conjunctivitis. *Informa Healthcare*, May 2009, Vol. 25, No. 5 , 1159-1169.

Mark S et al.The pharmacodynamic of azithromycin in a kinetics-of-kill model and implications for bacterial conjunctivitis treatment.. *Advances in Therapy*, 2008, Vol. 25, No.3, 208-17.

Ozcan, Altan A MD; Ersoz, T Reha MD; Dulger, Erol MD. Management of Severe Allergic Conjunctivitis With Topical Cyclosporin A 0.05% Eyedrops. *Cornea*, October 2007, Vol. 26, No. 9 , 1035-1038.

Papa V et al. Treatment of Acute Bacterial Conjunctivitis With Topical Netilmicin *Cornea*, 2002, Vol.21, No.1, 43-47.

Rose P. Management strategies for acute infective conjunctivitis in primary care:a systematic review. *Informa health care*, 2007, Vol.12,No.8, 1903-1921.

Santa JO,Mark BA.Allergic conjunctivitis:updates on patho-physiology and prospects for future treatment. *J Allergy & Cl immunology, 2005, Vol.115, 118-122.*

Sheikh A, Hurwitz B. Antibiotics versus placebo for acute bacterial conjunctivitis. *Cochrane Database Syst Rev.*, 2006 Apr, Vol.19, No.2,

Sherwin JI et al. A controlled trial of povidone-iodine to treat infectious conjunctivitis in children.*Am J Oph*, 2002, Vol.134, No.5 , 681-88.

7

Leukotriene Antagonist Drugs as Treatment of Allergic Conjunctivitis and Comorbidities in Children

Salvatore Leonardi[1], Giovanna Vitaliti[1], Giorgio Ciprandi[2], Carmelo Salpietro[3] and Mario La Rosa[1]
[1]*Department of Pediatrics, University of Catania*
[2]*Department of Pediatrics, University of Genova*
[3]*Department of Pediatrics, University of Messina*
Italy

1. Introduction

Allergy includes a variety of different illnesses (rhinitis, conjunctivitis, asthma, urticaria, and dermatitis) with a common pathological basis due to the release of chemical mediators such as histamine, platelet-activating factor, metabolites of arachidonic acid, and chemotactic factors from mastocytes, basophils, and eosinophils. The keyrole of leukotrienes (LTs) as mediators in allergic and inflammatory response justifies the new pharmacologic category of Cysteinil LT antagonists as possible therapeutic use in other allergic diseases beyond asthma (Leonardi et al., 2007).

Since 1938, known as slow-reacting substances of anaphylaxis (Feldberg & Kellaway, 1938), LTs have been products of the arachidonic acid methabolism pathway by the action of 5-lipoxygenase. LTs are generated by a number of cells including mast cells, eosinophils, basophils, and neutrophils, which appear in the airways of patients with asthma and in the skin of patients with chronic urticaria (CU). They mediate chemotaxis, vascular permeability, edema, eosinophils migration, airway constriction, and smooth muscle contraction (Samuelsson et al., 1997). As their effect has a long time efficacy , these molecules are defined as "slow reacting substances".

Among LTs, LTB4, LTC4, and LTD4 have particularly potent effects. LTB4 is a potent chemoattractant for leukocytes and is involved in the migration of granulocytes into tissues (Lewis et al., 1990; Wenzel et al., 1997). LTC4 evokes a wheal and flare reaction when intradermally injected. LTC4, LTD4, and LTE4 are chemical mediatoris of the inflammation involved in the pathogenesis of asthma, the overall biological effects of which are bronchial constriction and an increase in both mucus secretion and vascular permeability (Schleimer et al., 1986; Wenzel et al., 1990).

There are two different LT inhibitors/modifiers:

- LT receptos antagonists (LTRAs; montelukast, zafirlukast, and Pranlukast).
- 5-Lypoxigenase inhibitor of LT synthesis (zileuton).

Montelukast and zafirlukast block binding of cysteinil LTs to the cysLT1 receptor in the extracellular space. Zileuton inhibits 5-lipoxygenase and therefore all LT synthesis within

inflammatory cells. By blocking the actions of LTs, it promotes bronchodilation and decreases the inflammatory response.
Recent studies performed on adult patients suggest that anti-LTs can play an important role not only in the acute phase, but also in controlling the chronic development of bronchial asthma. Anti-LTs also have been used successfully by some authors to control allergic diseases such as rhinitis, atopic dermatitis, chronic urticaria and allergic conjuncitivitis. Moreover, recently, new reports have been published concerning other conditions (migraine prophylaxis, sleep disorders, inflammatory bowel disease, and nasal polyposis) that broaden the future range of clinical applications.

2. Leukotriene antagonists

2.1 Leukotriene synthesis

Leukotrienes are lipidic mediators, synthesised from arachidonic acid, by different reactions of the 5-lypoxigenase enzymatic pathway. The specific enzymatic pathway can be different in different cellular types and its activation depends on external cellular stimuli. However it is well established that the 5-lypoxigenase pathway is more frequently activated in cells deriving from the myeloid pathway (Henderson, 1994). The activation of 5-lypoxigenase pathway needs a signal of cell activation with mobilization of calcium and the availability of arachidonic acid as substrate. This process moreover requires the interaction with a protein called FLAP (protein activating the 5-lypoxigenase), important for the presentation of the arachidonic acid to the 5-lypoxigenase (Henderson WR Jr, 1994). The activation of the 5-lypoxigenase, on cellular and nuclear membranes, leads to the production of an instable intermediate molecule, known as LTA4, that could be transformed, according to the cellular type, in leukotriene B4 or in cysteinil-leukotriene (LTC4, LTD4, LTE4). Recently the gene codifying for LTC4 synthase was identified on the chromosome 5q, in a genetic region associated with bronchial asthma and atopic diseases (Bigby et al., 1996).

2.2 Leukotriene modifier drugs

Members of both types of LT blockers have been approved for use in the USA, Europe, and other nations (eg. Japan). The US Food and Drug Administration approved zileuton, a 5-LO inhibitor, in 1996, and two LT blockers, zafirlukast and montelukast, in 1996 and 1998 respectively; pranlukast was approved in Japan in 1995. the efficacy of montelukast, zafirlukast, pranlukast, and zileuton on bronchial asthma has been established in numerous randomized, controlled, multicenter clinical trials. LT modifiers reduce asthma symptoms, short-acting β2-antagonist (SABA) use, and asthma exacerbations, and improve all indexes of pulmonary function, as measured by the increases in forced expiratory flow at one second (FEV1), peak expiratory flow (PEF), quality of life, and indices of bronchial inflammation (blood eosinophils, inflammatory cells in the bronchial mucosa, exhaled nitric oxide, substance P, neurokin A, eosinophil cationic protein, and serum myeloperoxidase) (Riccioni et al., 2002; Lakomski & Chitre, 2004).

2.3 Leukotriene receptor antagonist drugs

Montelukast. Montelukast is an orally bioavailable Cys-LTRA that is usually administered once daily. This drug has been approved for long-term treatment of asthma in adults (10 mg/day) and children age 2 to 14 yr (using lower dosages, depending on the age of the child). Therapeutic concentrations do not inhibit cytochrome P450 isoenzymes. The most common adverse effects observed in adults at the 10 mg daily dosage were compatible with placebo, and included headache (18.4% vs 18.1%), abdominal pain (2.7% vs 2.4%), and cough (2.7% vs 2.4%). Elevations in liver enzymes occurred at a frequency that was generally comparable with placebo. The most common adverse effects that occurred in children at an incidence of 2% were slightly (but not significantly) higher than placebo. These included diarrhea, laryngitis, pharyngitis, nausea, otitis, sinusitis, and viral infections. The adverse event profile did not change with prolonged montelukast treatment (Jones et al., 1995; Spector & Antileukotriene Working Group, 2001).

Zafirlukast. Zafirlukast is a Cys-LTRA that is approved for the treatment of asthma in children aged 7 yr or older. It is administered orally twice daily and is metabolized by the liver; hepatic cytochrome P450 is inhibited by therapeutic concentrations. Therefore, there is a risk of drug interactions, and transient elevations of liver enzymes have been reported. The most common adverse effects that were comparable in incidence to placebo included headache (12.9% vs 11.7%), infections (3.5% vs 3.4%), nausea (3.1% vs 2.0%), and diarrhea (2.8% vs 2.1%). Other common adverse effects (eg, pharyngitis, rhinitis, flush syndrome, and increased cough) occurred at incidences identical to or lower than placebo (Accolate: Manufacturer's prescribing information, 1999; Spector & Antileukotriene Working Group, 2001).

Pranlukast. Pranlukast is an orally administered Cys- LTRA that is indicated for prophylactic treatment of chronic bronchial asthma in pediatric and adult patients. In clinical trials, pranlukast was well tolerated with an adverse event profile similar to that of the placebo. Gastrointestinal events and hepatic function abnormalities were the most common reported adverse effects, but were not significantly different from other LTRAs (Spector & Antileukotriene Working Group, 2001; Keam et al., 2003; Yanagawa et al., 2004).

Zileuton. Zileuton is the only marketed drug with a specific effect on Cys-LT synthesis via inhibition of the 5-LO enzyme. It is administered orally 4 times daily and is approved for treatment of asthma in patients 12 yr and older. It is metabolized by the cytochrome P450 isoenzymes and may, therefore, interact with other drugs metabolized by these enzymes, such as theophylline and warfarin. The use of zileuton is hampered by the dosing regimen and the requirement that liver enzymes be monitored. The adverse event profile in controlled clinical trials was generally similar to LTRAs. The most common adverse effects compared to placebo included headache (24.6% vs 24.0%), dyspepsia (8.2% vs 2.9%), unspecified pain (7.8% vs 5.3%), nausea (5.5% vs 3.7%), abdominal pain (4.6% vs 2.4%), and asthenia (3.8% vs 2.4%). Unlike the LTRAs, therapy with zileuton is associated with hepatotoxicity, and liver function enzymes should be monitored during treatment. Elevations of liver function tests may progress, remain unchanged, or resolve during continued treatment. At a dosage of 600 mg, 4 times daily, zileuton carries a pregnancy category C classification because of abnormalities noted in rabbit and rat fetuses (McGill & Busse, 1996; Spector & Antileukotriene Working Group, 2001).

3. Leukotriene antagonists in allergic diseases beyond asthma: Recent applications of antileukotriene drugs

Paranasal sinus disease. LTs are inflammatory mediators that have an important role in paranasal sinus disease (PSD) and the formation of nasal polyps (NP). Cys-LTs are overproduced in asthmatic subjects with chronic hyperplastic rhinosinusistis (CHR) and NP (Higashi et al., 2004). In view of the fact that these agents lead to symptoms in asthmatics patients, the use of LTRAs, particularly montelukast and zafirlukast, seems appropriate (Parnes, 2003; Steinke et al., 2003). A number of studies have indicated their role in inhibiting nasal symptoms in asthmatic patients. In addition, it has been suggested that many aspirin-intolerant asthma patients have NP and that treatment with the LTRAs results in improvement and resolution of the NP (Parnes & Chuma, 2000; Borish, 2002; Arango & Kountakis, 2002; Arango et al., 2002). The LTRAs might be good alternatives to the long-term administration of oral steroids, in view of their systemic anti-inflammatory effects and acceptable safety profiles (Parnes, 2002; Scadding, 2003; Haberal & Corey, 2003; Steinke et al., 2004).

Bronchiolitis. Many published studies have documented increased LTE4 levels in patients with infectious diseases due to respiratory syncytial virus (RSV), such as bronchitis, pneumonia, and bronchiolitis, suggesting that LTs may be involved. Cys- LTs, in fact, are released during RSV infection and may contribute to the inflammatory state (Takahashi et al, 2003). In a 36-months, double-blind trial, 130 infants (median age 9 months) who were hospitalized with acute RSV bronchiolitis were randomized into 2 parallel comparison groups of 5-mg montelukast chewable tablets or matching placebo given for 28 days starting within 7 days after the onset of symptoms. Infants in the montelukast group were free of symptoms on 22% of the days and nights, which was significantly lower than the placebo group, and there were significant reductions in daytime coughing and clinical exacerbations compared to the placebo (Khoshoo et al., 2002; Szefler & Simoes, 2003; Bisgaard, 2003, 2004).

Rhinitis. It is known that 4-11% of people have asthma and 10-30% have allergic rhinitis (AR) (Nathan et al., 1997; Von Mutius, 1998). Frequently comorbidities exists among these pathologies. Both conditions show the same allergic and proinflammatory mediators such as histamine, LTs, cytokines and eosinophils (Vignola et al., 2003).Moreover AR and asthma share common triggers as similar inflammatory cascade on exposure to allergen similar patterns of early and late-phase responses (Spector, 1997). Consequently, today, a combined approach in the managing of asthma and AR is recommended for an optimal strategy. On this regard, the new concept of "one-linked airway disease" between AR and asthma has led to LT modifiers being prescribed also for AR. In fact, it is well known that cysteinil LTs are common mediators as will in upper as in lower airway diseases, cysteinil LT challanges increase rhinorrhea in AR and a release of cysteinil LT reduces symptoms in AR (Howarth, 2000).

Allergic conjunctivitis. Allergic conjuctivitis (AC) is the most frequent form of ocular allergy in patients who consult ophthalmologists and allergists (Bhargava et al., 2004; Marmou and Raffard, 2004). The severity of the disease ranges from mild itching and redness, as seen in seasonal AC, to the serious, vision-threatening forms of ocular allergy that affect the cornea, such as atopic keratoconjunctivitis (AK). The pathogenesis of AC involves a complex mechanism that centers around IgE-mediated mast cell degranulation and release of multiple performed and newly formed inflammatory mediators. The diagnosis of AC is usually a clinical one that is made on a thorough history and careful examination (Epstein, 2003).

Treatment of ocular allergy should begin with conservative measures including allergen avoidance, environmental control, ocular irrigation, and cold compresses (Bhargava et al., 2004). Pharmacotherapy of AC consists of several classes of drugs: antihistamines, mast cell stabilizers, NSAIDs, topical steroids, and, in cases of AK, cyclosporine (Marmou and Raffard, 2004). Many studies have evaluated the signs and symptoms of coexisting vernal keratoconjunctivitis in asthmatic patients treated with oral montelukast. There were significant and persistent reductions of ocular signs and symptoms in asthmatic patients with vernal keratoconjunctivitis who were treated for 15 days with montelukast. This points to a need for double-blind, placebo-controlled trials to evaluate the potential of this new treatment in patients with vernal keratoconjuctivitis (Leonardi and Abelson, 2003; Lambiase et al., 2003).

4. Allergic conjunctivitis and the possible role of nasal allergy

Disorders of the conjunctiva, where an allergic component plays an important causal role are very common. However, the estimations of incidence of 'allergic conjunctivitis' and its particular forms vary (McGill et al., 1998; Bielory, 2000; Ziskin, 2006; Bielory & Friedlaender, 2008; Bielory, 2008; Uchio et al., 2008). Seasonal allergic conjunctivitis (SAC) occurs most frequently, followed by atopic keratoconjunctivitis (AKC), vernal keratoconjunctivitis (VKC) and perennial allergic conjunctivitis (PAC), whereas giant papillary conjunctivitis (GPC) may be seen only sporadically (McGill et al., 1998; Bielory, 2000; Ziskin, 2006; Bielory, 2008; Bielory & Friedlaender, 2008; Uchio et al., 2008). SAC and PAC appear in relatively milder form, whereas AKC and VKC occur in a more severe bilateral form, where the conjunctivae and cornea may also be affected (McGill et al., 1998; Bielory, 2000; Ziskin, 2006; Bielory, 2008; Bielory & Friedlaender, 2008; Uchio *et al.*, 2008).

The relationship between the conjunctiva and the nose is a well-known entity (McGill et al., 1998; Bielory, 2000; Ziskin, 2006; Bielory & Friedlaender, 2008; Uchio et al., 2008;). The coexistence of allergic rhinitis and conjunctivitis has repeatedly been reported in the literature (McGill et al., 1998; Bielory, 2000; Ziskin, 2006; Leonardi, 2005; Ono & Abelson, 2005; Bielory & Friedlaender, 2008; Bielory, 2008; Pelikan, 2009, 2010).

Nasal allergy could cohere with conjunctivitis in various ways. An allergic reaction occurring initially in the nasal mucosa may affect the conjunctiva in different ways upon involving diverse mechanisms: (i) this reaction leads to release of mediators, cytokines and other factors, which can then penetrate to the conjunctiva through the nasolacrimal duct (McGill et al, 1998; Bielory, 2000; Sirigu et al., 2000; Paulsen, 2003; Ono & Abelson, 2005; Pelikan, 2009 a, 2009 b); (ii) the released factors can also be transported to the conjunctiva by the local haematogenic ways (*a. maxillaris- pars pterygopalatina,v. facialis, plexus pterygoideus*) (Dua et al, 1995; Pelikan, 1996; Bielory, 2000; Pelikan, 2009 a, 2009 b); (iii) allergic reactions in the nasal mucosa can stimulate the local neurogenic network and released neuropeptides may reach conjunctiva along and/or through the appropriate nerves (*n. trigemini, n. nasociliaris, pterygopalatine* ganglion) (Pelikan, 1995; Fujishima et al., 1997; Calonge et al, 2005; Zoukhri, 2006; Motterle et al., 2006; Pelikan, 2009 a, 2009 b); and (iv) this reaction and released factors can stimulate the local nasal mucosal lymphatic system, 'nose-associated lymphatic tissue' (NALT), which is able to communicate with the lymphatic tissue of the lacrimal system, 'tear duct-associated lymphatic tissue' (TALT), 'lacrimal drainage-associated lymphoid tissue' (LDALT), 'eye-associated lymphatic tissue' (EALT) and that of the conjunctiva, called 'conjunctiva-associated lymphatic tissue' (CALT) (Pelikan, 1996; Sirigu et al, 2000; Knop & Knop, 2000; Knop & Knop, 2001, Paulsen et al, 2002; Paulsen et al, 2003; Zoukhri et al, 2006; Pelikan, 2009 a, 2009 b). In this way not only transmission of certain signals but also cellular traffic of various cell types, for example, T lymphocytes (Th1 and Th2) and B cells (plasma cells), can also be realized (Dua et al, 1995; Pelikan, 1996; Calder et al, 1999; Bacon, 2000; Magone et al, 2000.; Pelikan, 2002; Helintö, 2004; Ono & Abelson, 2005; Baudouin et al, 2005; Stern et al, 2005; Bielory, 2008; Pelikan, 2009 a, 2009 b). An additional mechanism that could also play a role in the cellular traffic among the particular organ-associated lymphatic tissues is the 'defective homing' of the B lymphocytes

(Pelikan, 1996; Mikulowska-Mennis et al, 2001; Pelikan, 2009 a, 2009 b). Diagnostic confirmation of hypersensitivity mechanism (s) in the nasal mucosa can be performed by various methods, such as skin tests and *in vitro* estimation of the specific immunoglobulin E antibody (Bielory, 2000; Leonardi, 2005; Radcliffe, 2006). However, these tests provide only general evidence for the possible existence of an allergic component somewhere in the body and not specifically in a particular organ or tissue. Moreover, these tests do not reflect the possible participation of local antibodies in the particular organ and do not provide data on the dynamic aspects of the hypersensitivity mechanism(s) (Pelikan, 2009).

Nasal provocation tests (NPTs) combined with registration of the conjunctival parameters are able not only to show the causal role of a certain allergen in the nasal mucosa and subsequently in the conjunctiva, but also to record quantitatively responses in their dynamic and time-related course. (Pelikan, 2009 a, 2009 b). Although the NPTs are a laborious, time-consuming technique and require special apparatus and facilities, they generate important clinical data that cannot be gathered by other tests. By combining of the recorded parameters, NPTs are also able to confirm a causal role of one organ in a response of another organ, in this case the causal relationship of nasal mucosa and nasal allergy in the reactions of the conjunctiva. Significant correlation of the first and repeated NPTs confirms reliable reproducibility of this technique (Pelikan 2009 a, 2009 b, 2010). NPTs can also discriminate between the participation of the allergy and the non-specific hypereactivity in the patient's complaints. (Pelikan, 2009 a, 2009 b, 2010) Another advantage of NPTs is their ability to follow relative parameter values, by comparing the post-challenge with the pre-challenge results. From this point of view the NPTs are independent of the absolute parameter values that regularly show high variability (Pelikan, 1996; Pelikan, 2002; Pelikan, 2009, 2010). Similar motivation is applicable for the conjunctival provocation tests (CPTs) with allergens showing an allergic reaction directly in the conjunctiva and its causal participation in the conjunctival complaints (Anderson, 1996; McGill et al, 1998). The results of Pelikan et al emphasize some important clinical implications. As nasal allergy can induce a secondary conjunctival response (CR), allergic rhinitis may not always be seen only as a coexisting disorder to allergic conjunctivitis, but in some patients as a causal trigger for the allergic conjunctivitis. This fact would implicate existence of two forms of allergic conjunctivitis, a 'primary or classical form' in which the initial allergic reaction and the subsequent steps (clinical symptoms) take place exclusively in the conjunctiva, whereas the 'secondary form' may be induced by an allergic reaction occurring initially in the nasal mucosa and only the consequences (clinical symptoms) are displayed by the conjunctiva (Pelikan, 1996; Pelikan, 2002; Pelikan, 2009 a, 2009 b). The involvement of various types of hypersensitivity in allergic conjunctivitis (Anderson, 1996; Pelikan, 1996; McGill, 1998; Calder et al, 1999; Bielory, 2000; Bacon, 2000; Magone et al., 2000; Pelikan, 2002; Bonini et al, 2003; Cook, 2004; Stahl & Barney, 2004; Baudouin et al., 2005; Ono & Abelson, 2005; Leonardi, 2006; Bielory & Friedlaender, 2008.; Bielory, 2008; Pelikan, 2009 a, 2009 b, 2010;) may result in three types of CR, immediate, late and delayed, analogous to the three basic types of nasal response (NR). (Pelikan, 1996; Pelikan, 2002).

5. The ocular allergic response and the role of LTs in allergic conjunctivitis

The burden of allergic conjunctivitis and related allergic diseases have been increasing worldwide. It is speculated that environmental factors are essentially responsible for this increase. Because of environmental degradation, especially in urban cities within developing countries, children are confronted with an array of new problems of allergic diseases including allergic conjunctivitis. Allergic conjunctivitis is a condition seldom associated with visual loss; however, it is important from the perspective of quality of life.

Particulate matter-pollutants, pollen, dust, mold, mite, animal dander, and other proteins, as well as dirt and sand, is meant to be blocked from reaching the eye by eyebrows, eyelashes, or eyelids. The particles that evade these barriers alight on the ocular surface and are buffered by the tear film, the most important barrier the eye has against foreign substances. Whatever is not washed away by the tear film eventually reaches the ocular surface. The ocular allergic response is caused by exposure of the conjunctiva, the mucus membrane that covers the posterior aspect of the eye, to an antigen. Immunologic recognition of intruders awakens the body's defenses, leading to antigen recognition and sensitization, antibody activation, and a full-blown over-reactive immunologic response.

Dry eye and allergic conjunctivitis are chronic inflammatory diseases of the cornea and conjunctiva (ocular surface). Dry eye affects 5 million individuals in the United States alone and is more prevalent in women than men (Smith et al, 2007). Allergy including seasonal allergic conjunctivitis, vernal keratoconjunctivitis, giant papillary conjunctivitis (also known as contact lens-induced papillary conjunctivitis), and atopic keratoconjunctivitis affects 20% of the population (Ono & Abelson, 2005). Hallmarks of these diseases are symptoms of ocular pain and discomfort, and signs of ocular surface inflammation that generate inflammatory cytokines and matrix metalloproteinases. These inflammatory mediators lead to death of the surface cells of the corneal and conjunctival epithelia (Lemp, 2007) (Figure 1).

The pathophysiological basis of conjunctivitis and other type I hypersensitivity disorders, such as, rhinitis, asthma and dermatitis, relies on the release of chemical mediators from inflammatory cells (Holgate 2000). Histamine plays a pivotal role in ocular hypersensitivity reactions of both immunological and non-immunological origin, by exerting its effects on blood vessels, nociceptive nerves, fibroblasts, epithelial and goblet cells, mainly *via* histaminergic receptor activation in the ocular surface (Abelson & Schaefer, 1993; Leonardi, 2000). Histamine, being the main early activating molecule of the inflammatory cascade leads to the release of late phase reaction mediators, such as nitric oxide (NO) (Meijer et al., 1996; Ko, 2000). Additionally, the de novo synthesized pro-inflammatory cysteinyl leukotrienes (cysLTs) seem to be equally important, their release in tears from patients with various forms of conjunctival inflammation having been documented

(Akman et al., 1998). Thus, histamine, cys-LTs and NO are involved in the inflammatory processes associated with type I hypersensitivity reactions, which have two well-defined periods. The early phase appears 5–30 min after challenge and it is characterized by vasodilatation and increased vascular permeability, attributed mainly to histamine, which initiates the production of other mediators, like prostaglandins, leukotrienes (LTs), NO and cytokines (Abelson & Schaefer, 1993; Meijer et al., 1996; Weimer et al., 1998). During the late phase response, which begins 2–6 h after challenge, overproduction of these secondary mediators exacerbates the inflammatory process.

The pathophysiology of allergic conjunctivitis is not a simple process. New findings suggest that a wide range of cytokines, chemokines, proteases and growth factors are involved by complex interrelated interactions (Leonardi *et al.*, 2008). In allergic conjunctivitis, there is increased tear levels of several chemical mediators such as histamine, tryptase, leukotrienes (LTs) and prostaglandins (Ono & Abelson, 2005). In addition, tear levels of LTB4 and LTC4 were found to be significantly higher in patients with vernal keratoconjunctivitis than in controls (Akman *et al.*, 1998). In fact, leukotrienes play a role in the development of seasonal allergic conjunctivitis as well as the more severe forms as vernal keratoconjunctivitis and atopic keratoconjunctivitis (Leonardi *et al.*, 2008).

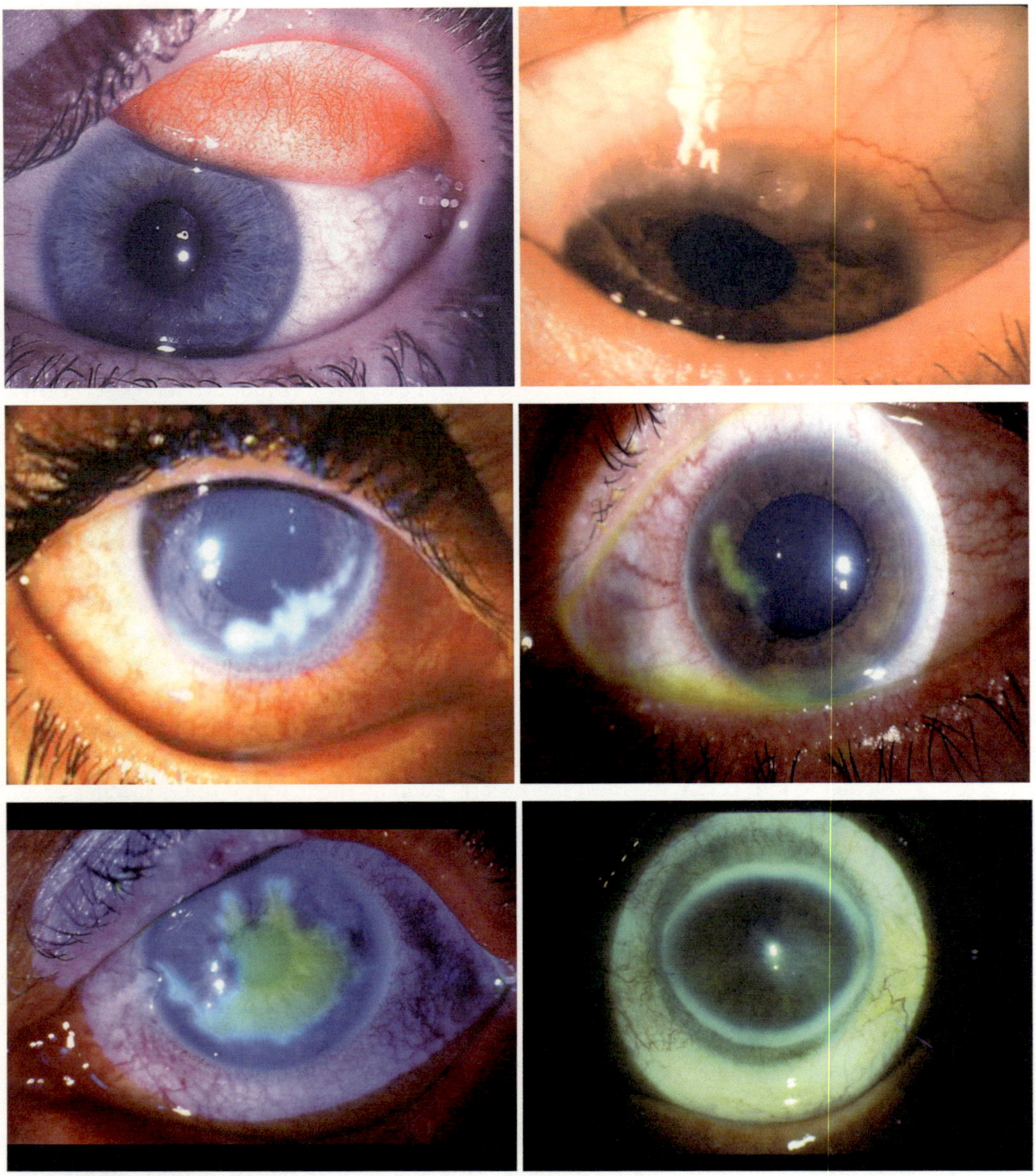

Fig. 1. Images of allergic conjunctivitis in pediatric patients. It is evident the presence of conjunctival hyperemia and oedema.

Dartt DA et al. (2011) showed that cysteinyl leukotrienes LTC4, LTD4, and LTE4 produced in the conjunctiva during ocular allergy, dry eye disease, or other inflammatory diseases of the ocular surface stimulate goblet cell mucous secretion that can contribute to the excess mucous seen in these diseases. The chronic inflammation in these ocular surface diseases damages the cornea and conjunctiva, causing chronic pain from exposed nerve endings. They demonstrated that cysteinyl-leukotriene-stimulated goblet cell secretion was completely blocked by the pro-resolution resolvins RvD1 and RvE1. Thus, resolution of inflammation by the production of pro-resolution mediators, namely, RvD1 and RvE1, can terminate excess goblet cell mucous secretion allowing the ocular surface to repair. These results also support the hypothesis that resolution of inflammation is an active process.

6. The use of leukotriene antagonist drugs in the treatment of allergic conjunctivitis

Allergic conjunctivitis, as described above, is a collection of hypersensitivity disorders that affect the lid, conjunctiva and cornea. It is characterized by immunoglobulin E (IgE-) mediated and/or T-lymphocyte-mediated immune hypersensitivity reactions (Chigbu de,2009). These reactions are initiated by binding of an allergen with specific IgE on the surface of mast cells. The resultant mast cell degranulation leads to early phase and late phase responses. The early phase response develops immediately after exposure to the allergen with clinical symptoms and signs such as itching, chemosis and congestion. This is followed by the late phase response after 8-24 hours which is characterized by conjunctival cellular infiltrations particularly eosinophilia and neutophilia (Miyazaki et al., 2008). The pathophysiology of allergic conjunctivitis is not a simple process, and a wide range of cytokines, chemokines, proteases and growth factors are involved by complex interrelated interactions (Leonardi et al., 2008).

Treatment of allergic conjunctivitis includes several drug groups such as antihistamines, mast cell stabilizers, non-steroidal anti-inflammatory drugs and corticosteroids in resistant cases (Bielory and Friedlaender, 2008). However, the increased worldwide prevalence of ocular allergy has stimulated expansion of management strategies towards physiologic and immunologic drug targets. One of these targets is the leukotrienes (Schultz, 2006). The pro-inflammatory effects of leukotrienes have been well described in asthma and rhinitis (Sacre Hazouri, 2008). Leukotriene receptor antagonists have emerged as important therapeutic options that show clinical efficacy in treatment of bronchial asthma

The ocular allergic response results from exposure of the conjunctiva to an environmental allergen and binding with specific IgE on the conjunctival mast cells. The resultant mast cell degranulation plays a key role in the pathogenesis of both the early and late phase responses of ocular allergy (Leonardi et al., 2008). Compound 48/80 is a non-immunogenic mast cell degranulating agent that produces manifestations of external allergic inflammation when applied topically to the ocular surface (Allansmith et al., 1989). The degranulation produced by the compound is less extensive but morphologically similar to that seen in vernal and giant papillary conjunctivitis. Therefore, it can serve as a useful tool for testing ocular anti-inflammatory agents (Udell et al., 1989). Studies with compound 48/80 applied topically to rabbit eyes, producing allergic inflammatory manifestations that were evident on clinical examination of the eye as well as on hystopathological examination of conjunctival specimens, have been described in literature to show the efficacy of anti-leukotrienes drugs efficacy in the treatment of allergic conjunctivitis. El-Hossary G.G. et al. demonstrated that pretreatment of allergic conjunctivitis model rabbits with 0.1% montelukast eye drops exhibited improvement of ocular inflammatory manifestations both clinically and by histopathological examination. The improvement was more evident after 24 hours of compound application. (El-Hossary et al., 2010). In agreement with the results of this study, it was before described that oral montelukast for 15 days produced significant and persistent reduction of ocular signs and symptoms in asthmatic patients with vernal keratoconjunctivitis (Lambiase et al., 2003). In addition, Oral montelukast combined with oral cetirizine were effective in decreasing orbital congestion and inflammation in patients with thyroid eye disease (Lauer et al., 2008). Moreover, oral zafirlukast, another leukotriene receptor antagonist similar to montelukast, could significantly attenuate the development of conjunctival oedema and inhibit the increase in the number of eosinophils in rats with experimental allergic conjunctivitis (Minami et al., 2004).

Regarding topical ocular application of these drugs, topical application of a leukotriene receptor antagonist in combination with a cyclooxygenase inhibitor could significantly improve inflammatory manifestations in rabbit eyes burned with sodium hydroxide (Struck et al., 1995) In addition, Papathanassiou et al. (2004) reported that topical application of zafirlukast to rat eyes, challenged with compound 48/80, produced significant inhibition of the late phase nitric oxide production of the conjunctival hypersensitivity response. The authors concluded that leukotriene receptor antagonists might contribute to the management of ocular inflammatory response (Papathanassiou et al., 2004). Outside the eye, inhaled montelukast could significantly inhibit the bronchial constriction induced by LTC4 and LTD4 with no injury to the lung tissue in an animal model of asthma (Muraki et al., 2009) and this demonstrates the therapeutic effectiveness and safety of locally applied montelukast.

Montelukast is a leukotriene receptor antagonist that is currently used to treat persistent asthma (Jarvis and Markham, 2000). Although leukotrienes play a role in development of allergic conjunctivitis, they are not the only mediators involved in this disease. Histamine, tryptase and prostaglandins are also involved in the immediate allergic response (Ono and Abelson, 2005). In addition, mast cell degranulation induces activation of vascular endothelial cells and thus the expression of several chemokines and adhesion molecules that finally lead to the ocular allergic late phase reaction (Leonardi et al., 2008). Moreover, conjunctival and corneal epithelial cells and fibroblasts may contribute to mounting the allergic inflammation by expressing and producing cytokines, chemokines, adhesion molecules and growth factors that maintain local inflammation and lead to tissue remodelling (Leonardi et al., 2006). Montelukast was reported to significantly attenuate LT-induced degranulation of bone marrow derived mast cells (Kaneko et al., 2009). The drug was also found to inhibit the expression of vascular endothelial growth factor and its receptors in lung tissue of experimentally induced asthma in rats. Vascular endothelial growth factor is over-expressed in vernal keratoconjunctivitis and may involve tissue growth and remodelling that occur in severe cases of this disease (Asano-Kato et al., 2005).

In El-Houssary's study, pre-treatment of allergic conjunctivitis model rabbits with 1% prednisolone produced more improvement of the allergic response than montelukast, this detected by significant decrease in the clinical scores at all time intervals of examination and by marked improvement of the histopathological picture as the conjunctiva appeared fairly normal after 24 hours of compound application. The result of this study is expected and logical, as topical corticosteroids are very effective in the treatment of allergic conjunctivitis. They have a variety of actions that play a role in suppressing the allergic diseases, and their role is well documented in both clinical and experimental situations (Reiss et al., 1996). Nevertheless, topical ocular montelukast can be a potential therapeutic drug with a new route of administration that can be used for treatment of allergic conjunctivitis.

Despite the number of pharmacological agents currently used to prevent the clinical manifestations of ocular hypersensitivity, there are still continuing efforts aiming at the development of more efficacious topical medications to control the most severe episodes of the disease (Yanni et al., 1999). Currently, anti-LT therapies are approved only for patients with asthma (Leff, 2001), though recent reports support the clinical efficacy of cysLT receptor antagonists in patients with rhinitis (Wilson,2001), and more recently in allergic conjunctivitis.

7. Conclusions

Allergic conditions are common in all pediatric age groups, and significantly affect the health and overall quality of life of children and their families. Although allergies seem relatively minor, they often cause considerable disruptions to daily life for pediatric patients, including sleep disturbances, limitation of activities, disrupted reading, computer work, or outside play, and impaired psychosocial functioning. Making certain that patients are properly treated with the appropriate therapy will help to improve their quality of life.

Familiarity with diagnosis, treatment, and potential complications of common pediatric ocular allergic conditions will increase the chances of early intervention and avert potentially serious consequences of these diseases.

Early and accurate detection of ocular allergy syndromes in children presents a challenge in the primary care setting, as young children are often unwilling participants in ocular examinations. Involvement of pediatric ophthalmologists with specialized training and equipment may be necessary to avoid preventable vision loss in more severe cases. It is the responsibility of all involved to optimize the treatment of these children suffering from allergic disease.

Topical ocular montelukast can be a potential therapeutic drug with a new route of administration that can be used for treatment of allergic conjunctivitis, as new therapeutic strategies an add-on therapy in resistant cases of ocular allergic diseases.

8. References

Abelson, M.B. & Schaefer, K. (1993). *Conjunctivitis of allergic origin: Immunologic mechanisms and current approaches to therapy*, Surv Ophthalmol, 38: 115–32.

Accolate: Manufacturer's prescribing information. (1999). Zeneca Pharmaceuticals, Carolina, Puerto Rico

Akman, A.; Irkec, M. & Orhan, M. (1998). *Effects of lodoxamide, disodium cromoglycate and fluorometholone on tear leukotriene levels in vernal keratoconjunctivitis,* Eye, 12: 291–95.

Allansmith, M.R.; Baird, R.S.; Ross, R.S.; Barney, N.P. & Bloch K.J. (1989). *Ocula anaphylaxis induced in the rat by topical ap- Placation of compound 48/80,* Acta Ophthamol, 67:145-153.

Anderson, DF. (1996). *The conjunctival late-phase reaction and allergen provocation in the eye,* Clin Exp Allergy, 26: 1105–7.

Arango, P.; Borish, L.; Frierson, H.F. & Jr, Kountakis, S.E. (2002). *Cysteinyl leukotrienes in chronic hyperplastic rhinosinusitis,* Otolaryngol Head Neck Surg, 127:512-515.

Arango, P. & Kountakis, S.E. (2002). *Presence of cysteinyl leukotrienes in asthmatic patients with chronic sinusitis,* Laryngoscope, 112:1190-1192.

Asano-Kato, N.; Fukugawa, K. & Okada, N. (2005). *TGF-beta1, IL-1 beta, and Th2 cytokines stimulate vascular endothelial growth Factor production from conjunctival fibroblasts,* Exp Eye Res, 80:555-560.

Bacon, A.S.; Ahluwalia, P.; Irani, A.M. et al. (2000). *Tear and conjunctival changes during the allergen-induced earlyand late- phase responses,* J Allergy Clin Immunol, 106: 948–54.

Baudouin, Ch.; Liang, H.; Bremond-Gignac, D. et al. (2005). *CCR4 and CCR5 expression in conjunctival specimens as differential markers of TH1/TH2 in ocular surface disorders,* J Allergy Clin Immunol, 116: 614–19.

Bhargava, A.; Jackson, W.B. & El-Defray, S.R. (1998) *Ocular allergic disease,* Drugs Today, 34:957-971.

Bielory, L. (2000). *Allergic and immunologic disorders of the eye; Part II: ocular allergy,* J Allergy Clin Immunol, 106: 1019–32.

Bielory, L. (2008). *Ocular allergy overview,* Immunol Allergy Clin North Am, 28: 1–23.

Bielory, L. & Friedlaender, M.H. (2008). *Allergic conjunctivitis,* Immunol Allergy Clin North Am, 28: 43–57.

Bigby, T.D.; Hodulik, C.R.; Arden, K.C. & Fu L. (1996). *Molecular cloning of the human leukotriene C4 synthase gene and assignment to chromosome 5q3,.* Mol Med, 2:637-646.

Bisgaard, H. & Study group on montelukast and respiratory syncytial virus. (2003) *A randomized trial of montelukast in respiratory syncytial virus post-bronchiolitis,* Am J Respir Crit Care Med, 167:379-383.

Bisgaard, H. (2004). *Montelukast in RSV-bronchiolitis,* Am J Respir Crit Care Med, 169:542-543.

Bonini, S.; Lambiase, A.; Sachhetti, M. & Bonini, S. (2003) *Cytokines in ocular allergy,* Int Ophthalmol Clin, 43: 27–32.

Borish, L. (2002). *The role of leukotrienes in upper and lower airway inflammation and the implications for treatment,* Ann Allergy Asthma Immunol, 88:16-22.

Calder, V.L.; Jolly, G.; Hingorani, M. et al. (1999). *Cytokine production and mRNA expression by conjunctival T-cell lines in chronic allergic eye disease,* Clin Exp Allergy, 29: 1214–22

Calonge, M.; De Salamanca, A.E.; Siemasko, K.F. et al. (2005). *Variation in the expression of inflammatory markers and neuroreceptors in human conjunctival epithelial cells,* Ocul Surf, 3: 145–8.

Chigbu de, G.I. (2009). *The pathophysiology of ocular allergy: a review,* Cont Lens Anterior Eye, 32:3-15.

Cook, E.B. (2004). *Tear cytokines in acute and chronic ocular allergic inflammation.* Curr Opin Allergy Clin Immunol, 4: 441–5.

Dartt, D.A.; Hodges, R.R.; Li, D.; Shatos, M.A.; Lashkari, K. & Serhan, C.N. (2011). *Conjunctival goblet cell secretion stimulated by leukotrienes is reduced by resolvins D1and E1 to promoteresolution of Inflammation,* J Immunol, 186:4455-4466.

Dua, H.S.; Gomes, J.A.; Donoso, L.A. & Laibson, P.R. (1995). *The ocular surface as part of the mucosal immune system: conjunctival mucosa-specific lymphocytes in ocular surface pathology,* Eye, 9: 261–7.

El-Hossary, G.G.; El-Hamid Rizk, K.A.; El-Shazly A.H.M. & Anafy L.K. (2010). *Montelukast as a new topical ocular therapeutic agent for treatment of allergic conjunctivitis: an experimental comparative study,* Australian Journal of Basic and Applied Sciences, 1:71-78.

Epstein, A.B. (2003). *Ocular allergy,* Optometry, 74:795- 797

Feldberg, W. & Kellaway C.H. (1938). *Liberation of histamine and formation of lysocythin like substances by cobra venom,* J Physiol, 94:187-191.

Fujishima, H.; Takeyama, M.; Takeuchi, T.; Saito, T. & Tsubota, K. (1997) *Elevated levels of substance P in tears of patients with allergic conjunctivitis and vernal keratoconjunctivitis,* Clin Exp Allergy, 27: 372–8.

Haberal, I. & Corey, J.P. (2003) *The role of leukotrienes in nasal allergy,* Otolaryngol Head Neck Surg, 129:274- 279.

Henderson, W.R. Jr. (1994) *The role of leukotrienes in inflammation,* Ann Intern Med, 121:684-697.

Helintö, M.; Renkonen, R.; Tervo, T. Et al. (2004). *Direct in vivo monitoring of acute allergic reactions in human conjunctiva,* J Immunol, 172: 3235–42.

Higashi, N.; Taniguchi, M.; Mita, H.; Kawagishi, Y.; Ishii, T.; Higashi, A.; Osame, M. & Akiyama, K. (2004) *Clinical features of asthmatic patients with increased urinary leukotriene E4 excretion (hyperleukotrienuria): involvement of chronic hyperplastic rhinosisusitis with nasal polyposis,* J Allergy Clin Immunol, 113:277-283.

Holgate, S.T. (2000). *Science, medicine, and the future. Allergic disorders,* Br Med J, 320: 231–34.

Howarth, P.H. (2000). *Leukotrienes in rhinitis,* Am J Respir Crit Care Med, 161:S133-S136.

Jarvis, B. & Markham, A. (2000). *Montelukast: a review of its therapeutic potential in persistent asthma,* Drugs, 59:891-928.

Jones, T.R.; Labelle, M.; Belley, M.; Champion E.; Charette, L.; Evans, J.; Ford-Hutchinson, A.W.; Gauthier, J.Y.; Lord, A. & Masson, P. (1995). *Pharmacology of montelukast sodium (Singulair), a potent and selective leukotriene D4 receptor antagonist,* Can J Physiol Pharmacol, 73:191-195.

Kaneko, I.; Suzuki, K.; Matsuo, H.; Kumagai, H.; Owada, Y.; Noguchi, N.; Hishinuma, H. & Ono, M (2009). *Cysteinil Leukotrienes enhance the degranulation of bone marrow-derived mast cells through the autocrine mechanism,* Tohoku J Exp Med, 217:185-191.

Keam, S.J.: Lyseng-Williamson, K.A. & Goa K.L. (2003). *Pranlukast: a review of its use in the management of asthma,* Drugs, 63:991-1019.

Khoshoo, V.; Ross, G. & Edell, D. (2002) *Effect of interventions during acute respiratory syncytial virus bronchiolitis on subsequent long term respiratory morbidity,* Pediatr Infect Dis J, 21:468-472.

Knop, N. & Knop, E. (2000). *Conjunctiva-associated lymphoid tissue in the human eye,* Invest Ophthalmol Vis Sci, 41: 1270–9.

Knop, E. & Knop, N. (2001). *Lacrimal drainage-associated lymphoid tissue (LDALT): a part of the human mucosal immune system,* Invest Ophthalmol Vis Sci, 42: 566–74.

Ko, S.M.; Kim, M.K. & Kim, J.C. (2000). *The role of nitric oxide in experimental allergic conjunctivitis,* Cornea, 19: 84–91.

Lakomski, P.G. & Chitre, M. (2004). *Evaluation of the utilization patterns of leukotriene modifiers in a large managed care health plan,* J Manag Care Pharm, 10:115-121.

Lambiase, A.; Bonini, S.; Rasi, G.; Coassin, M. & Bruscolini, A. (2003). *Montelukast, a leukotriene receptor antagonist, in vernal keratoconjunctivitis associated with asthma,* Arch Ophthalmol, 121: 615-620.

Lauer, S.A.; Silkiss, R.Z. &. McCormick, S. A (2008). *Oral montelukast and cetirizine for thyroid eye disease,* Ophthal Plast Reconstr Surg, 24: 257-261.

Leff, A.R. (2001). *Regulation of leukotrienes in the management of asthma: biology and clinical therapy,* Annu Rev Med, 52:1–14.

Lemp, M.; Baudoiin, C.; Baum, J.; Dogru, M.; Foulks, G.; Kinoshita, S.; Laibson, P.; McCulley, J.; Murube, J.; Pflugfelder, S. C., et al. (2007).*The definition and classification of dry eye disease: report of the Definition and Classification Subcommittee of the International Dry Eye WorkShop,* Ocul Surf, 5: 75–92.

Leonardi A. (2000). *Role of histamine in allergic conjunctivitis,* Acta Ophthalmol Scand, 230: S18–21.

Leonardi, A. & Abelson, M. (2003). *Double-masked, randomized, placebo-controlled, clinical study of the mast cellstabilizing effects of treatment with oloptadine in the conjunctival allergen challenge model in humans,* Clin Ther, 25:2539-2552.

Leonardi, A. (2005). *In-vivo diagnostic measurements of ocular inflammation,* Curr Opin Allergy Clin Immunol, 5:464–72.

Leonardi, A.; Fregona, I.A.; Plebani, M.;Secchi, A.G. & Calder VL. (2006). *Th1- and Th2-type cytokines in chronic ocular allerg,* Graefes Arch Clin Exp Ophthalmol, 244:1240–5.

Leonardi, A.; Motterle, L. & Bortolotti M. (2008). *Allergy and the eye,* Clin. Exp. Immunol, 153:17-21.

Leonardi, S.; Marchese, G.; Marseglia GL. & La Rosa M. (2007). *Montelukast in allergic diseases beyond asthma,* Allergy Asthma Proc, 28:287-291.

Lewis, R.A.; Austen, K.F. & Soberman, R.J. (1990). *Leukotrienes and other products of the 5-lipoxygenase pathway. Biochemistry and relation to pathobiology in human diseases,* N Engl J Med, 323:645-655.

Magone, M.T.; Whitcup, S.M.; Fukushima, A.; Chan, C.C.; Silver, P.B. & Rizzo, L.V. (2000). *The role of IL-12 in the induction of late-phase cellular infiltration in a murine model of allergic conjunctivitis,* J Allergy Clin Immunol, 105:299–308.

Marmou. S. & Raffard, M. (2004). *Allergic conjunctivitis: diagnosis and treatment,* Allergy Immunol, 36:25-29.

McGill, K.A. & Busse, W.W. (1996). *Zileuton*, Lancet, 348:519-524.

McGill, J.I.; Holgate, S.T.; Church, M.K.; Anderson, D.F.; & Bacon, A. (1998). *Allergic eye disease mechanisms,* Br J Ophthalmol , 82: 1203–14.

Meijer, F.; Van Delft, J.L.; Garrelds, I.M.; Van Haeringen, N.J. & Kijlstra, A. (1996). *Nitric oxide plays a role as a mediator of conjunctival edema in experimental allergic conjunctivitis,* Exp Eye Res, 62: 359– 65.

Mikulowska-Mennis, A.; Xu, B.; Berberian, J.M. & Michie, S.A. (2001). *Lymphocyte migration to inflamed lacrimal glands is mediated by vascular cell adhesion molecule-1/a4b1 integrin, peripheral node addressin/L-selectin, and lymphocyte function-associated antigen-1 adhesion pathways,* Am J Pathol, 159: 671–81.

Minami, K.; Fujii, Y. & Kamei, C. (2004). *Participation of chemical mediators in the development of experimental allergic conjunctivitis in rats,* Int. Immunopharmacol, 4: 1531-1535.

Miyazaki, D. ; Tominaga, T.; Yakura, K.; Cuo, C.; Komatsu, K.; Inoue, Y. & Ono, S.J. (2008). *Conjunctival mast cell as a mediator of eosinophilic response in ocular allergy,* Mol Vis, 14:1525-1532.

Motterle, L.; Diebold, Y.; De Salamanca, A.E. et al. (2006) *Altered expression of neurotransmitter receptors and neuromediators in vernal keratocinjunctivitis,* Arch Ophthalmol, 124: 462–8.

Muraki, M.; Imbe, S.; Sato, R.; Ikeda, Y.; Yamagata, S.; Iwanaga T. & Tohda, Y. (2009). *Inhaled montelukast inhibits cystinyl- leukotriene-induced bronchoconstriction in ovalbumin-sensitized guinea-pigs: the potential as a new asthma medication,* Int Immunopharmacol, 9: 1337-1341.

Nathan, R.A.; Meltzer, E.O.; Selner, J.C. & Storms, W. (1997). *Prevalence of allergic rhinitis in the United States,* J Allergy Clin Immunol, 99: S808-S814.

Ono, S.J. & Abelson, M.B. (2005). *Allergic conjunctivitis: update on pathophysiology and prospects for future treatment,* J Allergy Clin. Immunol, 115: 118-122.

Papathanassiou, M.; Giannoulaki V. & Tiligada, E. (2004). *Leukotriene antagonists attenuate late phase nitric oxide production during the hypersensitivity response in the conjunctiva,* Inflamm Res, 53: 373-376.

Parnes, S.M. (2002). *Targeting cysteinyl leukotrienes in the treatment of rhinitis, sinusitis, and paranasal polyps,* Am J Respir Med, 1:403-408.

Parnes, S.M. & Chuma, A.V. (2000). *Acute effects of antileukotrienes on sinonasal polyposis and sinusitis,* Ear Nose Throat J, 79:18-20, 24-25.

Parnes, S.M. (2003). *The role of leukotrienes inhibitors in patients with paranasal sinus syndrome,* Curr Opinion Otolaryngol Neck Surg, 11:184-191.

Paulsen, F. (2003). *The human nasolacrimal ducts,* Adv Anat Embryol Cell Biol, 170: 1–106.

Paulsen, F.P.; Paulsen, J.L.; Thale, A.B.; Schaudig, U.; Tillmann, B.N. (2002). *Organized mucosa-associated lymphoid tissue human nasolacrimal ducts,* Adv Exp Med Biol, 506: 873–6.

Pelikan, Z (1996). *The late nasal response. Thesis,* The Free University of Amsterdam, Amsterdam.

Pelikan, Z. (2002) .*The causal role of the nasal allergy in some patients with allergic conjunctivitis,* Allergy, 57: 230.

Pelikan, Z. (2009 a). *Seasonal and perennial allergic conjunctivitis: the possible role of nasal allerg,.* Clin Exp Ophtalmol, 37:448-457.

Pelikan, Z. (2009 b). *The possible involvement of nasal allergy in allergic keratoconjunctivitis,* Eye, 23:1653-1660.

Pelikan, Z (2010). *Allergic conjunctivitis and nasal allergy,* Curr Allergy Asthma Resp, 10:295-302

Radcliffe, M.J.; Lewith, G.T.; Prescott, P.; Church, M.K. & Holgate, S.T. (2006). *Do skin prick and conjunctival provocation tests predict symptom severity in seasonal allergic rhinoconjunctivitis?* Clin Exp Allergy; 36: 1488–93.

Reiss, J.; Abelson, M.B.; George, M.A.& Wedner, H.J. (1996). *Allergic conjunctivitis. In Ocular infection and immunity,* Eds, Pepose, J.S., G.N. Holland and K.R. Wilhelmus. Mosby-Year Book Inc.,pp:345-358.

Riccioni, G.; Santilli, F.; D'Orazio, N.; Sensi, S.; Spoltore, R.; De Benedictis, M.; Guagnano, M.T.; Di Illio, C.; Schiavone, C.; Ballone, E. & DellaVecchia R. (2002). *The role of antileukotrienes in the treatment of asthma,* Int J Immunopathol Pharmacol, 15:171-182.

Sacre Hazouri, J.A. (2008). *Leukotriene antagonists in the treatment of allergic rhinitis and comorbidities,* Rev Alerg Mex,55: 164-175.

Samuelsson, B.; Dahlén, S.E.; Lindgren, J.A.; Rouzer, C.A. & Serhan, C.N. (1987). *Leukotrienes and lipoxins: Structures biosynthesis, and biological effects,* Science, 237:1171-1176.

Scadding, G.K. (2003). *Recent advances in the treatment of rhinitis and rhinosinusitis,* Int J Pediatr Otorhinolaryngol, 67:S201-204.

Schleimer, R.P.; MacGlashan, D.W. Jr.; Peters, S.P. et al. (1986). *Characterization of inflammatory mediator release from purified human lung mast cells,* Am Rev Respir Dis, 133:614 -617.

Schultz, B.L. (2006). *Pharmacology of ocular allergy,* Curr Opin Allergy Clin Immunol, 6:383-389.

Sirigu, P.; Maxia, C.; Puxeddu, R.; Zucca, I.; Piras, F. & Perra, MT. (2000). *The presence of a local immune system in the upper blind and lower part of the human nasolacrimal dust,* Arch Histol Cytol, 63: 431–9.

Smith, J.; Albeitz, J.; Begley, C.; Caffery, B.; Nichols, K.; Schaumberg, D. A. & Schein, O. (2007). *The epidemiology of dry eye disease: report of the Epidemiology,* Subcommittee of the International Dry Eye WorkShop 2007. Ocul Surf, 5: 93–107.

Spector, S.L. (1997). *Overview of comorbid associations of allergic rhinitis,* J Allergy Clin Immunol, 99:S773-S780.

Spector, S.L. & Antileukotriene Working Group. (2001). *Safety of antileukotriene agents in asthma management,* Ann Allergy Asthma Immunol, 86:18-23.

Stahl, J.L. & Barney, N.P. (2004). *Ocular allergic disease,* Curr Opin Allergy Clin Immunol, 4: 455–9.

Stainke, J.W.; Bradley, D.; Arango, P.; Crouse, C.D.; Frierson, H.; Kountakis, S.E.; Kraft, M. & Borish, L. (2003). *Cysteinil Leukotriene expression in chronic hyperplastic sinusitis-nasal polyposis: importance to eosinophilia and asthma,* J Allergy Clin Immunol, 111:342-329.

Steinke, J.W.; Crouse, C.D.; Bradley, D.; Hise, K.; Lynch, .; Kountakis, S.E.& Borish, L. (2004). *Characterization of interleukin- 4-stimulated nasal polyp fibroblasts,* Am J Respir Cell Mol Biol, 30:212-219.

Stern, M.E.; Siemasko, K.F. & Niederkorn, J.Y. (2005). *The Th1/Th2 paradigm in ocular allergy,* Curr Opin Allergy Clin Immunol, 5: 446–50.

Struck, H.G.; Giessler, S. & Giessler, C. (1995). *Effect of non-steroidal anti-inflammatory drugs on inflammatory reaction. An animal experimental study,* Ophthalmologe, 92: 849- 853.

Szefler, S.J. & Simoes, E.A. (2003) *Montelukast for respiratory syncytial virus bronchiolitis: significant effect or provocative findings?* Am J Respir Crit Care Med, 167: 290-291.

Takahashi, Y.; Ichikawa, M.; Nawate, M.; Kamoshida, H. & Shikano, T. (2003). *Clinical evaluation of urinary leukotriene E4 levels in children with respiratory syncytial virus infection,* Arerugi, 52:1132-1137.

Taylor, F.; Hutchinson, S.; Graff-Radford, S. & Harris, L. *Diagnosis and management of migraine in family practice,* J Fam Pract, S3-S24.

Uchio, E.; Kimura, R.; Migita, H.; Kozawa, M. & Kadonosono, K. (2008) *Demographic aspects of allergic ocular diseases and evaluation of new criteria for clinical assessment of ocular allergy,* Graefes Arch Clin Exp Ophthalmol, 246: 291–6.

Udell, I.J.; Kenyon, K.R.; Hannien, L.A. & Abelson, M.B. (1989). *Time course of human conjunctival mast cell degranulation. In response to compund 48/80,* Acta Ophthalmol, 31,226-230.

Vignola, A.M.; Chanez, P. & Bousquet, J. (2003). *The relationship between asthma and allergic rhinitis: Exploring the basis for a common pathophysiology,* Clin Exp Allergy Rev, pp 3:63-68.

Von Mutius E. (1998). *The rising trend in asthma and allergic disease,* Clin Exp Allergy, pp 28, 45-49.

Yanagawa, H.; Sugita, A.; Azuma, M.; Ogawa, H.; Kitamuro, C.; Yoneda, K.; Shinkawa, K.; Tani, K.& Sone, S. (2004) *Long-term follow-up of pulmonary function in bronchial asthma in patients treated with pranlukast,* Lung, 182:51-58.

Yanni, J.M.; Sharif, N.A.; Gamache, D.A.; Miller, S.T.; Weimer, L.K. & Spellman, J.M. (1999). *A current appreciation of sites for pharmacological intervention in allergic conjunctivitis: effects of new topical ocular drugs,* Acta Ophthalmol Scan, 228: 33–7.

Weimer, L.K.; Gamache, D.A. & Yanni, J.M. (1998). *Histamine-stimulated cytokine secretion from human conjunctival epithelial cells: inhibition by the histamine H1 antagonist emedastine,* Int Arch Allergy Immuno, 115: 288–93.

Wenzel, S.E.; Szefler S.J.; Leung, D.Y.; Sloan, S.I.; Rex, M.D. & Martin R.J. (1997). *Bronchoscopic evaluation of severe asthma. Persistent inflammation associated with high dose glucocorticoids,* Am J Respir Crit Care Med. 156:737-743.

Wenzel, S.; Larsen, G.L.; Johnson, K. et al. (1990). *Elevated levels of leukotriene C4 in bronchoalveolar lavage fluid from atopic asthmatics after endobronchial allergen challenge,* Am Rev Respir Dis, 142:112-119.

Wilson, A.M.; Orr, L.C.; Sims E.J. & Lipworth, B.J. (2001). *Effects of monotherapy with intra-nasal corticosteroid or combined oral histamine and leukotriene receptor antagonists in seasonal allergic rhinitis,* Clin Exp Allergy, 31: 61–8.

Ziskin, A. (2006). *Allergic conjunctivitis,* Curr Allergy Clin Immunol, 19: 56–9.

Zoukhri, D. (2006) *Effect of inflammation on lacrimal gland function,* Exp Eye Res, 82: 885–98.

8

The Evaluation of Anti-Adenoviral Therapeutic Agents for Use in Acute Conjunctivitis

J.A. Capriotti[1], J.S. Pelletier[1], K.P. Stewart[1] and C.M. Samson[2]
[1]Ocean Ophthalmology Group, North Miami Beach, Fl
[2]New York Eye and Ear Infirmary, New York, NY
USA

1. Introduction

External ocular infections caused by adenoviruses are among the most common eye infections seen worldwide. They lead to highly infectious community epidemics, seasonal outbreaks, lost productivity, significant patient discomfort and in some cases permanent visual compromise from long-term immune-mediated sequelae[1]. Though several therapeutic agents have been evaluated for acute viral conjunctivitis in both animal models and human trials, none to date have been approved for therapeutic use in humans[2,3,4]. Both bacterial and viral pathogens cause acute infectious diseases of the ocular surface with similar clinical presentation. Key differences exist in the mechanism, host response and epidemiology of each etiologic agent. Consideration of these differences shapes our approach to treatment and our approach to the evaluation of therapeutic agents in clinical trials.

2. Clinical features of bacterial and adenoviral conjunctivitis

All acute conjunctivities share some common clinical features that aid in the design of appropriate clinical evaluations. Most cases involve conjunctival hyperemia with varying chemosis, some component of ocular discharge and a constellation of symptoms that can include foreign body sensation, pain and itching. A recent evidence-based review[5] examined several databases, including the Cochrane Controlled Trials Register, along with standard ophthalmology texts and concluded that signs and symptoms of acute bacterial and acute viral conjunctivitis are essentially identical. Measurement of the resolution of these symptoms is an essential part of the clinical evaluation of agents for use in acute conjunctivitis of any etiology. Analogy can be made with bacterial conjunctivitis for the clinical signs and symptoms of viral infection, and this analogy can guide in the selection of clinical endpoints. For this reason, the use of similar clinical criteria for one of the primary efficacy endpoints in both viral and bacterial clinical trials is suggested.

3. Differences in bacterial and adenoviral relationship to the healthy ocular surface

Bacterial conjunctivitis is commonly caused by normal ocular surface flora[6]. When the balance between host defense and microbial colonization on the ocular surface is somehow disrupted, the commensal relationship can proceed to frank infection[7]. Key factors that

affect this pathogenic conversion appear to be related both to host defense compromise and specific bacterial species present[8].
In contradistinction to bacteria, adenovirus species are not typically found among the normal ocular flora[9,10,11]. A definitive study employing tissue culture in ocular swab samples obtained from the conjuntival fornicies was unable to demonstrate the presence of adenovirus from even a single sample of over 200 collected in asyptomatic patients presenting for routine eye exam[12]. The absence of adenoviral colonization was similarly demonstrated in conjunctival specimens studied by tissue culture obtained from a series of patients with symptoms of non-infectious keratoconjunctivitis sicca[13]. The presence of adenovirus on the ocular surface would seem to indicate active or recent convalescent infection. This is a critical difference between bacterial and adenoviral conjunctivitis and must be considered when selecting efficacy endpoints for the evaluation of therapeutic agents. Anti-bacterials can clearly demonstrate their clinical utility by simply showing the resolution of clinical signs and symptoms in a shorter time period than would be expected with non-intervention. There is no need to show elimination of bacterial colonization as bacterial sterility is not a feature of the healthy ocular surface. Bacterial conjunctivitis is a much rarer cause of community outbreaks and is less likely to be associated with person-to-person transmission. Described below is the very different behavior of viral conjunctivitis and the relationship between transmissibility and viral shedding.

4. Viral transmission and shedding

The differences in the transmissibility of bacterial and viral conjunctivitities merit careful consideration. Ocular adenoviral infection represents a significant public health problem in the US and worldwide[14, 15] Although exact numbers are difficult to determine, estimates from a US survey of outpatient health encounters[4,9], comparison with epidemiological surveys completed in outside the US[15] and studies of incidence in military recruits[16] suggest that the number of cases of viral conjunctivitis may be as high as 15-20 million per year in the United States. Adenovirus conjunctivitis is a reportable infection in Germany[17] and is classified as a Category IV infectious disease by Japan's National Epidemiological Surveillance of Infectious Diseases (NESID) with mandated collection, analysis and publication of reports on occurrences[18].
Adenoviral transmission between infected and uninfected hosts is particularly efficient in areas of high population density, overcrowding or poor hygiene[19]. Studies on the rate of[20] horizontal transmission to asymptomatic family members and close contacts suggest transmissibility of up to 50%[21,22,23]. Adenovirus is spread through droplets from the respiratory tract, stool, saliva and tears. Through a process known as viral shedding, infectious particles are transferred from the extracellular environment of lytic infected cells through a variety of fomites[24]. Adenoviral particles, presumably shed from infected patients, have been isolated from multi-dose ophthalmic medications and diagnostic solutions[25,26] Recovery of infectious adenovirus has been reported from samples obtained from inanimate hard surfaces and objects for up to 49 days[27,28]. Actively infected persons readily transmit adenoviruses. Viral shedding persists for 12-14 days after onset of clinical signs and symptoms. Transmission can be prevented by personal hygiene measures including frequent handwashing; cleaning of towels, pillowcases and handkerchiefs; and disposal of contaminated facial tissues. Patients with adenoviral conjunctivitis may shed virus to these objects which can in turn infect other hosts Individuals who work with the public, in

schools, or in healthcare facilities in particular should consider a temporary leave of absence from work to prevent infection of others, especially those who are already ill[29]. This is common in hospital and clinic settings and can lead to systemic disease with or without conjunctivitis, particularly in immunocompromised patients[30]. The most effective measures for limiting the severity of adenoviral conjunctivitis outbreaks rely on reducing the contamination of objects, workspaces and surfaces by aggressive steps to remove shed virus particles[31,32]. It follows that reducing shedding at the source - the infected ocular surface- would be a highly effective strategy for epidemic prevention and control.

The clear relationship between shedding virus and infectivity necessarily affects our therapeutic options and our therapeutic requirements in acute viral conjunctivitis. The additional burden is placed on the evaluation of anti-adenoviral agents given their devastating potential to cause outbreaks. Proposed therapeutic agents should aim for a reduction in viral shedding in addition to the resolution of clinical symptoms. An evaluation of efficacy that incorporates both reduced viral infectivity and improvement in symptoms is required to fully demonstrate the utility of any proposed anti-adenoviral therapeutic agent.

Similar patterns of epidemic spread, droplet transmission and shedding are not typical features of bacterial conjunctivitis, though outbreaks have been reported in humans[33] and vector-dependent spread confirmed in animal models[34,35,36]. Bacterial conjunctivitis is a much less likely cause of outbreaks and is not a significant public health challenge (we acknowledge the enormous importance of bacterial conjunctivitis caused by *C. Trachoma* and defer its discussion as it is more commonly a chronic, endemic, recurrent infection with a distinct clinical course)[37]. Though vertical transmission remains an important aspect of neonatal bacterial conjunctivitis, these cases are rare in the industrialized world and do not share the features of epidemic infection. Furthermore neonatal conjunctivitis passed intra-partum from mother to newborn is easily eliminated through ocular administration of povidone-iodine at the time of birth[38].

5. Ocular immune response in bacterial and adenoviral infections

Components of both the innate and adaptive acquired immune systems play important roles in ocular defense.[39] While the predominantly extracellular bacterial pathogens are more effectively controlled by the innate ocular defense mechanisms, viral infections often lead to a more prolonged course. Viral exposures frequently involve a more robust acquired immune cascade with significant inflammatory damage[4041,42]. It is precisely this exuberant immune reaction that leads to the signs and symptoms of viral conjunctivitis and immune-mediated sequelae. It is often clinically beneficial to temper the ocular immune response in both viral and bacterial infections, with topical steroids frequently the agents of choice. Steroids have well characterized effects on both innate and adaptive immunity. The features of the immune responses to viral and bacterial pathogens need to be considered along with the relative effects of steroid on each system: Steroids have a more dramatic inhibitory effect on the adaptive system, and this is precisely the system that is most important at eliminating viral infections. In expected that steroids would have less of an effect on the eye's ability to counter bacterial pathogens than they would on the elimination of viral organisms. It has been demonstrated that co-administration of potent topical steroids along with antibiotics does not lead to higher bacterial counts (measured as CFU's)[43] in the normal bacterial conjunctival flora.

It has been repeatedly shown in ocular adenoviral infection that use of topical steroids can prolong the duration of viral shedding and therefore lengthen the period of transmissibility in these cases[44]. It is for this reason that topical steroid monotherapy in ocular adenovirus infections is ill-advised. It is well known that a short course of topical corticosteroids (and in some severe cases oral steroids) can limit patient discomfort and prevent some immune-related inflammatory complications of acute viral conjunctivitis. While this strategy may have some efficacy in the short-term amelioration of symptoms, even a short course of relatively low-potency corticosteroids without the addition of a suitable anti-viral agent can increase the duration of viral shedding and prolong the infectivity of affected patients[45]. The addition of topical steroids cripples the eye's immune response to viral pathogens. The effect on the ability to effectively clear viral infections is so pronounced that the addition of topical steroids can even reverse the effect of the most potent anti-virals[46]. This in turn can potentiate the occurrence of community outbreaks and epidemic transmission in schools, places of business and medical facilities[47]. As described above, this additionally requires that effects on infectivity be considered along with symptom resolution in the clinical evaluation of anti-adenoviral therapies[48].

6. Detection of adenoviral infectivity

There are several techniques available for the detection of adenovirus from ocular specimens. Despite recent advances in nucleic acid-based detection and the availability of a rapid point-of-care immunochromatographic tests for the presence of specific viral components, cell culture remains the only reliable method for the demonstration of viable, infectious virus.

Cell culture with confirmatory immunofluorescence (CC-IFA) is a highly sensitive and specific test and is considered the "gold standard" for the recovery of infectious virus from ocular samples. CC-IFA requires the presence of infectious virus and demonstrates unequivocally the ability of the recovered virus to cause a cytopathic effect (CPE) in a living cell. When combined with immunoflourescent staining, it provides a means to determine the presence, infectivity and identity of a viral specimen.

A sample from a conjunctival swab is inoculated in susceptible cell line and followed over time to measure the cytopathic effects (CPE). The "Shell Vial Culture" method is a specific cell culture technique that enables more rapid identification of CPE[49]. This test utilizes shell vials, centrifugation and visualization of adenovirus proteins inside host cells through binding of fluorescent dye. Shell vials are glass culture tubes that contain a coverslip coated with an A549 cell monolayer. The culture tube is inoculated with the clinical specimen and the tube is centrifuged at low speed and incubated. It is hypothesized that the centrifugation enhances the adenoviral entry into the susceptible cells. The visualization technique is indirect, where a secondary antibody labeled with fluorochrome is used to recognize a primary antibody directed towards a conserved adenoviral epitope. This test significantly shortens the time requirement and enhances the sensitivity and specificity. Positive results can be obtained from the visualization of even a single brightly stained cell, confirming that the adenoviral particles were capable of entering a cell, uncoating, replicating and producing infectious prodigy virions. In this way CC-IFA in general and the Shell Vial method specifically provide an unequivocal way to determine the infectivity of an ocular specimen. It is for this reason that we propose assessment of infectivity by CC-IFA as a second primary endpoint for clinical trials designed to evaluate the efficacy of anti-adenoviral therapeutic agents.

Single Active Ingredient Antibiotic Drugs

Besifloxacin (Besivance)
Ciprofloxacin (Ciloxan)
Neomycin (NeoSporin)
Erythromycin (Ilotycin)
Gatifloxacin (Zymar)
Tobramycin (AK_Tob, Tobrex)
Gentamycin (Gentak, Gentasol)
Moxifloxacin (Vigamox)
Polymyxin B and trimethoprim (Polytrim)
Bacitracin (Ak-Tracin, Bacitcin)
Ofloxacin (Ocuflox)
Sulfacetamide (Cetamide, Ocusulf_10)

Combination Antibiotic-Steroid Drugs

Tobramycin and dexamethasone (Tbradex)
betamethasone and neomycin
dexamethasone and neomycin/ polymixin B (Maxitrol)
Loteprednol / tobramycin (Zylet)
Prednisolone/polymyxin B/neomycin (PolyPred)
Prednisolone/gentamycin (PredG)
Prednisolone / sulfacetamide (Blephamide)

Though all of the above are commonly used to treat viral and bacterial conjunctivitis, none are approved by the FDA for use in acute viral conjunctivitis.

Table 1. Drugs commonly used to treat acute conjunctivitis

7. Proposed clinial study design for demonstrating utility of therapeutic agents in acute adenoviral conjunctivitis

The ideal treatment for adenoviral conjunctivitis would alleviate patient symptoms, resolve clinical signs, decrease inflammatory damage, shorten the clinical course of infection, reduce the duration of viral shedding and decrease the period of infectivity. The evaluation of all therapeutic agents for use in adenoviral conjunctivitis should include analysis of clinical and infectious parameters and consider effects on the individual patient and the community as a whole. The use of separate primary efficacy endpoints is proposed that can demonstrate the following:

1. Resolution of signs and symptoms associated with viral conjunctivitis.
2. Decrease in infectious viral shedding measured by CC-IFA at the test-of-cure visit.

Resolution of signs and symptoms of the disease is the most clinically meaningful assessment and derives from the similar clinical features shared by acute bacterial and acute viral conjunctivitis. Particularly from the patient's individual perspective, the resolution of signs and symptoms is the most important clinical outcome. Much can be learned and

borrowed from the myriad experience gained over decades of clinical trials in bacterial conjunctivitis. The use of standardized conjunctivial grading, scaled scoring for ocular discharge and conjunctival injection all have application in both bacterial and viral disease.
The required analysis of viral shedding, which derives from the differences in transmission between bacterial and viral conjunctivitis, is important to ensure that symptomatic relief in individuals doesn't lead to prolonged infectivity. The ideal therapeutic will radpidly decrease viral loads and shorten the overall length of time that active, replicating virus can be isolated from the ocular surface. This will ensure that the simple masking of symptoms cannot be substituted for a true viral cure. Though indivdual subjects may improve on symptom-alleviating therapy only, the requirement to reduce infectivity should ensure that no agents gain approval that could potentially lengthen epidemics or threaten the public health.
The requirement for all proposed agents to satisfy both of these endpoints is the most effective way to ensure that proposed ant-adenoviral therapies address both the infectious and inflammatory consequences of the disease.

8. References

[1] Ford E, Nelson KE, Warren D. Epidemiology of epidemic keratoconjunctivitis. *Epidemiol Rev,* 1987; 9:244–61.

[2] Hillenkamp J, Reinhard T, Ross R, *et. al.,* The effects of cidofovir 1% with and without cyclosporin A 1% as a topical treatment of acute adenoviral keratoconjunctivitis : A controlled clinical pilot study. *Ophthalmology,* 2002; (5):845-850.

[3] Teuchner B, Nagl M, Schidlbauer A, *et. al.,* Tolerability and efficacy of N-Chlorotaurine in epidemic keratoconjunctivitis—a double-blind, randomized, phase-2 clinical trial. *J Ocul Therapeut,* 2005; 21:157-164.

[4] Romanowski EG, Gordon YJ. Efficacy of topical cidofovir on multiple adenoviral serotypes in the New Zealand rabbit ocular model. *Invest Ophthalmol Vis Sci,* 2000; 41:460–3.

[5] Rietveld RP, van Weert HC, ter Riet G, Bindels PJ. Diagnostic impact of signs and symptoms in acute infectious conjunctivitis: systematic literature search. *BMJ.* Oct 4 2003;327(7418):789.

[6] Tabbara KF, Hyndiuk RA. *Infections of the Eye.* Little, Brown;1996.

[7] Smolin and Thoft's The Cornea: Scientific Foundations and Clinical Practice, 4th ed. Philadelphia: Lippincott Williams and Wilkins; 2005.

[8] Watanabe K, Watanabe KM, Hayasaka S. Methicilin-resistant Staphylococci and ofloxacin-resistant bacteria from clinically healthy conjunctivas. *Ophthalmic Res* 2001; 33: 136–139.

[9] Kaneko H, Maruko I, Iida T, et al. The possibility of human adenovirus detection from the conjunctiva in asymptomatic cases during nosocomial infection. *Cornea.* Jun 2008;27(5):527-530.

[10] Alvaregna L, Scarpi M, Mannis MJ. "Viral Conjunctivitis" In: Krachmer JH, Mannis MJ, Holland EJ.(eds.) Cornea (Vol.1): Fundamentals, Diagnosis, Management. 2nd Edition, Elsevier, Philadelphia, 2005, 629-639.

[11] Vastine D, Schwartz H, Yamashiroya H, Smith R, Guth S. Cytologic diagnosis of adenoviral epidemic keratoconjunctivitis by direct immunofluorescence. *Invest. Ophthalmol. Vis. Sci.* March 1, 1977 1977;16(3):195-200.

[12] Cambon E, Pollard M. Viral Studies of the Normal Eye *Arch Ophthalmol*, Oct 1959; 62: 562 - 565.

[13] Studies of the viral flora in keratoconjunctivitis sicca. *Br J Ophthalmol*. 1975 January; 59(1): 45–46.

[14] Ishii K, Nakazono N, Fujinaga K, et al. Comparative studies on aetiology and epidemiology of viral conjunctivitis in three countries of East Asia--Japan, Taiwan and South Korea. *Int J Epidemiol*. Mar 1987;16(1):98-103.

[15] D'Angelo LJ, Hierholzer JC, Holman RC, Smith JD. Epidemic keratoconjunctivitis caused by adenovirus type 8: epidemiologic and laboratory aspects of a large outbreak. *Am J Epidemiol*. Jan 1981;113(1):44-49.

[16] Heggie, AD. Incidence and etiology of conjunctivitis in Navy recruits. *Mil Med* 1990;155:1-3.

[17] Schrauder A, Altmann D, Laude G, Claus H, Wegner K, Köhler R, Habicht-Thomas H, Krause G. Epidemic conjunctivitis in Germany, 2004. *Euro Surveill*. 2006;11

[18] Aoki K, Tagawa Y. A twenty-one year surveillance of adenoviral conjunctivitis in Sapporo, Japan. *Int Ophthalmol Clin*. Winter 2002;42(1):49-54.

[19] Maranhao AG, Soares CC, Albuquerque MC, Santos N. Molecular epidemiology of adenovirus conjunctivitis in Rio de Janeiro, Brazil, between 2004 and 2007. *Revista do Instituto de Medicina Tropical de Sao Paulo*. Jul-Aug 2009;51(4):227-229.

[20] Cheung D, Bremner J, Chan JT. Epidemic kerato-conjunctivitis--do outbreaks have to be epidemic? *Eye*. Apr 2003;17(3):356-363.

[21] Schrauder A, Altmann D, Laude G, et al. Epidemic conjunctivitis in Germany, 2004. *Euro Surveill*. Jul 2006;11(7):185-187.

[22] Schepetiuk SK, Norton R, Kok T, Irving LG. Outbreak of adenovirus type 4 conjunctivitis in South Australia. *J Med Virol*. Dec 1993;41(4):316-318.

[23] Dawson CR, Hanna L, Wood TR, Despain R. Adenovirus type 8 keratoconjunctivitis in the United States. 3. Epidemiologic, clinical, and microbiologic features. *Am J Ophthalmol*. Mar 1970;69(3):473-480.

[24] Warren D, Nelson KE, Farrar JA, et al. A large outbreak of epidemic keratoconjunctivitis: problems in controlling nosocomial spread. *J Infect Dis*. Dec 1989;160(6):938-943.

[25] R. Kowalski, E. Romanowski, B. Waikhom, Y. Gordon The survival of adenovirus in multidose bottles of topical fluorescein. *Am J Ophthalmol*, 126:835-836

[26] Uchio E, Ishikio H, Aoki K, Ohno S. *Am J Ophthalmol* 2002, 134; 618-619.

[27] Nauheim RC, Romanowski EG, Araullo-Cruz T, et al. Prolonged recoverability of desiccated adenovirus type 19 from various surfaces. *Ophthalmology*. Nov 1990;97(11):1450-1453.

[28] Gordon YJ, Gordon RY, Romanowski E, Araullo-Cruz TP. Prolonged recovery of desiccated adenoviral serotypes 5, 8, and 19 from plastic and metal surfaces in vitro. *Ophthalmology*. Dec 1993;100(12):1835-1839; discussion 1839-1840.

[29] *External Disease and Cornea*. Basic and Clinical Science Course, 2004-2005. Section 8. San Francisco, Calif: American Academy of Ophthalmology; 2005:130–134.

[30] Hierholzer JC. Adenoviruses in the immunocompromised host. *Clin Microbiol Rev*. Jul 1992;5(3):262-274.

[31] Dart JKG, El-Amir AN, Maddison T et. al. Identification and control of nosocomial adenovirus keratoconjunctivitis in an ophthalmic department. *Br J Ophthalmo*200; 93: 918-920.
[32] Gottsch, J.D., Froggatt, J.W. III, Smith, D.M., et al. Prevention and control of epidemic keratoconjunctivitis in a teaching eye institute. *Ophthalmic Epidemiol*. 6:29–39, 1999.
[33] Dawson CR. Epidemic Koch-Weeks conjunctivitis and trachoma in the Coachella Valley of California. *Am J Ophthalmol* 1960;49:801-8
[34] Payne WJ Jr, Cole JR Jr, Snoddy EL, Seibold HR. The eye gnat Hippelates pusio as a vector of bacterial conjunctivitis using rabbits as an animal model. *J Med Entomol* 1977;13:599-603.
[35] The California eye gnat. *Science* 1929;69:14
[36] Dow RP, Hines VD. Conjunctivitis in Southwest Georgia. *Public Health Rep* 1957;72:441-8.
[37] World Health Organization (2003) Report of the 2nd global scientific meeting on trachoma. WHO/PBD/GET 03.1.
[38] Isenberg SJ, Apt L, Wood MA. A controlled trial of povidone-iodine as prophylaxis against ophthalmia neonatorum. *New England J Med*, 1995; 332:562-566.
[39] Mannis MJ, Smolin G. "Natural defense mechanisms of the ocular surface." In: Pepose JS, Holland GN, Wilhelmeus KR (eds.) Ocular Infection and Immunity. Mosby; St. Louis, MO, 1996, 185-190.
[40] Knop, E. and N. Knop, Anatomy and immunology of the ocular surface. *Chem Immunol Allergy*, 2007. 92: p. 36-49
[41] Smolin and Thoft's The Cornea: Scientific Foundations and Clinical Practice, 4th ed. Philadelphia: Lippincott Williams and Wilkins; 2005.
[42] Akpek, E.K. and J.D. Gottsch, Immune defense at the ocular surface. *Eye*, 2003. 17(8): p. 949-56
[43] Ermis SS, Aktepe OC, Inan UU, Ozturk F et. al. Effect of topical dexamethasone and ciprofloxacin on bacterial flora of healthy conjunctiva. *Eye*, 2004; 18: 249-252.
[44] Gordon YJ, Araullo-Cruz T, Romanowski EG. The effects of topical nonsteroidal anti-inflammatory drugs on adenoviral replication. *Arch Ophthalmol*. 1998; 116: 900-905.
[45] Romanowski EG. Yates KA. Gordon YJ. Short-term treatment with a potent topical corticosteroid of an acute ocular adenoviral infection in the New Zealand white rabbit. *Cornea* 2001; 20(6):657-60.
[46] Romanowski EG, Araullo-Cruz T, Gordon YJ. Topical corticosteroids reverse the antiviral effect of topical cidofovir in the Ad5-inoculated New Zealand rabbit ocular model. *Invest Ophthalmol Vis Sci*. Jan 1997;38(1):253-257.
[47] Romanowski EG, Roba LA, Wiley L, Araullo-Cruz T, Gordon YJ. The effects of corticosteroids on adenoviral replication. *Arch Ophthalmol*, 1996; 114:581-585
[48] Romanowski EG. Yates KA. Gordon YJ. Short-term treatment with a potent topical corticosteroid of an acute ocular adenoviral infection in the New Zealand white rabbit. *Cornea* 2001; 20(6):657-60.
[49] Kowalski RP, Karenchak LM, Romanowski EG, Gordon YJ. Evaluation of the shell vial technique for detection of ocular adenovirus *Ophthalmology*,106: 1324-1327.

9

Conjunctival Flora Before and After Application of 5% Povidone-Iodine Solution

Virginia Vanzzini-Zago[1], Jorge Villar-Kuri[2], Víctor Flores Alvarado[3], Alcántara Castro Marino[4] and Pérez Balbuena Ana Lilia[5]
[1]*Assistant to Laboratory of Microbiology*
[2]*Chief of staff of Surgery Service*
[3]*Assistant to Laboratory of Microbiology*
[4]*Assigned to Cornea Service*
[5]*Asociación para Evitar la Ceguera en México Hospital "Dr. Luis Sánchez Bulnes"*
Mexico

1. Introduction

Conjunctival flora is attached with protein links to conjunctival cells. For this reason, the resident flora, *Corynebacteria* and *Staphylococcus epidermidis* are almost always present in normal conjunctives of any age, and depuration mechanism like tears, blinking or even the antibiotic do not remove it [1]. *Staphylococcus epidermidis*, or other coagulasa negative *Staphylococcus, Corynebacteria* or *Propionibacterium acnes* resident in normal conjunctiva and eye lids are named as frequent post-surgical endophthalmitis cause [2], pathogen bacteria as *Staphylococcus aureus* and *Streptococcus pneumoniae* are also related to acute and severe endophthalmitis, reason why it is very important to diminish the conjunctival alive bacteria previous to cataract or other ocular surgery and since 1985 Apt had proposed the use of antiseptic solutions like povidone-iodine in ocular surface. [3]. Some years later, Speaker proved in one comparative study the efficiency of antisepsis using this solution with a statistical significance less endophtalmitis as surgical risk in anterior segment ocular surgeries [4].

The use of drops of aqueous 5 % solution of povidone-iodine (polivinil pirrolidonil iodine solution) is manadatory in all ocular surgeries and its efficacy has been proved and published [5] even when not all bacteria species are diminished to 0 CFU.

1.1 Problem statement

Prevention of an endophthalmitis event as post surgical complications in cataract or other ocular surgeries is very important for the eye preservation for a good visual acuity and integrity. The purpouse of this survey is to determine the efficacy of 2 drops of 5% povidone-iodine aqueous solution applied in conjunctival sacs 1 to 2 minutes before every cactarat surgery for to reduce conjunctival alive flora in 100 patients, and to know which bacteria are susceptible or resistent and remain alive in conjunctival sacs despite the antiseptic method.

1.2 Application area

In all ocular surgeries and applicaton of intravitreal injections.

1.3 Research course

This is a prospective, comparative and linear study in 100 patients that were submitted to cataract surgery.

1.4 Method used

In each patient immediately before the surgery was taken one sample (A) without antibiotic medical treatment of conjunctival sacs in the eye that will be submitted to surgery with a cotton swab for quantitative and qualitative determination of aerobic and anaerobic bacteria, mesured in count forming unit (CFU), and a second sample (B) 2 minutes after the application of 5% povidone-iodine aqueous solution and wash out with sterile saline solution. All patients were attended in an eye care hospital in México City, Asociación para Evitar la Ceguera en México "Dr. Luis Sánches Bulnes" IAP.

Collection of each specimen was performed by completely rotating the cotton swab through the lower conjunctival sac from the temporal to nasal conjunctival zone. We took care not to touch the eye lid margin or lashes. Immediately the cultures for aerobica and anaerobic bacteria were made by direct inoculation in 5% blood sheep agar with brain heart agar base, exposed on one swab side, then it was rotated 180 grades and inoculated on chocolate agar enriched plate media using the other swab side, by this technique bacteria collected in samples A and B have been distribuited equally in both solid culture media. After that, the cotton swab tip was put in thioglicolate broth an incubated at 37 centigrade for 7 days.

Blood agar plates were incubated for aerobic, hemolyitic and microaerophylic bacteria for 48 hours in a candle jar (5% CO2) , and chocolate agar plates were incubated for anaerobic bacteria in anaerobic bags for 7 days in 37 Centigrades incubator.

The enriched thioglycolate broth with 1% hemin and 0.001% vitamine K [6], was used for detection of even small amounts of living anaerobic, or microaerobic fastidious bacteria and incubated 7 days at 37C, and subcultured for anaerobic bacteria.

Multiple bacterial species were counted, selected and identified each one in the plates of blood agar and chocolate agar and expresed in CFU [7]. The same technique for the cultures was used for samples B, after two minutes of the action of antiseptic solution, and wash away with steril saline solution.

We used the sample A taken without any medical treatment as comparative sample, and samples B as problem sample for statistical calculations.

Aerobic and anaerobic bacteria were identified with semi-automated techniques by Crystal ® system (BBL Meryland USA) Gram stain, oxidase, catalase and indol reaction

2. Status

Inclusion criteria:

1. All patients that will be subbmitted to cataract surgery in a period of one month attended in Hospital para Evitar la Ceguera en México "Dr. Luis Sánchez Bulnes" IAP in surgeries performed by Anterior Segment Service
2. Patients of any age that were submitted to cataract surgery.

Exclusion criteria:

1. Patient that have been used topical antibiotic drops for prophylactic treatment before surgery.

2.1 Results

In the conjunctivas of 19 patients, sample A and B were negative for cultures of aerobic and anaerobic bacteria, 81 patients sowed 26 bacterial species.

The total CFU including all aerobic and anaerobic bacterial species isolated in all the samples A before the application of 5% povidone iodine solution was 5,701 and were diminished to 193 CFU including aerobic and anaerobic bacteria, with statistical significance calculated by Fisher method, of x= 0.033 as is shown in Fig 1.

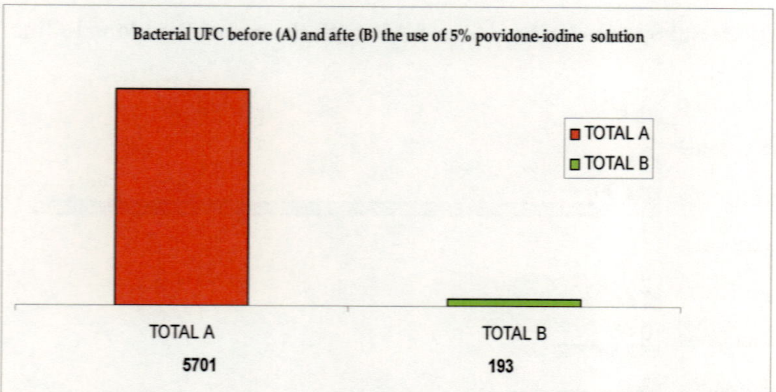

Fig. 1. The CFU of conjunctival sample A taken without antiseptic solution, Sample B after the application of 5% povidone-iodine solution.

Remained some anaerobic and aerobic bacteria as shown in Fig 2 with statistical significance by application of Fisher method with a value of x= 0,.035, for sample A and B.

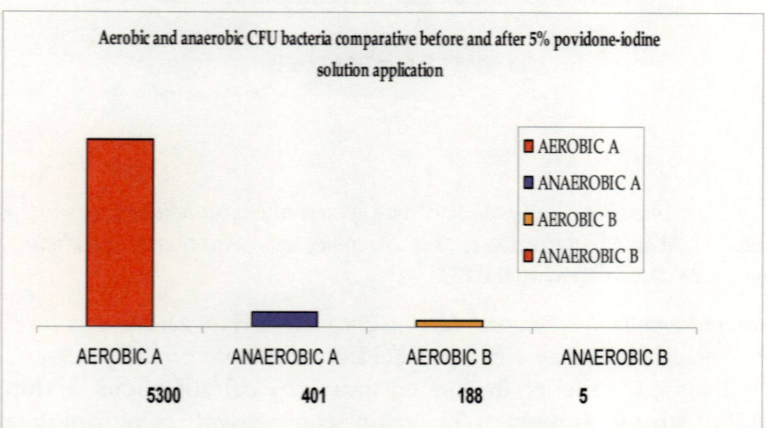

Fig. 2. Aerobic and anaerobic bacteria were diminished by 5% povidone-iodine solution.

Aerobic bacteria in sample A was 5,300 CFU and were diminished to 188 UFC in sample B, and for anaerobic bacteria samples A sowed 401 CFU and were diminished to 5 UFC in sample B, with Fischer statistical method value of x= 0.012.
Streptococcus pneumoniae and *Staphylococcus aureus* were the species more diminished, and in sample B was not found CFU of these two ocular pathogens as is showed in fig 3.
The action of 5% yodopovidone aqueous solution over the conjunctival flora in 100 patients samples mesuring the UFC and the species found was evaluated in Table 1 as shown:

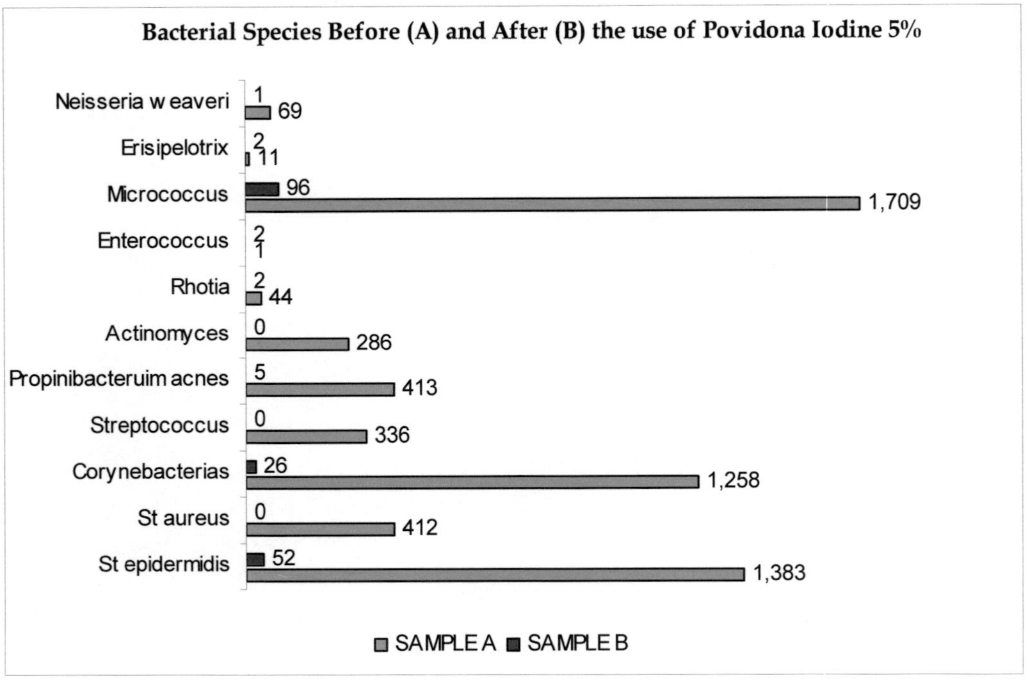

Fig. 3. Some aerobic bacteria like *Staphylococcus epidermidis* and *Micrococcus luteus* are isolated in high cuantities in samples A and *Streptococcus penumoniae, Staphylococcus aureus* and *Actinomyces* are diminished to 0 CFU

Staphylococcus epidermidis, Micrococcus luteus, Corynebacterium xerosis and *Propionibacterium acnes* were the bacteria most remained in UFC after antiseptic technique used.
None of the incuded patients developed post-surgical infectious endophtalmitis or corneal opacity during surgery. The main conjunctival colonization mesured by individuals were by *Staphylococcus epidermidis* in 53% of the patients and 18.5% by *Propionibacterium acnes.*

Bacterial genera	specie	Sample A (n=100) Total CFU	Sample B (n=100) Total CFU
Staphylococcus	*epidermidis*	1383	52
	aureus	487	0
Streptococcus	*pneumoniae*	335	0
	sanguis	1	0
Micrococcus	*spp*	79	0
	luteus	1630	96
Corynebacterium	*xerosis*	627	21
	bovis	116	1
	aquaticum	11	0
	propiqum	413	0
	Pseudo genitalium	4	1
	renale	4	0
	spp.	75	3
	diphteriae	6	1
	Pseudo diphteriae	2	0
Propionibacterium	*acnes*	112	5
Actinomyces	*meiyeri*	2	0
	odontolyticum	2	0
	pyogenes	286	0
Rothia	*dentocariosa*	44	2
Erisipelotrix	*rusiopathiae*	11	2
Bacillus	*subtilis*	1	0
Enterococcus	*faecalis*	1	2
Acinetobacter	*lwoffi*	0	6
Neisseria	*elongata*	1	0
	weaveri	68	1
Total		5701	193

Table 1. Bacterial CFU in samples A, and bacteria CFU eliminated, diminished or remained in samples B

The number of patients in whom have been diminished conjuntival flora by action of povidone-iodine 5 % solution are presented in Table 2

Genus and specie	n=Pateints before antisepsia	n=Patients after antisepsia	diminished frequency %
Staphylococcus epidermidis	60	32	46.7%
Staphylococcus aureus	8	0	100.0%
Streptococcus pneumoniae	1	0	100.0%
Streptococcus sanguis	1	0	100.0%
Micrococcus spp.	1	0	100.0%
Micrococcus luteus	1	1	0.0%
Enterococcus faecalis	1	2	0.0%
Corynebacterium xerosis	8	1	87.5%
Corynebacterium bovis	4	1	75.0%
Corynebacterium aquaticum	3	0	100.0%
Corynebacterium propiqum	6	0	100.0%
Corynebacterium pseudogenitalium	3	1	66.70%
Corynebacterium renale	1	0	100.0%
Corynebacterium spp.	2	2	0.0%
Corynebacterium diphteriae	6	1	83.30%
Corynebacterium pseudodifteriae	2	0	100.0%
Propionibacterium acnes	27	5	81.50%
Actinomyces meiyeri	1	0	100.0%
Actinomyces odontolyticum	2	0	100.0%
Actinomyces pyogenes	4	0	100.0%
Rothia dentocariosa	4	2	50.0%
Erisipelotrix rusiopathiae	1	1	0.0%
Bacillus subtilis	1	0	100.0%
Acinetobacter lwoffi	0	1	0.0%
Neisseria elongata	1	0	100.0%
Neisseria weaveri	1	1	0.0%

Table 2. Percentual disminution of conjunctival colonization, and number of patients with conjuntival colonization.

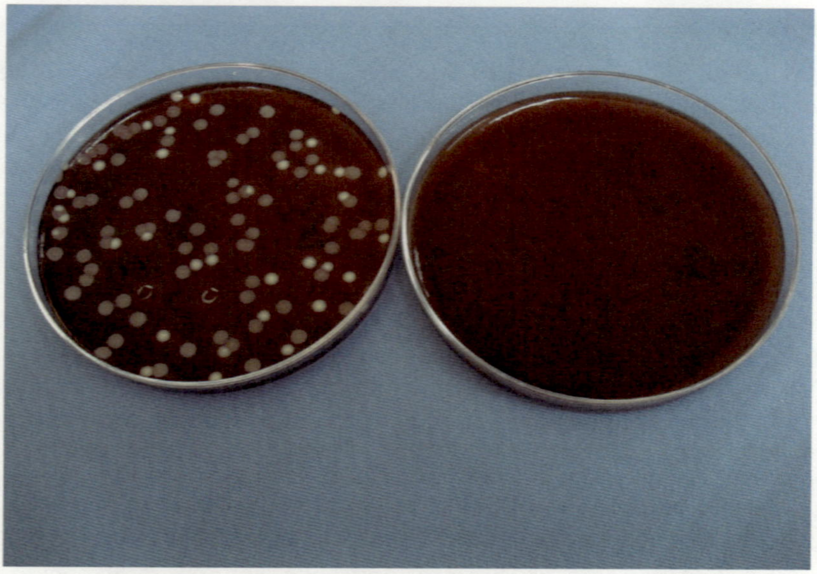

Fig. 4. *Staphylococcus aureus* 120 UFC, *Staphylococcus epidermidis* 104 UFC and *Corynebacterium diphteriae* 1 UFC in samples A in Blood agar. After the antiseptic 5 % povidone-iodine solution tecnique, *Staphylococcus epidermidis* 2 UFC in sample B

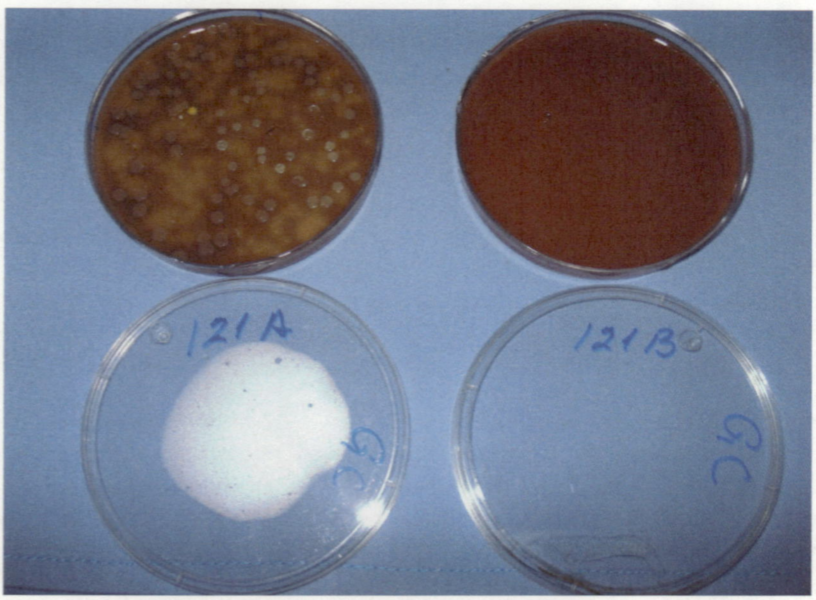

Fig. 5. *Staphylococcus epidermidis* 16 UFC, *Streptococcus penumoniae* 335 UFC, *Staphylococcus aureus* 74 UFC in samples A in Blood agar and after the antiseptic 5 % povidone-iodine solution tecnique in sample B *Staphylococcus epidermidis* 1 UFC

3. Further research

The contamination of aquous humor in anterior chamber by periocular flora from conjunctiva, Meibomian and Zies glands, or lids, was demonstrated by Saint-Blancart even with the application of topical antibiotic drops before the surgery [8] and the confirmation that are the same *Staphylococcus epidermidis* from conjunctival flora was maden by rPCR methods by pulse fields in gel [2].

In our survey the most numerous bacterial colonization was *Staphylococcus epidermidis* and *Micrococcus luteus* isolated in conjunctiva before the antiseptic solution application and remained some CFU from both species in the patients conjunctivas after the ansiseptic application, as it is described by Bausz [9].

We found *Corynebaterium diphteriae* in normal conjunctivas before the antiseptic application (sample A), with no clinical significance, because theydid not have in the bacterial cells DNA the structural Gen of Fago B that make it sinthetize its harmful toxin. *Rothia dentocariosa* were found in the sample A in two patients, and remained in one patient after the antiseptis method, this anaerobic bacteria, has been related as corneal pathogen [10] or as post-surgical endophtalmitis cause [11] in our patients did not have clinicals significance.

Survival bacterial in presence of universal antiseptic solution as 5% povidone-iodine mesured in comparative application methods [12] are indicative of some physical protective mechanism for bacteria as mucus, or tears proteins that capture the iodine molecules and its remaind in Henle conjunctival crypts, factors that have not been well studied.

There is no total conjunctiva surface asepsia using topical antibiotic drops alone or iodine compound as demonstrate Inoue. [13]

For this reason there are some antiseptic proposal using topical antibiotics drops in conjunctiva during three days before the anterior segment intraocular surgery [14] reaching an important reduction of bacterial CFU in the conjunctival surface and using 5% povidone iodine solution before the ocular surgeries.

Has been sugested the use of polyhexamethyl-biguanida as preoperative antiseptic for cataract surgery with equal microbicidal efficacy that povidone-iodine [15], this application have not further demonstrative studies. The comparison between povidone –iodine 16 times diluited from 10% concentration and 0.05% solution of chlorexidine gluconate, povidone iodine solution showed superior disinfectant effect. [16]

4. Conclusion

This survey demonstrate the effectivness of 5% povidone-iodine aqueous solution for the erradication of pathogenic bacteria like *Streptococcus pneumoniae, Staphylococcus aureus, Actinomyces pyogenes, A meiyeri,* and *A odontolyticus* in conjuntival surface.

The largest population of *Staphylococcus epidermidis* and *Micrococcus luteus* in conjuntival isolated in sample A remained in low quantities in sample B with statistical significance.

There were two patients with colonization after antiseptic technique method used as described, with a different bacterial genus in sample A that in sample B, the colonization was caused by *Acinetobacter lwoffi* and *Enerobacter faecalis.*

With the exception of *Micrococcus luteus* and *Corynebacterium xerosis* others bacterial species were present in conjunctiva after the antisepsis in very low quantities as 1 or 2 colonies.

5. References

[1] M.S. Osato, Normal ocular flora. En Pepose JS, Holland GN, Wilhelmus KR. Ocular Infection and Immunity Mosby Co. 2a ed. 1998, pp. 191-199.

[2] T. L. Bannerman, D. L. Rhoden, S. K. Mc Allister, J. M.Millar, L. A. Wilson. The source of coagulasa-negative staphylococci in the Endophthalmitis Vitrectomy Study. A comparison of eyelid and intraocular isolates using pulsed-field gel electrophoresis. Arch Ophthalmol. no 115: 357-361. Mar. 1997.

[3] L. Apt, S. Isenberg, R. Yoshimori, J. H. Paez. Chemical preparation of the eye in ophthalmic surgery. III. Effect of povidone-iodine on the conjunctiva. Arch Ophthalmol no 102 pp 728- 729. May 1984.

[4] M. G. Speaker, J. A. Menikoff. Prophylaxis of endophthalmitis with topical povidone-iodine. Ophthalmology. no 98 pp1769-75, Dec. 1991.

[5] T.A. Ciulla, M. B. Starr, S. Masket. Bacterial endophtalmitis prophylaxis for cataract surgery an evidence-base update. Opthalmology; vol. 1 no. 109 pp 13-24. Jan. 2002.

[6] D. B. Jones, T. J. Liesegang, M. N. Robinson, Cumitech 13 Laboratory diagnosis of ocular infections. Amer. Soc. for Microbiology Washington D.C. pp 1-27. 1981.

[7] M. H. Kaspar, R. T. Chang, K. Singh, P. R. Eghert, M. S. Blumenkranz, C. N. Ta. Prospective randomized comparison of 2 different methods of 5% povidone-iodine applications for anterior segment intraocular surgery. Arch Ophthalmol. Vol. 123 pp 161-165. Feb. 2005.

[8] P. Saint-Blancart, C. Burucoa, M. Boissonnot, F. Gobert, J. F. Risse. Search of bacterial contamination of the aquous humor during cataract surgery with and whitout local antibiotic prophylaxis. J. Fr Ophthalmol no 18 vol 11 pp. 650 sup. Nov 1995.

[9] M. Bausz, E. Fodor, M.D. Resch, K. Kristóf. Bacterial contamination in the anterior chamber after povidona-iodine application and the effect of the lens implantation device. Cataract Refract Surg no. 32 vol. 10 pp. 1691 sup.S. Oct. 2006.

[10] Morley AM, Tuft SJ. Rothia dentocariosa isolated from a corneal ulcer. Cornea no 25 vol 9 pp 1128-9 Oct 2006.

[11] M. M. MacKinnon, M. R. Amezaga, J. R. McKinnon. A case of Rothia dentocariosa enophthalmitis. Microbiol Infect Dis no. 20 vol. 10 pp. 756-7. Oct. 2001.

[12] H. Miño de Kaspar, R. T. Chang, K. Singh , P. R. Egbert, M. S. Blumenkranz, C. N. Ta. Prospective randomized comparison of 2 different methods of 5% povidone-iodine applications for anterior segment intraocular surgery. Arch Ophthalmol no 123 pp. 161-165 Feb. 2005.

[13] Y. Inoue, M. Usui, Y. Ohashi, H. Shiota, T. Yamazaki. Preoperative disinfection of the conjunctival sac with antibiotic and iodine compounds: A prospective randomized multicenter study. Jpn J. Ophthalmol no. 52 vol. 3 pp. 151-61 May-Jun. 2008.

[14] C. N. Ta, R. C. Lin, G. Singh, H. Miño de Kaspar. Prospective study demonstrating the efficacy of combined preoperative three-day application of antibiotic and povidone-iodine irrigation. Ann Ophthalmol. (Skokie) no. 39 vol. 4 pp. 313-7. Dec. 2007.

[15] Hasmann F, Kramer A, Ohgke H, Strobel H, Müller M, Geerling G. Ophthalmologe. No. 101 vol 4:pp 377-83. Apr. 2004.

[16] Yokohama Y, Makino S, Ibaraki N. Comparison in effectivness of sterilization between chlorexidine gluconate and povidone iodine. Nippon Ganka Gakkai Zasshi no 12. vol 2. pp. 148-51. Feb. 2008.

Part 4

Special Forms of Conjunctivitis

10

Ophtalmia Neonatorum

Flora Abazi, Mirlinda Kubati, Blerim Berisha, Masar Gashi,
Dardan Koçinaj and Xhevdet Krasniqi
University Clinical Centre of Kosovo
Republic of Kosovo

1. Introduction

Sexually transmitted infections (STIs) or sexually transmitted diseases (STDs) are common in low- income countries. Among adult women STIs (excluding HIV) represent around 9% of the disease burden (World Bank, 1993). This group of disease (Table 1) can lead to infertility, abortion, neonatal blindness and sometimes death. Furthermore in up to 75% of women STIs are thought to be asymptomatic, knowing also that vaginal discharge might be caused by non-sexually transmitted changes in vaginal flora (Sloan et al., 2000; Lush et al., 2003).

Common STI syndrome	Possible cause
Genital ulcer disease	Chancroid, Syphilis, Chlamydia, Herpes simplex virus, Donovanosis
Urethral discharge	Gonorhoea, Chlamydia
Vaginal discharge	Gonorhoea, Chlamydia, Herpes, trichomonas, Candida, Bacterial vaginosis
Pelvic inflammatory disease	Gonorhoea, Chlamydia
Ophtalmia neonatorum	Gonorhoea, Chlamydia

Table 1. Common STI syndromes and possible causes Modified from Lush L, Walt G, Ogden J. (2003) Transferring policies for treating sexually transmitted infections: what's wrong with global guidelines? Health Policy and planning 18(1): 18-30.

Ophtalmia neonatorum (neonatal conjunctivitis) is an ocular redness, swelling and drainage (sometimes even purulent) due to a pathogenic organism or even chemical irritant occurring in infants less than 4 weeks of age with potentially serious ocular and systemic consequences (Merck Manual 2006, Rudolph's 2002). The frequency of this disease varies up to 19% and is related to prenatal care (Rudolph's 2002).

Bacterial infection is acquired from infected mother during delivery. The most common bacteria is Chlamydia trachomatis causing Chlamydial ophtalmia occurring in 2 to 4% of births. This entity accounts for about one third to half of all conjunctivitis in neonates, characterizing developed countries (Current, 2009), while the prevalence of maternal chlamidial infection ranges from 2 to 20% (Mohile et al., 2002) with the incidence increasing dramatically through years (Miller, 2006).

Streptococcus pneumoniae and Haemophilus influenze as other bacteria responsible account for another 15% of cases. On the other hand, the incidence of conjunctivitis due to Neisseria gonorrhoeae (gonorrheal ophtalmia) in the USA is 2 to 3 per 10,000 births.
Usually the isolation of other bacteria than mentioned above (e.g. Staphylococcus aureus) represents colonization.
Herpetic kerato- conjunctivitis caused by herpes simplex virus types 1 and 2 represents the major viral infection, while chemical conjunctivitis is generally secondary to the instillation of ocular drops (e.g. silver nitrate) for prophylaxis purpose.

2. Etiology

Ophtalmia neonatorum may be caused by microorganisms (infectious etiology), or may be sterile (non infectious etiology) from chemical irritants (Table 2). Sterile or non infection ophtalmia neonatorum usually is caused by silver nitrate during prophylaxis of this entity. As far as infectious etiology concerns there are different bacteria and viruses known to cause this disease. The most commonly isolated bacteria are: Chlamydia trachomatis and Neisseria gonorrhoeae; but also: Staphylococcus aureus, Streptococcus pneumoniae, Streptococcus viridians, Staphylococcus epidermidis, Escherichia coli, Klebsiella pneumoniae, Serratia marcescens, Proteus, Enterobacter, and Pseudomonas species. Also, Eikenella corrodens has been reported as a cause of neonatal conjunctivitis (Chhabra et al., 2008). The most commonly viral cause is Herpes simplex virus (HSV) associated most often with a generalized herpes simplex infection.

Etiology	Percentage (%)	Incubation period	Associated problems
Chemical	Varies	1	---
Chlamydia trachomatis	2-40	5-14	Pneumonia
Neisseria gonorrhoeae	<1	2-7	Disseminated infection
HSV	<1	6-14	Disseminated infection

Table 2. Pathogens of neonatal conjunctivitis

Modified from "Red Book-Report of the Committee on Infectious Diseases, 29th Edition. The American Academy of Pediatrics.".http://aapredbook.aappublications.org/.

2.1 Silver nitrate solution

Silver nitrate solution is one the most common sterile causes of ophtalmia neonatorum. It was used for prophylaxis of ocular gonococcal infections as the most effective agent in prevention of ophtalmia neonatorum by direct inactivating of Gonococi. Crede's method was a major advance in preventing of ophtalmia neonatorum using 2% drops of Silver nitrate (Jatla et al., 2009). Later silver nitrate was found to be toxic for conjunctiva, causing chemical neonatal conjunctivitis, usually lasting 2-4 days. Because of replacement of silver nitrate with neomycin and chloramphenicol eye drops, and erythromycin ointment the incidence of chemical neonatal ophtalmia in the most countries have significantly decreased.

2.2 Chlamydia trachomatis

It was postulated that unknown agent acquired from the genital tract of mother, is a cause of abacterial ophthalmia neonatorum (Kroner, 1884). Lindner comes to conclusion that inclusion of blennorrhoea was due to the trachoma agent, and after techniques evolution in Ophtalmology the first isolation was performed by Tang et al. This was realized by using the yolk sac of embryonated eggs and latter followed by isolating chlamydia from the babyes eyes with inclusion of blennorrhoea, and also from cervix of mother (Linder, 1909; T'ang et al., 1957; Jones et al., 1959).

Chlamydia trachomatis is an intracellular parasite, one of the common causes of ophtalmia neonatorum 2-4% of births. Chlamydia trachomatis, based on immunogenic epitope analysis of the major outer membrane protein (MOMP), differentiates in 18 serovars. D to K serovars are common urogenital and ocular pathogens. Genotype classification correlates with the serovar classification previously mentioned (Rodriguez et al., 1993). Even though this classification is practical and accepted among researchers, it is found increased frequency of C. trachomatis genotype E in neonatal conjunctivitis (Lucía et al., 2010).

It is thought that infants may acquire infection from their immediate surroundings, not only from mother birth canals. The high incidence of caesarean sections with high incidence of early onset conjunctivitis suggests in a possibility of intrauterine Chlamydial infection due to rupture of membrane. These kind of infections with Chlamydia trachomatis are sexually transmitted and WHO estimated 90 million new cases in 1999 (World Health Organisation, 2010). The developing risk of the Chlamydial infection as a conjunctivitis or pneumonia at birth is increased with an incidence up to 15% (Schachter et al., 1986; Numazaki et al., 2003; Rosenman et al., 2003).

In some newborns with Chlamydia conjunctivitis, the infection persists too long with panus and scarring formation and after this, if this infection is left untreated it may be complicated even with pneumonia. Prevalence of this conjunctivitis is 8%. (Hobson, 1977; Valencia et al., 2000; Olatunji, 2004).

Chlamydial conjunctivitis occurs after three days of life but may occur up to two weeks of life with mucopurulent and less inflamed discharge. Chlamydial conjunctivitis is associated with low risk of blindness compare to Gonorrheal conjunctivitis.

2.3 Neisseria gonorrhoeae

Neisseria gonorrhoeae was identified by Albert Neisser in 1879 in stained smears of exudates. Availability of Sulfonamides and Penicillin in 1943 was effective in treating of Gonorroheae (Kampmeier, 1978; Morton, 1977).

In the past N. Gonorroheae was a common cause of conjuctivitis, but after 1881 based on observations of Crede (using the silver nitrate) the prevalence as a causative agent of ophtalmia is decreased, in the industrial zones from 10 to 0.3% (Di Bartolomeo et al., 2001).

Neisseria species are aerobic, gram negative, non motile and non spore forming. Gonococci occurs in pairs as diplococcal and have outer membrane overlying, a thin peptidoglycan and cytoplasmic membrane. The species lacks a true polysaccharide capsule but produces a surface polyphosphate that provides a hydrophilic, negatively charged surface. The microbes frequently are seen within phagocytes in Gram stains of clinical specimens (Noegel et al., 1983).

Gonococci have ability to adhere to mucosal epithelial cells and thus can survive, activating nuclear factor kappa B and activator protein 1, with release of numerous of cytokines and chemokines (Nauman et al., 1997; Ramsey et al., 1995).
The individual gonococci can invade, replicate intracellulary, and by exocytosis can exit into the submucosal space (Alexey et al., 2000; Nauman et al., 1999). This lead in a chemotactic influx of neutrophils resulting in formation of micorabscesses and exudation of purulent material into lumen of infected tissues. Infection can persist for weeks to months if untreated because of escape immune response (Gergg et al., 1983; Casey et al., 1986; Shafer et al., 1986; Kallstrom et al., 1997).
Incubation period of Neisseria gonorrhoeae in eye infection is 2 to 5 days and in some cases may arise 2 to 3 weeks (Gutman, 2001). Gonococcal conjunctivitis begins as benign and bilateral with eyelid edema, followed by chemosis. The discharge in the beginning is sero-sanguineous, later becomes thick and purulent, and may contain also blood. The infection can spread if treatment is delayed causing complications such as corneal ulceration and perforation, iridocyclitis, and panophtalmitis. From conjunctiva gonococcus can spread to cause gonococcus septicemia, arthritis, and other manifestations (Friendly, 1969).
Staphylococcus aureus can cause ophtalmia neonatorum with purulent discharge. The treatment consists in topical or systemic antibiotic. In some cases spontaneous resolution can occur. Also, in Ophtalmia neonatorum are verified methicillin and erythromycin resistant S. aureus, but serious ophtalmologic infection was not found. In case of erythromycin-resistant Staphylococcus aureus conjunctivitis is used erythromycin ointment to prevent ophtalmia neonatorum (Cimolai, 2006; Hedberg et al., 1990).
The group B Streptococcus also may causes ophtalmia neonatorum, and is resolved after 7 days of treatment (Pöschl et al., 2002).
Eikenella corrodens is a gram-negative bacillus, fastidious, slow growing, and facultative anaerobic bacterium. It is found as the normal flora of the human mouth, nasopharynx, gut, and genitourinary tract. In the last two decades has been recognized as cause of head and neck infections. It is presented as a cause of neonatal conjunctivitis (Chhabra et al., 2008).
Neonatal conjunctivitis also is caused from other bacteria such as: Staphylococcus epidermidis, Streptococcus pneumoniae, Haemophilus species, Klebsiella pneumoniae, Pseudomonas aeruginosa, and Escherichia coli (Martinez et al., 1993; Olatunji et al., 2007).

2.4 Herpes simplex virus

Herpes simplex virus (HSV) can lead to neonatal keratoconjuctivitis passing to the baby during childbirth. Although it is rare it might be associated with a generalized herpes simplex infection (Overall, 1994).

2.5 Risk factors of neonatal conjuctivitis

Risk factors of neonatal conjunctivitis may include:

- Maternal infections
- Exposure of the infant to infectious organisms
- Increased birth weight
- Inadequacy of ocular prophylaxis immediately after birth (Gichuhi et al., 2009)
- Premature Rupture Of Membranes (Wu et al., 2009)

- Ocular trauma during delivery
- Mechanical ventilation
- Prematurity
- Poor prenatal care
- Poor hygienic delivery conditions
- Post-delivery infection due to direct contact with health care workers or by environment
- Silver nitrate exposure

3. Clinical findings

The Clinical presentation of Neonatal Conjuctivitis varies depending upon the severity and the type of infection. The signs and symptoms of ophthalmia neonatorum are similar for most of the infectious agents (Foster, 1995). Diffuse unilateral or bilateral redness due to injection of conjuctival vessels is the hallmark. Other common findings incude conjuctival oedema and discharge. More serious finding include keratitis and orbital celulitis, but also serious systemic involvement if left untreated (Woods, 2005; Zar, 2005). It is necessary to make accurate diagnosis in order to begin appropriate treatment which can help to reduce complications (Table 3).

3.1 Chemical conjunctivitis

It is present with mild injection of conjunctiva with minimal discharge. It is important that these occur within few hours after application of irritant. Sometimes the persistent redness of the eye might be folowed by purulent discharge and in that case there is a need for further laboratory investigation.

3.2 Bacterial conjunctivitis

The occurrence time and severity of clinical features depend on the type of microorganism.

Gonococal conjunctivitis

During this infection there is a severe redness, swelling of conjunctiva and eyeleads, and a lot of purulent drainage presenting few days after birth (Woods 2005), but may occur later as hyperacute conjunctival injection and chemosis, lid oedema and severe purulent discharge. Corneal ulceration and perforation may be associated features (Jackson, 2008).
Hyperacute conjunctivitis has the incubation period 1-7 days (Isenberg et al., 1996; Chandler et al., 1990), often bilateral and signs are more severe. Serosanguinous exudate may be replaced by mucopurulent discharge, with development of membranes. A disseminated gonococcal infection with arthritis, meningitis, pneumonia and sepsis that may lead to death of an infant is very rare.

Chlamydial conjunctivitis

Cervical infection with Chlamydia carries a risk to the neonate of 18-50% (Vaz et al., 1999; Schachter et al., 1986; Hollier et al., 2009; Roberts, 2009). The clinical features present at 5 to 14 days after birth with gradually worsening. Eyelids and conjunctiva are redness and swollen (Figure 1), and mucopurrulent drainage is present. It may also occur severe swelling and discharge with a course of 6 to 12 weeks (if left untreated) leading to scars of conjunctiva and cornea. In this case, if untreated or even only topically treated, may worsen with upper respiratory infection, in severe cases with afebrile pneumonitis usually presenting at 2 to 20 months of age (Darville, 2005). Approximately 50% of infants with chlamydial pneumonitis have concurrent conjunctivitis or a recent history of conjunctivitis (Tarabishy et al., 2008).

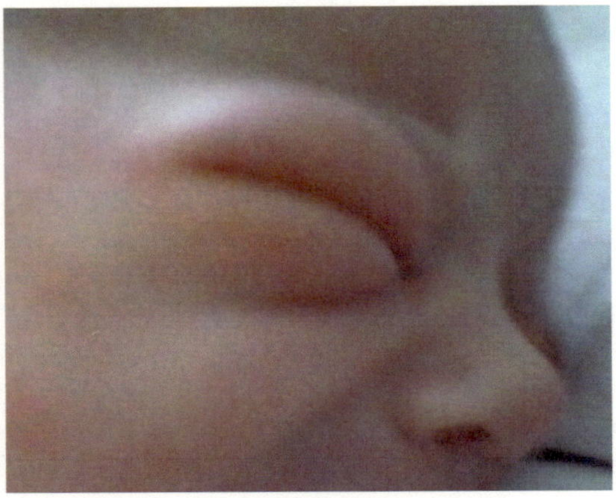

Fig. 1. Neonatal conjuctivitis due to chlamydia trachomatis in a five days old infant

Staphylococcus conjunctivitis. Staphylococcus aureus can cause neonatal conjuctivitis with redness, swollen purulent discharge (Figure 2).

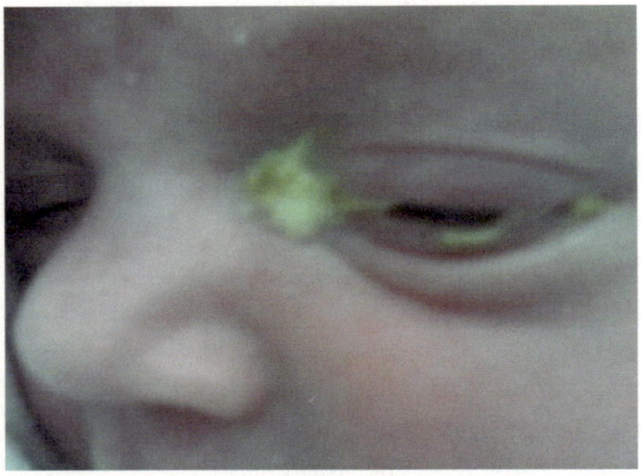

Fig. 2. Neonatal conjuctivitis due to staphylococcus aureus infection in an one week old infant.

3.3 Herpetic conjunctivitis

It is present usually the first two weeks of life with moderate injection, edema of conjuctiva and nonpurrulent discharge after vesicular skin lesions which can precede the eye involvment. In some cases it may be complicated with corneal clouding with dentritic or geographic corneal ulcers or upper respiratory infection (Rudolph, 2002). Systemic infection can cause jaundice, hepatosplenomegaly, pneumonitis, meningoencephalitis and disseminated intravascular coagulation.

Etiology	Onset after birth	Clinical findings
Chemical	3-36 hours	Mild injection, watery dicharge
Gonnococal	1-7 days	Injection and lead edema, purulent discharge
Chlamydial	5-14 days	Mild- severe injection, watery-purulent discharge, psudomembranes, chronicity, associated pneumonia
Herpetic	1-14 days	Watery discharge, injection and lead edema, associated keratitis

Table 3. Clinical findings of neonatal conjunctivitis by etiological factor modified from Rudolph's fundametntals of Pediatrics, 2002

4. Diagnosis

Prompt diagnosis is key in establishing proper treatment and minimizing potential serious complications of disease. An accurate diagnosis of conjunctivitis centers on taking a patient history to learn when symptoms began, how long the condition has been going on, the symptoms experienced, and other predisposing factors, such as upper respiratory complaints, allergies, sexually transmitted diseases, herpes simplex infections, and exposure to persons with pink eye. It may be helpful to learn whether an aspect of an individual's occupation may be the cause.

A thorough examination of the globe and periocular structures of a neonate suspected to have neonatal conjunctivitis is crucial. Corneal involvement should be investigated closely with and without fluorescein and blue cobalt light. Non-specific signs of neonatal conjunctivitis include conjunctival injection, tearing, mucopurulent or non-purulent discharge, chemosis, and eyelid swelling.

Diagnostic tests are usually not indicated unless initial treatment fails or an infection with gonorrhea or chlamydia is suspected. In such cases, the discharge may be cultured and stained to determine the organism responsible for causing the condition. Cultures and smears are relatively painless (Jackson, 2008).

Laboratory studies for suspected infectious etiology should include the following (Table 4 and 5):

- Conjunctival scraping, stains for Chlamydia. C. trachomatis is an obligate intracellular organism and exudates are not adequate for testing so conjunctival specimens for chlamydia testing must include conjunctival epithelial cells;
- Culture on chocolate agar for N gonorrhoeae ;

- Culture on blood agar for other strains of bacteria;
- Culture for HSV if vesicles present or is supicious of viral etiology;
- Direct antibody testing or Polymerase Chain Reaction (PCR) may also be indicated.

The laboratory studies may need to be repeated if symptoms worsen or recur following treatment.

Etiology	Laboratory diagnosis
Chemical	-
Gonnococal	Stain and cultures
Chlamydial	Stain, cultures, enzyme immunoassay, direct fluorescent antibody assay
Herpetic	Stain, cultures, antigen or DNA assay

Table 4. Laboratory diagnosis based on etiology

Modified from Rudolph's fundametntals of Pediatrics, 2002

Etiology	Conjuctival Scraping
Chemical	Minimal reactive cells to few polymorphonuclears
Gonococcal	Many reactive cells with gram negative intracellular dyplococci
Chlamydial	Many reactive cells with stain for basophilic cytoplasmic inclusion bodies or direct immunofluorescent assay
Other bacteria (Staphylococcus, Streptococcus, Haemophilus)	Stain for bacteria
Herpes simplex virus	Variable reactive cells with multinucleated giant cells

Table 5. Conjuctival scraping findings in ophtalmia neonatorum

Modified from Duane's Clinical Ophthalmology, 2008

5. Differential diagnosis

The differential diagnosis of neonatal conjunctivitis includes:

- Cellulitis (Orbital, Preseptal)
- Dacryocystitis
- Glaucoma, Primary or Secondary Congenital
- Keratitis, Bacterial, Fungal or Herpes Simplex

6. Complications

Complications usually can be divided concerning eye and/or systemic complications.
Ocular complications of neonatal conjunctivitis include pseudomembrane formation, corneal edema, thickened palpebral conjunctivia, peripheral pannus formation, corneal opacification, staphyloma, corneal perforation, endophthalmitis, loss of eye, and blindness.
Systemic complication due to Chlamydia infection
Systemic complications of chlamydia conjunctivitis include pneumonitis, otitis, pharyngeal and rectal colonization. Pneumonia has been reported in 10-20% of infants with chlamydial conjunctivitis.
Systemic complications due to gonococcal infection
Complications of gonococcal conjunctivitis and subsquent systemic involvement include arthritis, meningitis, anorectal infection, septicemia, and death.
The complications can be avoided if the proper treatment is initiated at time.

7. Treatment

7.1 Initial therapy

Ophtalmia neonatorum is treated with a broad-spectrum antibiotic e.g. ofloxacin 0.3% qds. When the microbiological results is present the treatment is based on microbiological cause (Jackason, 2008).

7.2 Chemical ophtalmia neonatorum

Chemical neonatal conjunctivitis usually disappears spontaneously within 2-4 days, and no treatment is required. The use of artificial tear is preferred.

7.3 Chlamydial ophtalmia neonatorum

The recommended regimen for chlamydial neonatal conjunctivitis is erythromycin base or ethylsuccinate, as a systemic therapy, 50mg per kg per day orally, divided into four doses per day for two weeks (Table 6). A follow-up of infants is recommended to determine whether initial treatment was effective because the efficacy is only approximately 80% and a second course of therapy might be required. Also, the evaluation of concomitant chlamydial pneumonia should be considered (Sexually transmitted disease treatment guidelines, 2010; Lippincott Williams & Wilkins, 2008; Yanoff & Duker, 2008).
The systemic treatment is administred as additional to topical treatment. (Sexually transmitted disease treatment guidelines, 2010). From local antibiotics usually are applied erythromycin 0.5% or tetracycline 1% eye ointment.
The mother and her sexual partners also should be treated with erythromycin base or ethylsuccinate (Sexually transmitted disease treatment guidelines, 2010).

7.4 Gonococcal ophtalmia neonatorum

The immediate treatment is needed because of complications such as corneal perforation and blindness. Gonococcus conjunctivitis is treated with ceftriaxone 25-50mg/kg IV or IM in a single dose (Table 6), not to exceed 125mg. An alternative regimen is cefotaxime 100mg/kg/24 hours IV or IM divided in two doses for seven days or 100mg/kg as a single dose. The irrigation with saline is preferred until the purulent discharge is cleared. The local

antibiotics such as bacitracin or erythromycin eye ointment are applied as additional therapy because topical antibiotic alone is inadequate. The atropine sulphate ointment should be applied if the cornea is involved (Sexually transmitted disease treatment guidelines, 2010; Lippincott Williams & Wilkins, 2008; Yanoff & Duker, 2008).
The mothers of infants and mother's sex partners should be evaluated and treated according to the recommendations for treating gonococcus infections in adults (Sexually transmitted disease treatment guidelines, 2010).
Neonatal conjunctivitis due to other bacteria usually respond to topical ointments containing bacitracin for gram positive stain bacteria, and tobramycin or ciprofloxacin for gram negative stain bacteria.

Type of bacteria	Drug	Dose for day	Duration
Chlamydia trachomatis	Erythromycin	50mg/kg	14 days
Nesseria gonorrhoeae	Ceftriaxone	25-50mg/kg	A single dose

Table 6. Recommended regimens for bacterial neonatal conjuctivitis

Modified from Sexually transmitted disease treatment guidelines 2010. Centers for Disease Control and Prevention, MMWR Recomm Rep 2010; 59 (RR-12): 53-54.

7.5 Herpetic ophtalmia neonatorum

Herpetic neonatal conjunctivitis is recommended to be treated with acyclovir 45-60mg/kg/day in three doses for 14 days in non disseminated disease and 21 days in disseminated disease. Local antiviral therapy is 1% trifluridine or 3% vidarabine or 0.1% iododeoxyuridine (drops or ointment) (Lippincott Williams & Wilkins, 2008).

8. Prophylaxis

8.1 Silver nitrate prophylaxis

German obstetrician Credé', in 1881, has applied 2% silver nitrate solution for prophylaxis of neonatal ophtalmia, resulting in a reduction of incidence from 7.8% to 0.17%. Thereafter was started instillation of silver nitrate, based on legislation, in most European countries and most of North America states in the first half of last century (Schneider, 1984; Crede CSR, 1881; Barasam, 1966). Latest in 1970s approximately half the United States specified 1% silver nitrate solution as the sole agent (Hammerschlag MR et al., 1908). In the United Kingdom the procedure has been discontinued, and in Japan and Australia, it was never used (Shaw EB, 1977). The mother usually can be representative consent of using of Credé's method in Sweden (Wahlberg V, 1982). The decision for changing of the Wisconsin law in 1980 that tetracycline and erythromycin could be used for prophylaxis against GON was based on a previous ruling by US Supreme Court (Whittaker N et al., 1981).
The siver nitrate, which by law is instilled within 1 hour after birth, may cause chemical conjunctivitis pain and visual impairment. The silver nitrate does not prevent all cases of gonococcal neonatal conjunctivitis. The chemical conjunctivitis caused by silver nitrate may mask the onset of gonococcus neonatal conjunctivitis (Shaw, 1977; Snowe et al., 1973).

Since 1940s, when antibiotics were developed the incidence of gonococcal neonatal conjunctivitis was decreased dramatically (Butterfield et al., 1981).

Recommendations of the US Centers for Disease Control (CDC) are supported from American Academy of Pediatrics in 1986 and 1988. According to these recommendations 1% tetracycline ointment and 0.5% erythromycin ointment were equally acceptable in preventing of gonococcus ophtalmia neonatorum. Although it was felt that silver nitrate might be the best agent in areas where the incidence of penicillinase-producing neisseria gonorrhoeae (PPNG) was appreciable (Peter, 1988).

The CDC's 1989 guidelines on the treatment of sexually transmitted diseases were unchanged with respect to the prevention of ophthalmia neonatorum (Sexually Transmitted Diseases Treatment Guidelines, 1989).

In Canada the incidence of PPNG among reported cases of gonorrhea increased from 0.5% in 1985 to 5.5% in 1989 (Status of penicillinase-producing Neisseria gonorrhoeae in Canada, 1991).

In 1989 the US Preventive Services Task Force recommended that 1% tetracycline ointment or 0.5% erythromycin ointment have to be applied topically to the eyes of all newborns as soon as possible after birth and no later than 1 hour after birth (Preventive Services task Forces, 1989). Silver nitrate was not recommended since it is locally irritating, frequently causing chemical conjunctivitis, and has limited efficacy in preventing chlamydial ophthalmia neonatorum.

8.2 Povidon-iodine prophylaxis

In 1995, is reported the use of a 2.5% povidone-iodine solution for prophylaxis of ophtalmia neonatorum in Kenya, and was found to be more effective than treatment with erythromycin or silver nitrate for prophylactic purposes. Also, the povidone-iodine was less toxic and it costs less (Isenberg et al., 1995).

The povidone-iodine prophylaxis against ophtalmia neonatorum, applied twice in the first postnatal day over a single application at birth, revealed with no advantage. It was supported the original notion of Crede in 1881 that a single drop of an effective medication given at birth is the best way to prevent the development of ophtalmia neonatorum. The povidone-iodine applications approximately 24 hours later were with no further benefit.

8.3 Antibiotics prophylaxis

The procedure for prevence of gonococcal ophthalmia neonatorum is required by law in most states. Prophylactic agent should be instilled into the eyes of newborns. But, the efficacy of prophylactic agents in preventing chlamydial ophthalmia is clearless, and they do not eliminate nasopharyngeal colonization by C. trachomatis.

This preparation should be instilled into both eyes of every neonate as soon as possible after delivery. Ideally, ointment should be applied using single-use tubes or ampoules rather than multiple-use tubes. If prophylaxis is delayed (i.e., not administered in the delivery room), a monitoring system should be established to ensure that all infants receive prophylaxis. All infants should be administered ocular prophylaxis, regardless of whether they are delivered vaginally or by cesarean section.

Antibiotics that are applied in prevention of gonococcal ophtalmia are tetracycline and erythromycin and are more effective than silver nitrate (Rothenberg, 1979; American Academy of Pediatrics, 1980). Erythromycin is less effective than tetracycline against sensitive isolates of N. gonorrhoeae in vitro. Canadian Paediatric Society in 2010 has revised recommandations for the prevention of neonatal ophthalmia due to N gonorrhoeae (Table 7).

Recommendation	Category	Grade
Prophylaxis to prevent neonatal ophthalmia due to N gonorrhoeae should be provided to all infants.	A	1
Physicians and their patients may choose among the recommended prophylactic agents - that is, 1% silver nitrate solution in single-dose ampoules, or an ointment containing 0.5% erythromycin base or 1% tetracycline hydrochloride in single-dose tubes.	A	1
The use of povidone-iodine for ophthalmia prophylaxis.	C	1
To prevent potential cross-contamination, a separate ampoule or tube should be used for each eye. Ampoules and tubes should be discarded after use.	A	3
When 1% silver nitrate solution is used, each eyelid should first be wiped gently with a sterile cotton ball to remove foreign matter and permit adequate eversion of the lower lid. Two drops of solution are placed in each lower conjunctival sac. The closed eyelids can be massaged gently to help spread the solution to all areas of the conjunctiva. After 1 min, any excess silver nitrate should be gently wiped from the eyelids and surrounding skin with sterile cotton.	A	3
When an ophthalmic ointment (tetracycline or erythromycin) is used, the eyelids should be prepared as for the application of silver nitrate. A line of ointment 1 to 2 cm long is placed in each lower conjunctival sac, if possible covering the whole lower conjunctival area. Care is needed to prevent injury to the eye or the eyelid from the tip of the tube. The closed eyelids can be massaged gently to help spread the ointment. After 1 min, any excess ointment should be wiped gently from the eyelids and surrounding skin with a sterile cotton.	A	3
The eyes should not be irrigated after instillation of a prophylactic agent. Irrigation may reduce the efficacy of the agent and probably does not decrease the incidence of chemical conjunctivitis caused by silver nitrate.	A	3
Prophylaxis should be given as soon as possible after birth. However, delaying prophylaxis for up to 1 h after birth probably does not impair the agent's efficacy.	B	3
A check system should be established to ensure that all infants are treated.	A	3
Infants born by caesarian section should also receive prophylaxis.	B	3
Pregnant women should be screened for infection by N gonorrheoae and C trachomatis during pregnancy and their identified infections should be treated during pregnancy.	A	3
Infants born to women with gonococcal infection discovered during labour or at the time of delivery should be given a single dose of ceftriaxone (25 to 50 mg/kg) or cefotaxime (100 mg/kg) in addition to topical prophylaxis.	A	2

Table 7. Recommandations for the prevention of neonatal ophthalmia due to N gonorrhoeae

Modified from Canadian Pediatric Society. Revised Recommandations for the prevention of neonatal ophtalmia, 2010.
Classification used to determine the strength of the recommendations and the quality of the evidence on which the recommendations are based.

Category	Definition
A	Good evidence to support a recommendation for use
B	Moderate evidence to support a recommendation for use
C	Insufficient evidence to support a recommendation for or against use
D	Moderate evidence to support a recommendation against use
E	Good evidence to support a recommendation against use
Grade	
1	Evidence from at least one properly randomized, controlled trial
2	Evidence from at least one well-designed clinical trial without randomization, from cohort or case- controlled analytic studies, preferably from more than one centre, from multiple time series, or from dramatic results in uncontrolled experiments
3	Evidence from opinions or respected authorities on the basis of clinical experience, descriptive studies or reports of expert committees

Source. Canadian Pediatric Society. Revised Recommandations for the prevention of neonatal ophtalmia, 2010.

Table 8.

Tetracycline as silver nitrate does not prevent completely chlamydial ophtalmia neonatorum (Laga et al., 1988, Canadian Task Force on the Periodic Health Examination, 1992). There were no significant differences between the rates of chlamydial ophtalmia neonatorum when prophylaxis with erythromycin was compared with prophylaxis with tetracycline or silver nitrate. For a modest reduction in chlamydial ophtalmia neonatorum now are recommended the agents for gonococcal prophylaxis.
Erythromycin 0.5 % is the only antibiotic ointment recommended for use in neonates in each eye in a single application. Silver nitrate and tetracycline ophthalmic ointment are no longer manufactured in the United States, bacitracin is not effective, while povidone iodine has not been studied adequately (Sexually Transmitted Diseases Treatment Guidelines, 2010).
If erythromycin ointment is not available, infants at risk for exposure to N. gonorrhoeae (especially those born to a mother with untreated gonococcus infection or who has received no prenatal care) can be administered ceftriaxone 25-50 mg/kg IV or IM, not to exceed 125 mg in a single dose (Sexually Transmitted Diseases Treatment Guidelines, 2010).
The diagnosis and treatment of gonococcal and chlamydial infections in pregnant women is the best method for preventing neonatal gonococcal and chlamydial disease. Also preventative measures include proper hand-washing techniques by peripartum and nursery staff.

9. Prognosis

- Chlamydial infection: good - 80% fully recover after one course of treatment.
- Bacterial infection: rarely fails to respond to appropriate treatment.
- Viral infection: the ocular prognosis can be poor and the systemic sequelae may be fatal.
- Chemical irritation: good - full spontaneous recovery expected after 24-36 hours.

10. References

[1] World Bank. (1993) World development report: investing in health. Oxford. Oxford University Press.

[2] Sloan NL, Winikoff B, Haberland N, Coggins C, Elias C. (2000) Screening and syndromic approach to identify gonorrhhoea and chlamydial infection among women. Studies in Family Planning 31: 55-68.

[3] Lush L, Walt G, Ogden J. (2003) Transferring policies for treating sexually transmitted infections: what's wrong with global guidelines? Health Policy and planning 18(1): 18-30.

[4] Beers MH, Porter RS, Jones TV, Kaplan JL, Berkwits M. (2006) The Merck Manual of Diagnosis and Therapy. Merck Research Laboratories.

[5] Rudolph AM, Kamei RK, Overby KJ. (2002) Rudolph's Fundamentals of Pediatrics. McGraw-Hill.

[6] Hay WW, Levin MJ, Sondheimer JM, Deterding RR. (2009) Current Diagnosis & Treatment pediatrics. Lange.

[7] Mohile M, Deorari A, Satpathy G, Sharma A, Singh M.(2002) Microbiological study of neonatal conjunctivitis with special reference to Chlamydia trachomatis. Indian J Ophtalmol 50:295-99.

[8] Miller K. (2006) Diagnosis and treatment of Chlamydia trachomatis infection. Am Fam Physician 73:1411-6.

[9] Jatla et al. (2009) Conjuctivitis, Neonatal, Medscape.

[10] Kroner, T. (1884) ZurAetiologie der Opthalmoblennorrhoea Neonatorum. Zentrablattfiir Gyndkologie 8, 643-645.

[11] Lindner, K. (1909) Uebertragungsversuche von gonokokkenfreier Blennorrhoea neonatorum auf Affen. WienerKlinische Wochenschrift 22, 1554; 1659-1660.

[12] T'ang, F. F., Chang, H. L., Huang, Y. T., and Wang, K. C. (1957) Studies on the aetiology of trachoma with special reference to isolation of the virus in chick embryo. ChineseMedical Journal 75, 429-447.

[13] Jones, B. R., Collier, L. W., and Smith, C. H. (1959) Isolation of virus from inclusion blennorrhoea. Lancet 1, 902-905.

[14] Rodriguez P, B de Barbeyac K, Persson K, Dutilh B, Bebear C. (1993) Evaluation of molecular typing for epidemiological study of Chlamydia trachomatis genital infections. J Clin Microbiol 31:2238-2240.

[15] Lucía Gallo Vaulet1, Carolina Entrocassi, Ana I Corominas, Marcelo Rodríguez Fermepin. (2010) Distribution study of Chlamydia trachomatis genotypes in symptomatic patients in Buenos Aires, Argentina: association between genotype E and neonatal conjunctivitisBMC Research Notes 3:34.

[16] World Health Organisation. (2001) Global prevalence and incidence of selected curable Sexually Transmitted Infections: overview and estimates. Geneva: WHO.

[17] Schachter J, Grossman M, Sweet RL, Holt J, Jordan C, Bishop E. (1986) Prospective study of perinatal transmission of Chlamydia trachomatis. JAMA 55:3374-3377.

[18] Numazaki K, Asanuma H, Niida Y. (2003) Chlamydia trachomatis infection in early neonatal period. BMC Infect Dis 4;3(1):2.

[19] Rosenman MB, Mahon BE, Downs SM, Kleiman MB. (2003) Oral erythromycin prophylaxis vs watchful waiting in caring for newborns exposed to Chlamydia trachomatis. Arch Pediatr Adolesc Med 157(6):565-71.

[20] Hobson D. (1977) Chlamydial infection in neonates. New Eng J Med 1977:296:398.

[21] Valencia C, Prado V, Rios M, Cruz MA, Pilorget JJ. (2000) Prevalence of the Chlamydia trachomatis in neonatal conjunctivitis determination by indirect fluorescente and gene amplification. Rev Med Chil. 128(7):758-65. 8.

[22] Olatunji FO. (2004) A case control study of ophthalmia neonatorum in Kaduna II: causative agents and their antibiotic sensitivity. West Afr J Med. 23(3):215-20.

[23] Kampmeier RH. (1978) Identification of the gonococcus by Albert Neisser. Sex Transm Dis 5:71-72.

[24] Morton RS (ed). (1977) Gonorrhoea [Vol. 9 in the series Major Problems in Dermatology]. Philadelphia, W.B. Saunders.

[25] Di Bartolomeo S, Mirta DH, Janer M, et al. (2001) Incidence of Chlamydia trachomatis and other potential pathogens in neonatal conjunctivitis. Int J Infect Dis 5(3);139-43.

[26] Noegel A, Gotschlich EC. (1983) Isolation of a high molecular weight polyphosphate from *Neisseria gonorrhoeae*. J Exp Med 157:2049-2060.

[27] Naumann M, Wessler S, Bartsch C, et al. (1997) *Neisseria gonorrhoeae* epithelial cell interaction leads to the activation of the transcription factors nuclear factor kappaB and activator protein 1 and the induction of inflammatory cytokines. J Exp Med 186:247-258.

[28] Ramsey KH, Schneide H, Cross AS, et al. (1995) Inflammatory cytokines produced in response to experimental human gonorrhea. J Infect Dis 172:186-191.

[29] Alexey JM, So M. (2000) Interactions of pathogenic *Neisseriae* with epithelial cell membranes. Ann Rev Cell Dev Biol 16:423-57.

[30] Naumann M, Rudel T, Meyer TF. (1999) Host cell interactions and signaling with *Neisseria gonorrhoeae*. Curr Opin Microbiol 2:62-70.

[31] Gregg CR, Melly MA, Hellerqvist CG, et al. (1983) Toxic activity of purified lipopolysaccharide as *N. gonorrhoeae* for human fallopian tube mucosa. J Infect Dis 143:432-439.

[32] Casey SG, Shafer WM, Spitznagel JK. (1986) Neisseria gonorrhoeae survive intraleukocytic oxygen-independent antimicrobial capacities of anaerobic and aerobic granulocytes in the presence of pyocin lethal for extracellular gonococci. Infect Immun 52:384-389.

[33] Shafer WM, Onunka VC, Martin LE. (1986) Antigonococcal activity of human neutrophil cathepsin G. Infect Immun 54:184-188.

[34] Kallstrom H, Liszewski MK, Atkinson JP, et al. (1997) Membrane cofactor protein (MCP or CD46) is a cellular pilus receptor for pathogenic *Neisseria*. Mol Microbiol 25:639-647.

[35] Gutman LT. (2001) Gonococcal infections, in Remington JS, Klein JO (eds): Infectious Diseases of the Fetus and Newborn Infant (ed 5). Philadelphia, W.B. Saunders Co., pp 1199-1215.

[36] Friendly DS. (1969) Gonococcal conjunctivitis of the newborn. Clin Prac Child Hosp 25:1-9.

[37] Cimolai N. (2006) Ocular methicillin-resistant Staphylococcus aureus infections in a newborn intensive care cohort. Am J Ophthalmol 142(1): 183-4.

[38] Hedberg K, Ristinen TL, Soler JT, White KE, Hedberg CW, Osterholm MT, MacDonald KL.(1990) Outbreak of erythromycin-resistant staphylococcus conjunctivitis in a newborn nursery. Pediatr Infect Dis J 9(4):268-73.

[39] Pöschl JM, Hellstern G, Ruef P, Bauer J, Linderkamp O. (2002) Ophtalmia neonatorum caused by B Streptococcus. Scand J Infect Dis 34(12):921-2.

[40] Chhabra MS, Motley WW 3rd, Mortensen JE. (2008) Eikenella corrodens as a causative agent for neonatal conjunctivitis.JAAPOS 12(5): 524-5.

[41] Martinez Ruiz MT, Ascaso Puyuelo FJ, Navales Bertol, Palomar Gómez MT, Garcia Garcia C, Olivares López JL. (1993) Neonatal conjunctivitis: microbiologic study and antibiotic sensitivity. An Esp Pediatr 39(1);42-5.

[42] Olatunji FO, Fadeyi A, Ayanniyi AA, Akanbi AA 2nd. (2007) Non-gonococcal bacterial agents of conjunctivitis and their antibiotic susceptibility patterns in llorin, Nigeria. Afr J Med Sci 36(3):243-7.

[43] Overall JC Jr. (1994) Herpes simplex virus infection of the fetus and newborn. Pediatr Ann 23: 131-136.

[44] Gichuhi S et al. Risk factors for neonatal conjunctivitis in babies of HIV-1 infected mothers. (2009) Ophthalmic Epidemiol 16(6):337-45.

[45] Wu J et al. (2009) Influence of premature rupture of membranes on neonatal health. Zhonghua Er Ke Za Zhi 47(6):452-6. 5.

[46] Foster A, Klauss V. (1995) Ophtalmia neonatorum in developing countries. N Engl J Med 332: 600-601.

[47] Woods, CR. (2005) Gonococcal infections in neonates and young children. Semin Pediatr Infect Dis 16: 258-270.

[48] Zar HJ. (2005) Neonatal chlamydial infections: prevention and treatment. Paediatr Drugs : 103-110.

[49] Isenberg SJ, Apt L, Wood M. (1996) The influence of prenatal factors on ophthalmia neonatorum. J Pediatr Ophthalmol Strabismus 33:185-188.

[50] Chandler JW, Rapoza PA. (1990) Ophtalmia neonatorum. Int Ophthalmol Clin 30: 36-38.

[51] Vaz FA, Ceccon ME, Diniz EM. (1999) Chlamydia trachomatisinfection in the neonatal period: clinical and laboratory aspects. Experience of a decade: 1987- 1998. Rev Assoc Med Bras 45: 303-311.

[52] Schachter J, Grossman M, Sweet RL, Holt J, Jordan C, et al. (1986) Prospective study of perinatal transmission of Chlamydia trachomatis. JAMA 255: 3374-7.

[53] Hollier LM, Wendel GD. (2009) Third trimester antiviral prophylaxis for preventing maternal genital herpes simplex (HSV) recurrences and neonatal infection. Cochrane Database Syst Rev 1:CD004946.
[54] Roberts S. (2009) Herpes simplex virus: incidence of neonatal herpes simplex virus, maternal screening, management during pregnancy and HIV. Curr Opin Obstet Gynecol 21: 124-130.
[55] Tarabishy AB, Jeng BH. (2008) Bacterial conjunctivitis: areview for internists. Cleve Clin J Med 75: 507-512.
[56] Yip PP et al. (2008) The use of polymerase chain reaction assay versus conventional methods in detecting neonatal chlamydial conjunctivitis. J Pediatr Ophthalmol Strabismus 45(4):234-9.
[57] Rubenstein JB, Virasch V. (2008) Conjunctivitis: infectious and noninfectious. In: Yanoff M, Duker JS, eds. *Ophthalmology*. 3rd ed. Philadelphia, Pa: Mosby Elsevier.
[58] Jackson TL. (2008) Moorfields Manual of Ophtalmology, Mosby.
[59] Ophthalmia neonatorum (Newborn conjunctivitis). (2008) Wills Eye Manual. Philiadelphia.PA: Lippincott Williams & Wilkins 181-183.
[60] Ophthalmia neonatorum. (2008) Yanoff & Duker: Ophthalmology, 3rd edition. Mosby.
[61] Sexually transmitted disease treatment guidelines 2010. (2010) Centers for Disease Control and Prevention, MMWR Recomm Rep; 59 (RR-12): 47-48.
[62] Schneider G. (1984) Silver nitrate prophylaxis. Can Med Assoc J 131(3): 193–196.
[63] Crede CSR. (1881) Die Verhutung der Augentzundung der Neugeborenen. Arch Gynakol 18: 367-370.
[64] Barsam PC. (1966) Specific prophylaxis of gonorrheal ophthalmia neonatorum; a review. N Engl J Med 274: 731-734.
[65] Hammerchlag MR, Chandler JW, Alexander ER et al. (1980) Erythromycin ointment for ocular prophylaxis of neonatal chlamydial infection. JAMA 244: 2291-2293.
[66] Shaw EB. (1977) Comment on silver nitrate prophylaxis [C]. Pediatrics 60: 773.
[67] Wahlberg V. (1982) Reconsideration of Credé prophylaxis. Introduction. Acta Pediatr Scand [Suppl] 295: 9-25.
[68] Whittaker N, Strasser J. (1981) The silver nitrate challenge. Mother Mag 27-30.
[69] Snowe RJ, Wilfert CM. (1973) Epidemic reappearance of gonococcal ophthalmia neonatorum. Pediatrics 51: 110-114.
[70] Butterfield PM, Ende RN, Svejda MJ. (1981) Does the early application of silver nitrate impair maternal attachment? Pediatrics 67: 737-738.
[71] Peter G (ed). (1988) 1988 Red Boot Report of the Committee on Infectious Diseases, 21st ed, Am Acad Pediatr, Elk GroveVillage, Ill.
[72] 1989 Sexually Transmitted Diseases Treatment Guidelines. (1989) MMWR 38 (S-8): 27.
[73] Status of penicillinase-producing Neisseria gonorrhoeae in Canada- 1989. (1991) Can Dis Wkly Rep. 17: 49-50.
[74] US Preventive Services Task Force. (1989) Guide to Clinical Preventive Services, Williams & Wilkins, Baltimore, 136.
[75] Isenberg SJ, Apt L, Wood M. (1995) A controlled trial of povidone-iodine as prophylaxis against ophthalmia neonatorum. New Eng J Med 332:562–6.
[76] Rothenberg R. (1979) Ophthalmia neonatorum due to Neisseria gonorrhea: prevention and treatment. Sex Trans Dis 6(Suppl 2):187-91.

[77] American Academy of Pediatrics. (1980) Prophylaxis and treatment of neonatal gonococcal infections. Pediatrics 65:1047-50.

[78] Laga M, Plummer FA, Piot P, et al. (1988) Prophylaxis of gonococcal and chlamydial ophthalmia neonatorum. A comparison of silver nitrate and tetracycline. N Engl J Med 318:653-7.

[79] Canadian Task Force on the Periodic Health Examination. (1992) Periodic health examination, 1992 update: 4. Prophylaxis for gonococcal and chlamydial ophthalmia neonatorum. CMAJ 147:1449-54. Jatla, 2009; Sexually Transmitted Diseases Treatment Guidelines.

11

Trachoma and Conjunctivitis

Imtiaz A. Chaudhry[1], Yonca O. Arat[2] and Waleed Al-Rashed[3]
[1]Senior Academic Consultant, Ophthalmic Plastic Reconstructive Surgeon
Oculoplastic and Orbit Division, King Khaled Eye Specialist Hospital, Riyadh
[2]Department of Ophthalmology, University of Wisconsin
School of Medicine, Madison, Wisconsin
[3]Senior Consultant Ophthalmologist, Division of Anterior Segment
King Khaled Eye Specialist Hospital and Vice Dean for Medical Services
Al-Imam Muhammad ibn Sauid Islamic University Faculty of Medicine, Riyadh
[1,3]Saudi Arabia
[2]USA

1. Introduction

Trachoma remains the leading cause of preventable corneal blindness worldwide and especially in the developing countries. It afflicts some of the poorest regions of the globe, predominantly in Africa and Asia. The disease is initiated in early childhood by repeated infection of the ocular surface by Chlamydia trachomatis. Initial clinical manifestation is a follicular conjunctivitis which if not treated on timely basis, may lead to conjunctival and eyelid scarring that may eventually result in corneal scarring and loss of vision. Despite the remarkable progress in our understanding of Chlamydial infection, the basic mechanisms involved in tissue damage, scarring and repeated episodes of conjunctivitis remain to be elucidated. However, over the past 2 decades, a remarkable reduction in the prevalence of active trachoma in poor countries has occurred due to the World Health Organization's (WHO) program GET 2020 for the elimination of trachoma, with adoption of the SAFE strategy incorporating Surgery, Antibiotic treatment, Facial cleanliness and Environmental hygiene. Immunohistochemical studies of conjunctival biopsies from children with active trachoma demonstrate the presence of both humoral and cell-mediated immune responses. Recurrent chronic inflammatory episodes cause conjunctivitis which leads to the development of conjunctival scarring/contractures, distorting the eyelids in the form of trichiasis and entropion. This compromises the cornea and blinding opacification often ensues. Since trachoma is a disease of poverty, overcrowding, and poor sanitation, active disease affects mainly children, but adults are at increased risk of scarring. Its prevalence is disproportionately high among women and children in poor rural communities.

Improvement in socio-economic status/health facilities within the last 20 years has lead to the public awareness, prevention and treatment of bulk of active trachoma. In the active trachomatous conjunctivitis, macrophages may play an active role in conjunctival scarring by upregulated local production of extracellular matrix by the expression of the fibrogenic and angiogenic connective tissue growth factor. It is believed that the chronic trachomatous follicular conjunctivitis may lead to canaliculitis, canalicular obstruction, dacryocystitis and nasolacrimal duct obstruction. Entropion has been found to be the most significant predictor of corneal opacity. Among the lacrimal complications of trachoma, dry eye syndrome, punctal phimosis, punctal occlusion, canalicular occlusion, nasolacrimal-duct obstruction, dacryocystitis, dacryocystocele, and dacryocutaneous fistula are the most common findings. Trachoma may cause dryness of the eye by decreasing mucus production and aqueous secretions. Severe cases of trachoma may lead to contracture of the conjunctiva, deeper tissues including Müller muscle and the tarsal plate, which supports the insertion of the levator aponeurosis. The upper eyelid of these patients may show eyelid retraction which also may show eyelid lag on patient's down-gaze. Four major eyelid complications: cicatricial entropion, eyelid retraction, secondary blepharospasm and brow ptosis may be seen. Entropion/trichiasis may be the most common with significant blinding complication. Eyelids of patients with inactive trachoma may be thickened. This thickening could be attributed to trachomatous changes in the conjunctiva and tarsus. Light microscopy studies of tarsal plates obtained during biopsies of tarsal plates and palpebral conjunctivae obtained from upper eyelids of patients with inactive trachoma show a thick and compact subepithelial fibrous membrane adherent to the tarsal plate. Other histopathologic findings include atrophy of the meibomian glands with thickening of the acinar basement membrane, loss of goblet cells, retention cysts, and hyaline degeneration of the tarsal plate with focal replacement by adipose tissue.

The prevalence of active trachoma infection has dropped significantly in some African countries attributable to both improvements in socioeconomic standards and the training of village health workers and traditional birth attendants in eye care. Azithromycin oral single dose has been found to be safe and effective in children with active trachoma. However, patients who already have infection at young age continue to present with adnexal related complications of trachomatous scarring which continue to cause corneal scarring and visual loss. Management of trachomatous cicatricial entropion of the upper eye lid causing chronic conjunctivitis presents a difficult problem. Many surgical approaches have been developed to address it. Most effective surgery is full-thickness incision of the tarsal plate and rotation of the terminal tarsal strip 180 degrees. With the modified surgical technique, a combination of bilamellar tarsal margin rotation procedure with blepharoplasty may be advocated. With this technique, the eye lids as well as the normal eyelashes can be rotated away from the surface of the eye and eyes have adequate lid closure and regular lid margin. The modified technique prevents any overhanging baggy fold of skin at operation site. In developing countries, where manpower and other resources are limited and patient-load high, ophthalmic surgeons are recommended to choose a procedure that is simple, quick and effective. Surgery for entropion results in healing of superficial keratopathy, improved tear film stability. The realigned eyelid margin may spread tears evenly and efficiently, thus contributing to improvement of chronic conjunctivitis and vision.

2. Trachoma in history

The word "trachoma", derived from ancient Greek, means "rough eye", due to the "cobblestone" appearance of the conjunctival lining of the globe as a result of reactive lymphoid follicles.[1] Treatment of trachoma and its complications have been recorded in the ancient Egyptian writings. It is reported that both Hippocrates and Galen, had access to ancient Egyptian methods of treating both acute as well as chronic complications of trachoma.[1]

2.1 Trachoma: Extent of the problem

Trachoma remains the leading infectious cause of ocular morbidity in some parts of the world.[2,3] The disease is caused by an obligate intracellular bacterium *Chlamydia trachomatis (C. trachomatis)*.[4] The transmission of the disease occurs primarily in children during their early years of life.[5] Repeated episodes of re-infection within the family members cause chronic conjunctivitis resulting in scarring in later years and continued loss of vision. The scarring is mostly in the conjunctiva and cornea but can affect nasolacrimal drainage system causing ocular complications as a result of its blockage. Eyelid scarring may result in distortion of the upper tarsal plate leading to trichiasis, entropion of eyelids and conjunctivitis. Chronic abnormality of the eyelids may cause corneal scaring, recurrent infections and decreased vision.[6]

2.2 Clinical presentation of trachomatous conjunctivitis

The initial response of an eye to infection with C. trachomatis is conjunctivitis involving the palpebral and bulbar conjunctiva.[7,8] In these eyes, the conjunctiva may be inflamed, swollen along with papillary hypertrophy prominent in the palpebral conjunctiva (Figure 1). The initial conjunctival response may be followed by lymphoid follicle formation, most

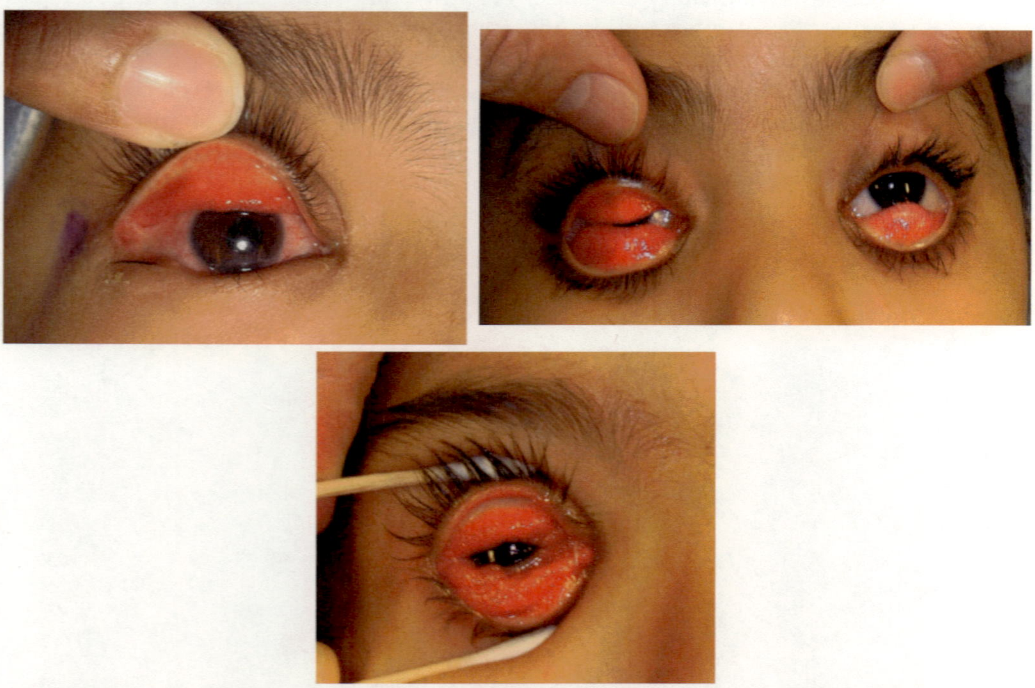

Fig. 1. Right upper eyelid of a child showing follicular reaction due to trachomatous conjunctivitis (upper right). Bilateral trachomatous conjunctivitis in another child with discharge (upper left). Intense follicular reaction in the right eye of a young child with trachomatous conjunctivitis (bottom figure).

commonly found on the palpebral conjunctiva as well as on the bulbar conjunctiva especially on at the limbus.[6] After healing, these conjunctival follicles may result in Herbert's pits, named after an English ophthalmologist. These patients may be more prone to infection by other bacterial species resulting in secondary conjunctivitis and discharge.

Active trachoma is characterized by a mucopurulent keratoconjunctivitis (Figure 1). The conjunctival surface of the upper eyelid shows a follicular and inflammatory response.[9] The cornea may have limbal follicles, superior neovascularization (pannus), and punctate keratitis. Infection with *C. trachomatis* concurrently occurs in other extraocular mucous membranes, commonly the nasopharynx, leading to a nasal discharge. Follicular trachoma (designated TF in the WHO simplified trachoma grading scheme), is defined as the presence of 5 or more follicles at least 0.5 mm in diameter in the central part of the upper tarsal conjunctiva. Follicular trachoma indicates active disease. This form is most commonly found in children, with prevalence in those aged between 3 to 5 years of age children. The prevalence rapidly decreases in school-aged children as they leave the pool of re-infection. Follicles are germinal centers that primarily consist of lymphocytes and monocytes.[10] Involution of follicles at the limbus (corneoscleral border) give rise to the pathognomonic lesion of past active trachoma, Herbert's pits. Intense inflammatory trachoma (designated TI in the WHO simplified trachoma grading scheme), is defined as pronounced inflammatory thickening of the upper tarsal conjunctiva that obscures more than one half of the normal deep tarsal vessels.

During the intense inflammatory response, normally thin tarsal conjunctiva develops a velvety thickening. Papillae are visible under slit lamp examination (Figures 1). Intense inflammatory trachoma indicates an increased potential for significant conjunctival scarring and, hence, a higher ultimate risk of blinding disease. Surveying the prevalence of intense inflammatory trachoma in children can help in predicting the risk of future blinding trachoma in that cohort of children.[5] Trachomatous scarring (designated TS in the WHO simplified trachoma grading scheme), indicates presence of easily visible scars in the tarsal conjunctiva (Figures 2,3). Trachomatous scarring indicates past inflammatory disease and a

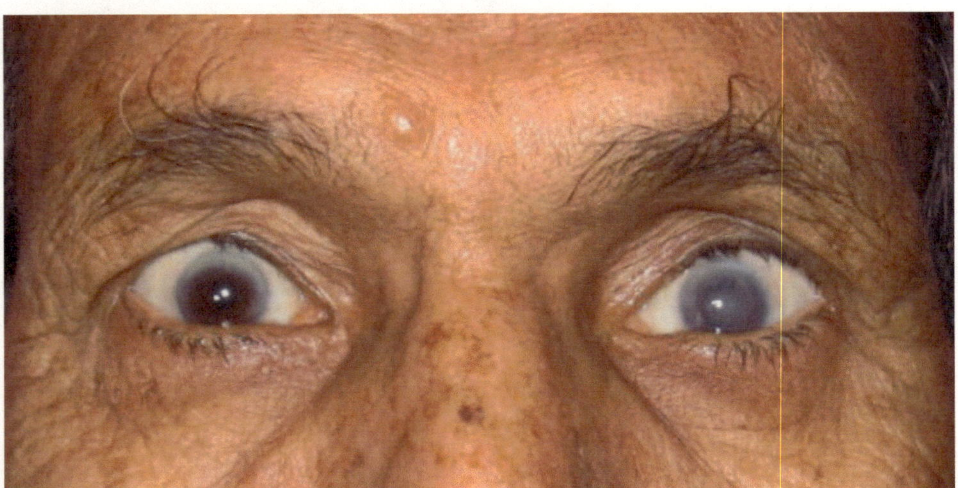

Fig. 2. An elderly patient with bilateral corneal scarring and upper eyelid retraction due to old trachoma

risk of future trichiasis. In the setting of more severe scarring, there is higher risk of subsequent trichiasis.[8] This form may be associated with the development of dry eye syndrome and picture of chronic conjunctivitis. However, chronic, low-grade bacterial conjunctivitis and dacryocystitis may also lead to a weeping eye.[6] Trichiasis (designated TT in the WHO simplified trachoma grading scheme), is defined when at least one eyelash rubs on the eyeball or evidence of recent removal of in-turned eyelashes. This condition is a potentially blinding situation that may lead to chronic conjunctivitis and corneal opacification (Figtures 2-4). Trichiasis is due to subconjunctival fibrosis over the tarsal plate that leads to lid distortion. Some vision can be restored with the successful correction of trichiasis. Corneal opacity (designated CO in the WHO simplified trachoma grading scheme), is defined as easily visible corneal opacity over the pupil that is so dense that it blurs at least part of the pupillary margin when it is viewed through the opacity (Figures 2-4). Corneal opacity or scarring reflects the prevalence of vision loss and blindness resulting from trachoma.[11] This condition includes pannus, epithelial vascularization, and infiltration only if it involves the central cornea.

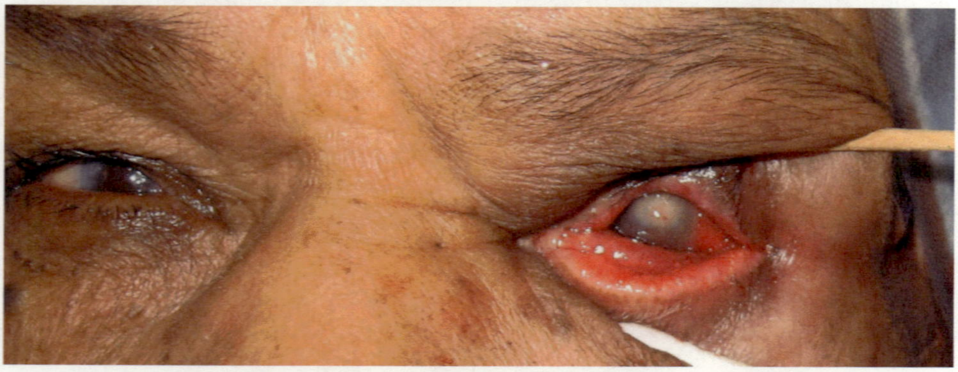

Fig. 3. An elderly patient with old trachomatous corneal scarring and chronic conjunctivitis due to abnormalities of eyelids

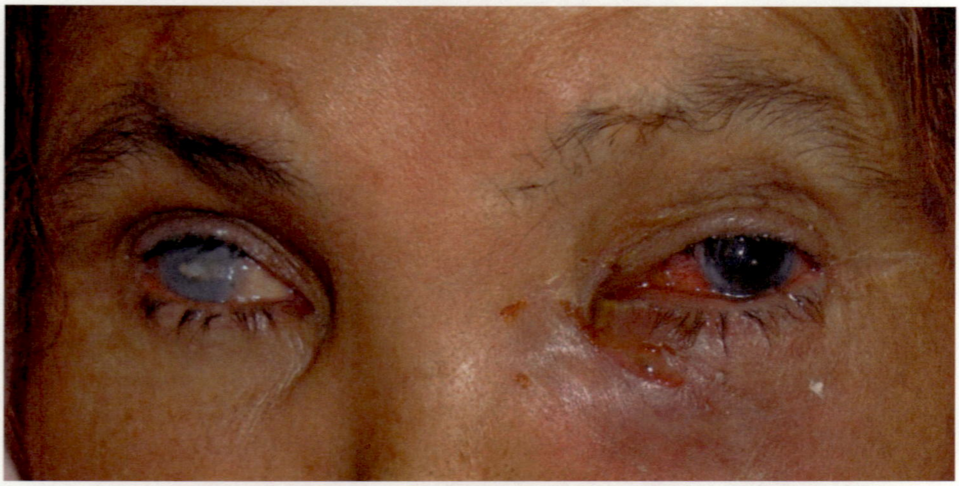

Fig. 4. Patient with long-standing bilaterl trachomatous scarring and left-sided nasolacrimal duct obstruction causing chronic conjunctivitis

2.3 Epidemiology of trachomatous conjunctivitis

Despite the fact that trachoma has been eradicated from the well-developed countries of the World, it still persists in hot, dry regions throughout many parts of Africa, Southern Asia, Middle East, Brazil, Mexico and some parts of Australia. [12-15] According to some rough estimates, worldwide, trachoma infects 84 million people in 55 countries, blinding over 8 million.[16] According to the WHO estimates, if appropriate measures are not taken, over 75 million may become legally blind over the next twenty years.

Trachoma is caused by the eye to eye transmission of infection with *C. trachomatis*. Flies are considered a major factor in the spread of trachoma in many parts of the World.[17] Flies may be more attracted to children with eye discharges or nasal discharges in the setting of dirty environment. Spread of active trachomatis cases can be reduced by controlling the population of flies in the known endemic areas.[18,19] Over 50% of the household of an infant infected with trachomatous infection may have active trachoma. Cases of active trachoma may be predominantly clustered in families who share communal housing of interconnecting roof spaces through which flies could freely fly. Obviously a close contact with infected ocular secretions within the family is considered to be a significant channel of trachoma transmission. Chronic infection in older women from repeated exposure from their children may be the reason for severe trachomatous scarring, dry eye syndrome and chronic conjunctivitis.[20] In the endemic trachoma areas such as North Africa, the Middle East and northern India, most infants become infected by age 2 or 3 and the condition is primarily a disease of childhood.[21-23]

3. Differential diagnoses for trachomatous conjunctivitis

The differential clinical diagnosis for *C. trachomatis* conjunctivitis may include adult inclusion conjunctivitis, adenovirus conjunctivitis, herpes simplex virus conjunctivitis, vernal conjunctivitis, other bacterial conjunctivitis, toxic follicular conjunctivitis, ligneous conjunctivitis and allergic conjunctivitis (Figures 5-7).[24] Patients having inclusion

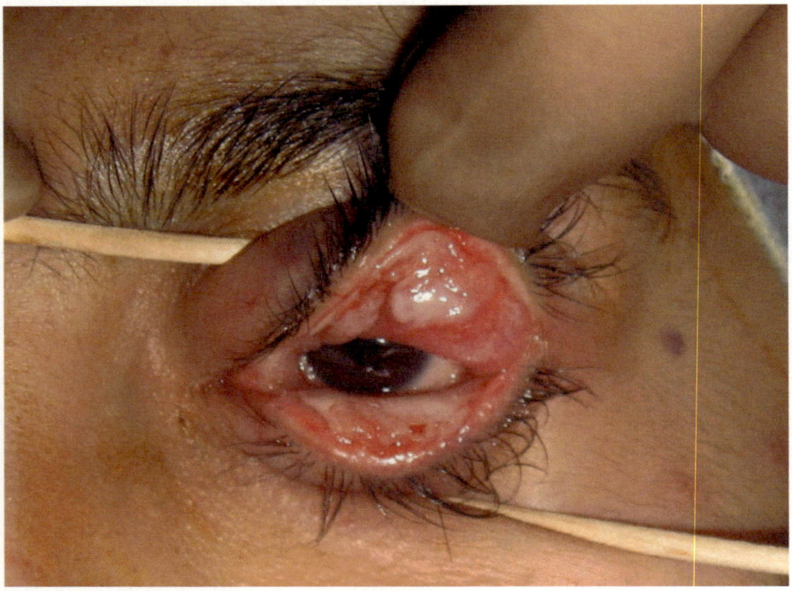

Fig. 5. A young patient with ligneous conjunctivitis

conjunctivitis may present with a history of a red, uncomfortable eye with a mucupurulent discharge. On examination, one may find signs of large lymphoid follicles and conjunctivitis.[25,26] Majority of these patients have associated urinary tract infections. Chlamydial inclusion conjunctivitis is caused by genital tract serotype D-K of C. trachomatis.[25] It is thought that eye is infected through transmitting organisms from genital tract secretions by the hands.[27] Conjunctival chlamydial infection can be demonstrated by staining a conjunctival smear with C. trachomatis-specific fluorescent monoclonal antibody, or by the use of commercial nucleic acid-based diagnostic kits.[25]

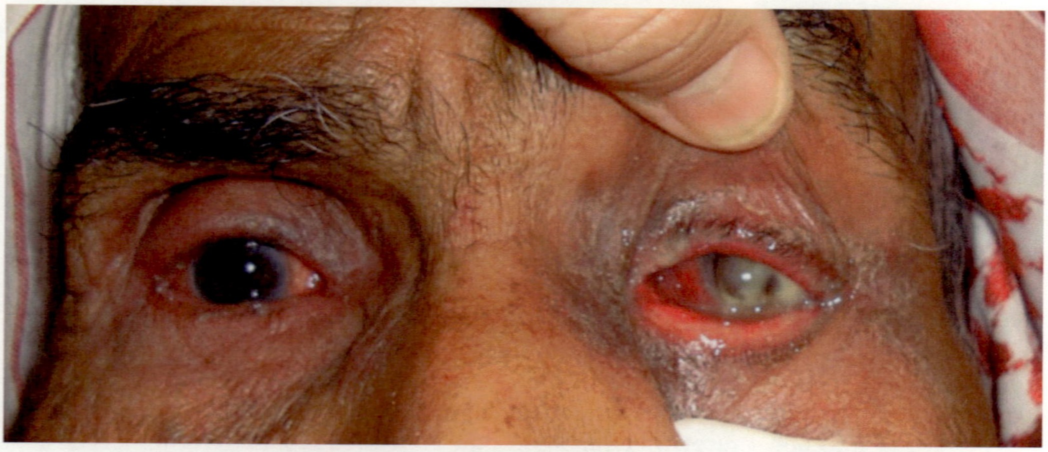

Fig. 6. An elderly patient with old trachomatous scarring and recent bacterial conjunctivitis

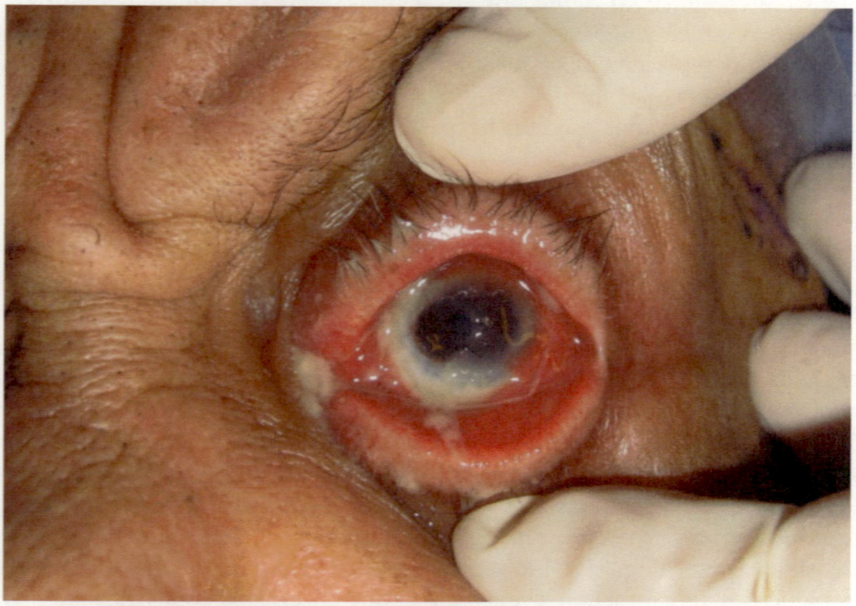

Fig. 7. An older patient having old trachoma and chronic dacryocystitis causing mucupurulent discharge

4. Workup for trachomatous conjunctivitis

The laboratory tests for ocular C. trachomatis confirmation for the clinical diagnosis of active trachoma conjunctivitis are based on techniques for the nucleic acid amplification tests, of which the polymerase chain reaction (PCR) is one example.[25,28] These tests have high specificity and sensitivity. Patients may have infection for several weeks prior to the appearance of any specific clinical signs and symptoms. These patients may have persistent conjunctivitis for few weeks to months after the infection may have resolved. Some of the other useful techniques for laboratory identification of C. trachomatis include, direct fluorescein-labeled monoclonal antibody (DFA) assay and enzyme immunoassay (EIA) of smears obtained from conjunctival tissue. These tests are less sensitive than PCR. In Giemsa cytology, microscopic examinations of the stained conjunctival scrapings for intracytoplasmic inclusions may be useful.

5. Pathophysiology of trachomatis conjunctivitis

Chlamydiae are gram-negative, obligate intracellular bacteria. The species *C. trachomatis* causes trachoma and also genital infections (serovars D-K) and lymphogranuloma venereum (serovars L1-L3).[25] Serovars D-K occasionally cause a chronic follicular conjunctivitis that is clinically indistinguishable from trachoma, including follicular conjunctivitis with pannus and, at times, conjunctival scarring. However, these genital serovars do not typically enter stable transmission cycles within communities. Therefore, they are not involved in trachomatous conjunctivitis and blindness.

Trachomatous infection causes inflammation, that is, a predominantly lymphocytic and monocytic infiltrate with plasma cells and macrophages in follicles. The follicles are typical germinal centers with islands of intense B-cell proliferation surrounded by T cells.[29] Recurrent conjunctival reinfection causes the prolonged inflammation that leads to conjunctival scarring. Scarring is associated with atrophy of the conjunctival epithelium, loss of goblet cells, and replacement of the normal, loose, vascular subepithelial stroma with thick compact bands of collagen.

Active trachoma most commonly occurs in preschool children of both sexes and their (usually female) care providers. Trichiasis and blindness may be 2-4 times more common in women than men. Trachoma is endemic in parts of Africa, Asia, the Middle East, Latin America, the Pacific Islands, and aboriginal communities in Australia.[15,16,30,31] In endemic areas, most members of nearly all families may have active disease. Active trachoma may be seen in clusters in some families. In 1 of 5 families, most children may have active trachoma (as opposed to 1 in 5 children in most families). This clustering becomes more apparent in communities as the prevalence decreases.[5,32] Active disease most commonly occurs in preschool children, with the highest prevalence in children aged 3-5 years. Cicatricial disease is most common in middle-aged adults. The age group in which cicatricial disease begins to appear depends on the intensity of transmission in the community. In areas of extremely high recurrent infections, trichiasis may occur in children younger than 10 years of age. Young children may have follicular trachoma with intense conjunctival inflammation, while their mothers may have trachomatous scarring; and middle-aged patients or grandparents may have trichiasis and corneal opacity. Individuals may have episodes of follicular trachoma with intense conjunctival inflammation even after cicatricial complications develop. The active phase resembles many other diseases in which follicular conjunctivitis is a feature. Without laboratory facilities, the diagnosis is solely based on the clinical appearance of active trachoma in someone living in a community where trachoma is endemic or suspected to be endemic. Many patients with active trachoma may remain relatively asymptomatic.

The duration of disease and infection in active trachoma decreases markedly as the child grows. More rapid disease resolution is found to be the main source of reduction in the prevalence of active trachoma and ocular C. trachomatis infection with age. The serious sequelae of repeated infection may result from conjunctival scarring. Although a severe primary childhood infection may result in conjunctival scarring, the evidence is that re-infection is the most important factor. With increasing age, there is an increasing exposure to infection and increasing immunity which may also increase the likelihood of severe sequelae. Poor hygiene increases the likelihood of a high chlamydial load. In some villages of Africa, familial cattle ownership, facial cleanliness and living less than two hours from a source of clean water may be associated with reduced severity of trachoma. [33,34] Host genetic factors affecting the cellular immune response to trachoma agents may be important in determining disease severity.

In active trachoma, the inflammatory infiltrate is organized as lymphoid follicles in the underlying stroma and cytoplasmic inclusion bodies can be seen in the conjunctival epithelia. In follicular trachoma (grade TF) there is a strong local IgA antibody response to the infecting chlamydiae and this is associated with elevated levels of antibody secreting cells with specificity for chlamydial antigens in the blood. However in the most severe cases with intense inflammation (grade TI) there is a substantial suppression of chlamydia-specific antibody secreting cells for all isotypes, including IgA.[8,34] The suppression may be a contributory factor leading to local tissue damage with ensuing scarring.

In scarring trachoma there are more marked pathological changes in the tissue of the eye lid. These include: subepithelial fibrous membrane formation, squamous cell metaplasia, loss of goblet cells, pseudogland formation in the conjunctiva, degeneration of the orbicularis occuli muscle fibers, sub-epithelial vascular dilatation and lymphocytic infiltration and localized peri-vascular amyloidosis.[34,35] Accessory lacrimal glands and the ducts of glands are compromised by sub-epithelial infiltration and scarring. Contraction of the sub-epithelial fibrous tissue formed by collagen fibers and anterior surface drying are considered some of the main factors contributing to the chronic scarring and distortion of the eyelid.[36] Ocular C. trachomatis infection stimulates local cytokines which favor a strong cell-mediated and pro-inflammatory response in both the acute active and chronic forms of trachoma.

6. Ophthalmia neonatorum (neonatal conjunctivitis)

Often known by its Latin name of Ophthalmia neonatorum, it is conjunctivitis of the eyes of the new born caused by bacterial infection. Usually the infection is derived from the mother's genital tract at birth, in which case the causative organism is either the gonococcus or the genital serotype D to K of C. trachomatis (Figure 8).[37,38] Other bacterial species may also cause conjunctivitis in the newborn, including Neisseria, Pneumococci, Klebsiella Pneumoniae and Streptococcus mitis. Some of these organisms are probably acquired after birth, as the mode of delivery has little influence.

In the developing countries, C. trachomatis is a much commoner cause of sexually acquired neonatal conjunctivitis than the Gonococcal conjunctivitis. Approximately a third to a half of infants born through a chlamydial infected birth canal may develop neonatal conjunctivitis.[38] Chlamydial neonatal conjunctivitis is a significant, but little diagnosed problem in the developing world. Typically, neonatal chlamydial conjunctivitis has an

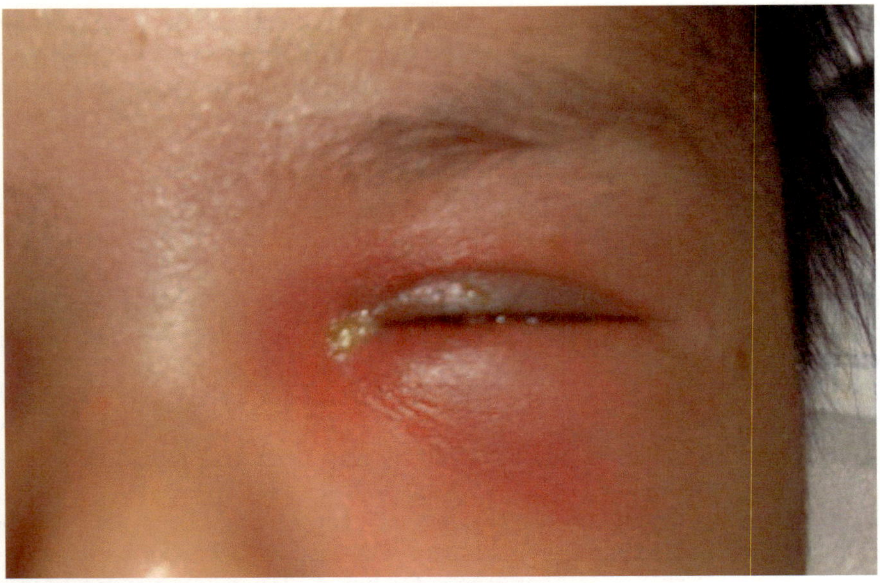

Fig. 8. New born with neonatal conjunctivitis due to Chlamydia

incubation period of 10 to 14 days compared with the much shorter 2 to 3 days incubation for Gonococcal ophthalmia. The conjunctiva of the eye in these patients may be significantly swollen with much mucoid discharge that may be less purulent than that usually seen with overt Gonococcal ophthalmia. The infection is particularly common in pre-mature babies, who are often born to women at particular risk of C. trachomatis infection.[24] Conjunctival swab obtained from the cul-de-sac of these patients stained with C. trachomatis specific fluorescent monoclonal antibody often shows the presence of chlamydial elementary bodies, looking like the "star-spangled sky at night". In neonatal conjunctivitis, the nasopharynx is also commonly infected with C. trachomatis, presumably via drainage from the oto-lacrimal duct, so it is important to treat the infants with systemic rather than topical antibiotic. If left untreated, up-to 20% of infants may develop neonatal pneumonia.[39]

6.1 Laboratory diagnosis of neonatal trachomatous conjunctivitis and pneumonia

A chlamydial aetiology should be considered in all infants aged less than thirty days with conjunctivitis. There have been no modern studies of commercial nucleic acid amplification based tests for the diagnosis of neonatal conjunctivitis. Commercial tests are not specifically licensed for use on ocular specimens from neonates. An alternative is the identification of chlamydial elementary bodies by direct immunofluorescence. Swabs should be collected from the everted eyelid using a swab. It is important that specimens contain conjunctival cells, not just exudates. The diagnosis of neonatal C. trachomatis infection confirms the need for treatment of the mother and her sexual partner as well as the infant.

7. Adult inclusion conjunctivitis

The trachoma serovars of C. trachomatis and the oculo-genital serovars associated with adult inclusion conjunctivitis do not appear to differ greatly in their virulence. In trachoma, the complications arise from the fact that, where the disease is endemic repeated infection may be common that may lead to increased severity. In adult inclusion conjunctivitis secondary to genital tract infection, there is not the same likely-hood of re-infection.[25] Furthermore, in developed countries there is a greater likelihood that the infection will be treated promptly. Thus conjunctival scarring is rarely a complication of adult inclusion conjunctivitis, although micro-pannus, and micro ulceration of the cornea following punctate keratitis may occur.

7.1 Laboratory diagnosis of adult conjunctivitis

Laboratory testing is usually required to establish, with any certainty, the cause of follicular conjunctivitis in the adult. This is because other agents, most notably adenovirus, may cause a similar clinical appearance. Very occasionally, adenoviral and chlamydial co-infection occur together. This should be considered in patients with prolonged follicular keratoconjunctivitis.[40]

8. Treatment

Prevention of trachoma-related ocular complications may require early intervention and treatment. The WHO endorses the SAFE strategy for trachoma control. At the community level, adequate water access for personal hygiene, sanitation, and fly control determine the risk of endemic trachoma. Infants with untreated chlamydial pneumonia shed C. trachomatis and are symptomatic for many weeks. Erythromycin, azithromycin and clarithromycine may be effective for halting transmission to the baby and treating neonatal conjunctivitis.[41,42] Prophylaxis, however, may be ineffective in some new born patients. Erythromycin base or ethyl succinate 50 mg/kg/day may be given orally divided into four doses daily for 14 days. Data on the use of other macrolides (e.g., azithromycin and clarithromycin) for the treatment of neonatal chlamydial infection are limited although a short course of azithromycin, 20 mg/kg/day orally, one dose daily for 3 days, may be effective.

It is essential that all patients with chlamydial conjunctivitis and their sexual partners be examined and treated for concomitant chlamydial genital tract infection.[43] Inclusion conjunctivitis generally responds well to the kind of regimens of macrolide or doxycycline used for treating chlamydial genital tract infection.[44] In the case of doxycycline, treatment with a weekly dose of 300 mg for three weeks or a daily dose of 1.5 mg/kg for one week may produce a clinical and microbiological response in vast majority of patients with adult chlamydial conjunctivitis. Mild to moderate papillary responses may persist in some patients for several months after completion of their treatment. The best results may be obtained with a daily dose of 100 mg Doxycycline for fifteen days, which may produce rapid clinical and microbiological response in most of the patients. The use of azithromycin for the treatment of trachoma suggests that it is likely to be a convenient and effective drug for use in treating adult chlamydial inclusion conjunctivitis.[45]

Azithromycin is a long-acting antibiotic that has been widely sold in the United States and other industrialized nations since the late 1980s under the name Zithromax. The key to the treatment of trachoma is the SAFE strategy developed by the WHO.[33] In the SAFE strategy. "S" stands for trichiasis surgery. The antibiotics ("A"), facial cleanliness ("F"), and environmental improvement ("E") components of this strategy are described in Medical Care. The WHO recommends 2 antibiotics for trachoma control: oral azithromycin and tetracycline eye ointment. Azithromycin is better than tetracycline, but it is more expensive. National trachoma control programs in a number of countries are beneficiaries of a philanthropic donation of azithromycin. Azithromycin is the drug of choice because it is easy to administer as a single oral dose. Its administration can be directly observed. Therefore, compliance is higher than with tetracycline and can actually be measured, whereas, with the home administration of tetracycline, the level of compliance is unknown. Azithromycin has high efficacy and a low incidence of adverse effects. When adverse effects occur, they are usually mild; gastrointestinal upset and rash are the most common adverse events. Infection with *C. trachomatis* occurs in the nasopharynx; therefore, patients may re-infect themselves if only topical antibiotics are used. Beneficial secondary effects of azithromycin include its treatment of genital, respiratory, and skin infections.[45]

The aim of treatment is to reduce the amount *C trachomatis* in the infection reservoir in the family. Treating an individual and not treating infected family members leaves the individual at risk for repeat infection. All family members, including infants, should be treated. The antibiotic of choice for treating active trachoma is azithromycin. The dose for children is 20 mg/kg in a single dose; adults receive a single dose of 1 g. The second-line treatment is topical tetracycline eye ointment 1%. Topical tetracycline is applied to both eyes twice a day for 6 weeks. If the patient lives in a hyperendemic area, the whole district (or whole community) is eligible for antibiotic treatment.

Antibiotic therapy is part of the WHO SAFE strategy for trachoma.[46] Azithromycin (Zithromax) 1 g PO as a single dose is recommended. Although, plasma concentrations may be low, because of long-tissue life and higher tissue concentrations, it may be valuable in treating intracellular organisms. For pediatric patients, a dose of 20 mg/kg PO once may be sufficient. Current WHO recommendations for antibiotic treatment of trachoma are as follows: Determine the district-level prevalence of follicular trachoma in 1- to 9-year-old children. If the prevalence is 10% or higher, conduct mass treatment with antibiotic of all people throughout the district. If the prevalence is less than 10%, conduct assessment at the community level in areas of known disease. If assessment at the community level is undertaken in communities where the prevalence of follicular trachoma in 1- to 9-year-old children is 10% or more, conduct mass treatment of all people with antibiotics. If assessment at the community level is undertaken in communities where the prevalence of follicular trachoma in 1- to 9-year-old children is 5% or more but less than 10%, targeted treatment should be considered. Targeted treatment involves the identification and treatment of all members of any family in whom one or more members have follicular trachoma.[47] If assessment at the community level is undertaken in communities where the prevalence of follicular trachoma in 1- to 9-year-old children is less than 5%, antibiotic distribution may not be necessary, though targeted treatment can be considered.

Epidemiologic studies and community-randomized trials have shown that facial cleanliness in children reduces both the risk and the severity of active trachoma.[8] To be successful, health education and promotion activities must be community based and require considerable effort. Environmental change activities may include the promotion of improved water supplies and improved household sanitation, particularly methods for safe disposal of human feces. These activities should be prioritized. The flies that transmit trachoma preferentially lay their eggs on feces lying exposed on the soil. Controlling fly populations by spraying insecticide is difficult. Studies on the impact of fly control on trachoma have had variable results. Trials undertaken to evaluate the installation of pit latrines suggest that the prevalence of trachoma may be reduced but may not demonstrate a statistically significant effect. Nevertheless, the general improvements in personal and community hygiene are almost universally associated with a reduction in the prevalence and eventually the disappearance of trachoma. This may be true not only in Europe, the Americas, and Australia but also in Africa and Asia.

8.1 Surgical care

Eyelid surgery to correct trichiasis is important in people with trichiasis, who are at high-risk for trachomatous visual impairment and blindness. Eyelid surgery to correct entropion and/or trichiasis may prevent blindness in individuals at immediate risk (Figure 9).[48-50] Eyelid rotation limits the progression of corneal scarring. In some cases, it can result in improvement in visual acuity due to restoration of the visual surface and reductions in ocular secretions and blepharospasm.[51] The WHO has produced a training manual on the bilamellar tarsal rotation procedure. This procedure involves a full-thickness incision of the scarred lid and external rotation of the distal margin by using 3 sutures. In regions where access to ophthalmologists is limited, well-trained and well-supported health workers can perform bilamellar tarsal rotation. Results of randomized clinical trials have confirmed the superiority of this method over other techniques. Even after successful surgery, patients remain at risk for recurrence. Therefore, long-term follow-up care and intermittent screening are important after surgery. Recurrence rates vary greatly between surgeons. Evidence supports the adjuvant use of single-dose azithromycin to patients at the time of surgery. Patients experiencing recurrent episodes of chronic dacryocystitis and/or canaliculitis may benefit from surgical intervention (Figures 4,7,10).

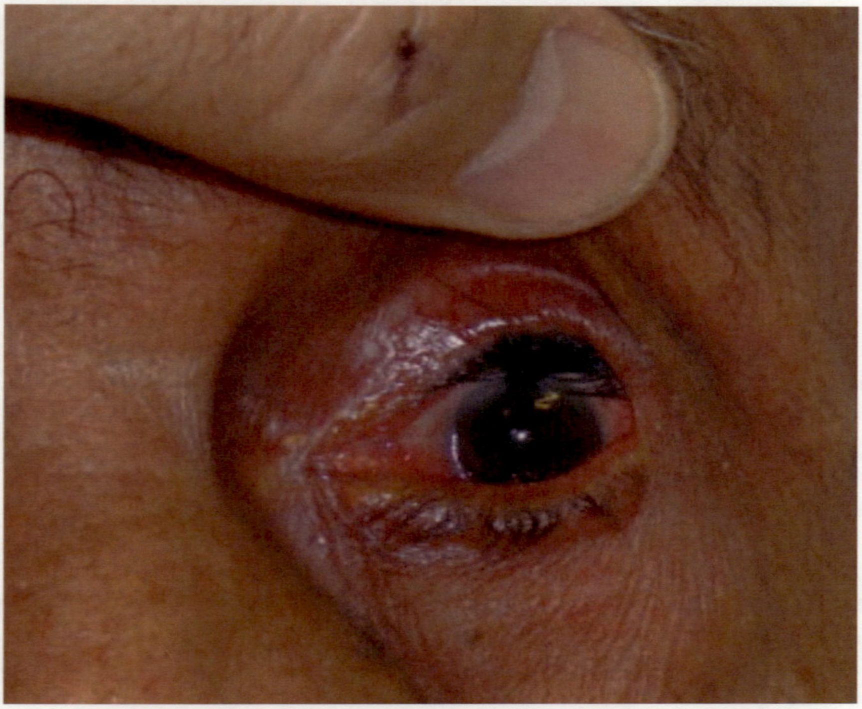

Fig. 9. An elderly patient with old trachomatous scarring and upper eyelid entropion causing chronic conjunctivitis

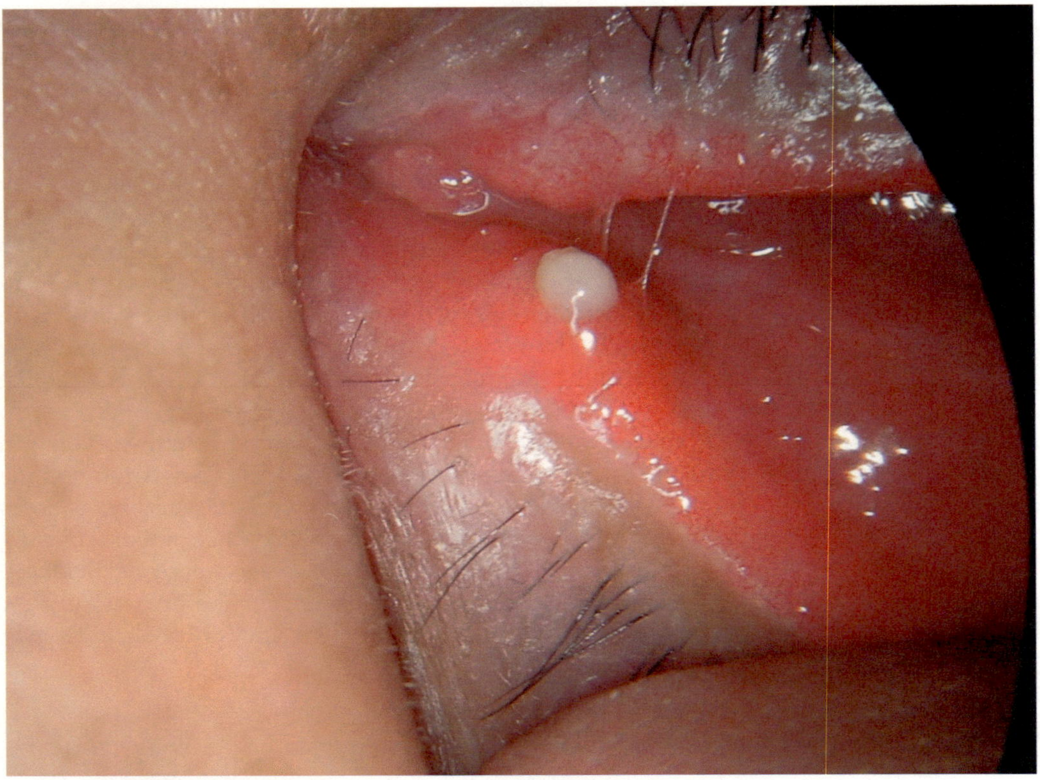

Fig. 10. Patient with chronic trachomatous scarring and canaliculitis and conjunctivitis

9. Trachoma preventive strategies

In the mid 1990s, WHO announced a program called Vision 2020, to tackle the world's major causes of blindness. Approximately 45 million people in the world are blind, with a further 135 million visually disabled. Some 90% of these people live in the developing world. Cataract, trachoma, childhood blindness and onchocerciasis account for roughly 70% of the global burden of blindness, much of it preventable.[52] Part of this program includes the Global Elimination of Trachoma by the year 2020, the acronym for which is GET 2020. Key to this has been the international trachoma initiative (ITI), a partnership between the pharmaceutical company Pfizer and the Edna MacConnell Clarke Foundation, a philanthropic organization. [53] The foundation has already funded much valuable work on trachoma field studies and basic science including some key studies which indicated the efficacy of simple intervention measures, such as face washing, in the prevention of trachoma. Pfizer has provided their anti-chlamydial drug, azithromycin, free of charge for use in pilot studies in some countries of trachoma prevention by antibiotic treatment. These are key elements in the SAFE strategy for GET 2020.

Among the SAFE strategy, Surgery (to correct eyelid defects that lead to blindness), Antibiotic therapy, Facial cleanliness and Environmental improvement (including clean water supplies), surgery and antibiotic therapy dominate most programmes that have been implemented.[46] Surgery has a sustained effect in preventing an individual going blind, but it has no effect on trachoma transmission. Prophylactic antibiotic reduces the transmission of infection but, unless frequently repeated, has no sustained effect on disease eradication.[46] Of the antibiotics most commonly used, oral azithromycin is far easier to administer and thus achieves better patient compliance.[23,54] Antibiotic treatment might be successful if it is targeted at all children in an endemic area under 10 years of age. Mathematical models suggest that antibiotic therapy should be given to communities twice a year in areas with hyperendemic trachoma (>30% of children infected) and once a year in communities where trachoma is only moderately prevalent (<30% of children infected).[47]

Sustainable reductions in transmission may be more likely through the F and E components of SAFE. Environmental improvement with improved hygiene, better access to water and better sanitation and education reduce trachoma transmission which must eventually lead to the disappearance of blinding sequelae. Evidence from intervention studies indicates that the promotion of face-washing yields modest gains for intense educational effort, raising the question for how long the effect will be sustained once health educators have left a village. Other studies have shown that latrines, improved access to water or reduction in eye-seeking flies are associated with a lower prevalence of active trachoma or with reduced transmission. This suggests that the beneficial effects of a combination of improved water supplies, provision of latrines, facial hygiene promotion through established infrastructure and control of eye-seeking flies may be long term and sustainable. Each of these interventions offers other tangible public health benefits. While the main aim of the SAFE program is to reduce trachoma infection to a level where blindness would be minimal, multiple mass antibiotic treatments alone may be sufficient to eliminate infection in an area with modest disease.

10. References

[1] al-Rifai K M. Trachoma through history. *International Ophthalmology* 1988;12:9-14.

[2] Evans TG, Ranson MK. The global burden of trachomatous visual impairment: II. Assessing burden. *International Ophthalmology* 1996;19:271-280.

[3] Ranson MK, Evans TG. The global burden of trachomatous visual impairment: I. Assessing prevalence. *International Ophthalmology* 1996;19:261-270.

[4] Schachter J. Infection and disease epidemiology. In Chlamydia. Intracellular biology, pathogenesis and immunity (Stephens RS, ed.) *American Society of Microbiology Press*, 1999, pg139-169, Washington DC, USA.

[5] Bobo LD, Novak N, Munoz B, Hsieh YH, Quinn TC, West S. Severe disease in children with trachoma is associated with persistent Chlamydia trachomatis infection. *Journal of Infectious Diseases* 1997;176:1524-1530.

[6] Taylor HR, Johnson SL, Schachter J, Caldwell HD, Prendergast RA. Pathogenesis of trachoma: the stimulus for inflammation. *J Immunol*. 1987;138:3023-7.

[7] Abu el-Asrar AM, Geboes K, Missotten L. Immunology of trachomatous conjunctivitis. Bull Soc Belge Ophtalmol. 2001;280:73-96.

[8] Mabey DC, Solomon AW, Foster A. Trachoma. *Lancet*. 2003;362:223-9.

[9] el-Asrar AM, Geboes K, al-Kharashi SA, Al-Mosallam AA, Missotten L, Paemen L, Opdenakker G. Expression of gelatinase B in trachomatous conjunctivitis. British Journal of Ophthalmology 2000;84:85-91.

[10] Bobo L, Novak N, Mkocha H, Vitale S, West S, Quinn TC. Evidence for a predominant proinflammatory conjunctival cytokine response in individuals with trachoma. *Infection and Immunity* 1996;64:3273-3279.

[11] Schachter J, Dawson CR. The epidemiology of trachoma predicts more blindness in the future. *Scandinavian Journal of Infectious Diseases Supplement.* 1990;69:55-62.

[12] Tabbara KF, Ross-Degnan D. Blindness in Saudi Arabia. JAMA. 1986;255:3378-84. Tabbara KF, al-Omar OM. Trachoma in Saudi Arabia. Ophthalmic Epidemiol. 1997;4:127-40.

[13] Burton MJ. Trachoma: an overview. Br Med Bull. 2007;84:99-116.

[14] West SK, Munoz B, Turner VM, Mmbaga BB, Taylor HR. The epidemiology of trachoma in central Tanzania. Int J Epidemiol. 1991;20:1088-92.

[15] Landers J, Kleinschmidt A, Wu J, Burt B, Ewald D, Henderson T. Prevalence of cicatricial trachoma in an indigenous population of Central Australia: the Central Australian Trachomatous Trichiasis Study (CATTS). Clin Experiment Ophthalmol. 2005;33:142-6.

[16] Chaudhry IA. Eradicating blinding trachoma: what is working? Saudi J Ophthalmol. 2010;24:15-21. Available on-line at http://dx.doi.org/10.1016/j.sjopt.2009.12.008.

[17] Emerson PM, Bailey RL, Mahdi OS, Walraven GE, Lindsay SW (2000) Transmission ecology of the fly Musca sorbens, a putative vector of trachoma. *Transactions of the Royal Society of Tropical Medicine and Hygiene* 94, 28 - 32.

[18] Emerson PM, Lindsay SW, Walraven GE, Faal H, Bogh C, Lowe K, Bailey RL. Effect of fly control on trachoma and diarrhoea. *Lancet.* 1999;353:1401-1403.

[19] West S, Munoz B, Lynch M, Kayongoya A, Chilangwa Z, Mmbaga BB, et al. Impact of face-washing on trachoma in Kongwa, Tanzania. *Lancet.*1995;345:155-8.

[20] Abou-Gareeb I, Lewallen S, Bassett K. Courtright P. Gender and blindness: a meta-analysis of population-based prevalence surveys. *Ophthalmic Epidemiology* 2001; 8: 39 - 56.

[21] Haddad NA. Trachoma in Lebanon: observations on epidemiology in rural areas. *American Journal of Tropical Medicine and Hygiene.* 1965;14:652-655.

[22] Courtright P, Sheppard J, Lane S, Sadek A, Schachter J, Dawson CR. Latrine ownership as a protective factor in inflammatory trachoma in Egypt. *British Journal of Ophthalmology.* 1991;75:322-825.

[23] Dawson C, Schachter J. Can blinding trachoma be eliminated world wide? *Archives of Ophthalmology.*1999;117:974.

[24] Krohn MA, Hillier SL, Bell TA, Kronmal RA, Grayston JT. The bacterial etiology of conjunctivitis in early infancy. Eye Prophylaxis Study Group. American Journal of Epidemiology. 1993;138:326- 32.

[25] Isobe K, Aoki K, Itoh N, Ohno S, Takashima I, Hashimoto N. Serotyping of Chlamydia trachomatis from inclusion conjunctivitis by polymerase chain reaction and restriction fragment length polymorphism analysis. *Japanese Journal of Ophthalmology.*1996;40: 279-285.

[26] Mellman-Rubin TL, Kowalski RP, Uhrin M, Gordon YJ. Incidence of adenoviral and chlamydial coinfection in acute follicular conjunctivitis. *American Journal of Ophthalmology.* 1995;119:652-554.

[27] Postema EJ, Remeijer L, van der Meijden WI. Epidemiology of genital chlamydial infections in patients with chlamydial conjunctivitis; a retrospective study. *Genitourinary Medicine.*1996;72:203-205.

[28] Solomon AW, Holland M J, Burton MJ, West SK, Alexander ND, Aguirre A, *et al.* Strategies for control of trachoma: observational study with quantitative PCR. *Lancet.* 2003; 362:198-204.

[29] Ghaem-Maghami S, Bailey RL, Mabey DC, Hay PE, Mahdi OS, Joof HM, Whittle H. C, Ward ME, Lewis DJ. Characterization of B-cell responses to Chlamydia trachomatis antigens in humans with trachoma. *Infection and Immunity.* 1997;65:4958-4964.

[30] Courtright P, Sheppard J, Schachter J, Said ME, Dawson CR. Trachoma and blindness in the Nile Delta: current patterns and projections for the future in the rural Egyptian population. *British Journal of Ophthalmology* 1989;73:536 - 540.

[31] Dolin PJ, Faal H, Johnson GJ, Ajewole J, Mohamed AA, Lee PS. Trachoma in The Gambia. *British Journal of Ophthalmology* 1998;82: 930 - 933.

[32] Dawson CR, Schachter J, Sallam S, Sheta A, Rubinstein RA, Washton H. A comparison of oral azithromycin with topical oxytetracycline/polymyxin for the treatment of trachoma in children. *Clin Infect Dis.* Mar 1997;24:363-8.

[33] Kuper H, Solomon AW, Buchan J, Zondervan M, Foster A, Mabey D. A critical review of the SAFE strategy for the prevention of blinding trachoma. *Lancet Infectious Diseases.* 2003;3:372–381.

[34] Solomon AW, Taylor HR. Trachoma. eMedicine Updated: Sep 5, 2007. Downloaded March, 13th 2011.

[35] el-Asrar AM, Geboes K, Tabbara KF, al-Kharashi SA, Missotten L, Desmet V. Immunopathogenesis of conjunctival scarring in trachoma. *Eye.* 1998;12: 453-460.

[36] al-Rajhi AA, Hidayat A, Nasr A, al-Faran M. The histopathology and the mechanism of entropion in patients with trachoma. Ophthalmology. 1993;100:1293-6.

[37] Black-Payne C, Ahrabi MM, Bocchini JA Jr, Ridenour CR Brouillette RM. Treatment of Chlamydia trachomatis identified with Chlamydiazyme during pregnancy. Impact on perinatal complications and infants. *Journal of Reproductive Medicine.* 1990;35:362-367.

[38] Francois P, Hirtz P, Rouhan D, Favier M, Gratacap B, Beaudoing A. Maternal-child transmission of Chlamydia trachomatis. A prospective inquiry in 168 pregnant women. *Presse Medicale.*1989;18:17-20.

[39] Herieka E, Dhar J. Acute neonatal respiratory failure and Chlamydia trachomatis. *Sexually Transmitted Infections.* 2001;77:135-136.

[40] Mellman-Rubin TL, Kowalski RP, Uhrin M, Gordon YJ. Incidence of adenoviral and chlamydial coinfection in acute follicular conjunctivitis. *American Journal of Ophthalmology* . 1995;119: 652-554.

[41] Black-Payne C, Ahrabi MM, Bocchini JA Jr, Ridenour CR Brouillette RM. Treatment of Chlamydia trachomatis identified with Chlamydiazyme during pregnancy. Impact on perinatal complications and infants. *Journal of Reproductive Medicine.* 1990; 35:362-367.

[42] Hammerschlag MR, Gelling M, Roblin PM, Kutlin A, Jule JE. Treatment of neonatal chlamydial conjunctivitis with azithromycin. *Pediatric Infectious Diseases Journal.* 1998;17:1049-1050

[43] Garland SM, Malatt A, Tabrizi S, Grando D, Lees MI, Andrew JH, Taylor HR. Chlamydia trachomatis conjunctivitis. Prevalence and association with genital tract infection. *Medical Journal of Australia.* 1995; 162:363-866.

[44] Stenberg K, Mardh PA. Treatment of concomitant eye and genital chlamydial infection with erythromycin and roxithromycin. *Acta Ophthalmology* (Copenhagen). 1993;71:332-335.

[45] Negrel AD, Mariotti SP. WHO alliance for the global elimination of blinding trachoma and the potential use of azithromycin. *International Journal of Antimicrobial Agents.* 1998;10:259-262.

[46] Emerson PM, Cairncross S, Bailey RL, Mabey DC. Review of the evidence base for the 'F' and 'E' components of the SAFE strategy for trachoma control. *Tropical Medicine and International Health.* 2000;5:515-527.

[47] Lietman T, Porco T, Dawson C, Blower S. Global elimination of trachoma: how frequently should we administer mass chemotherapy? *Nature Medicine.* 1999;5:572-576.

[48] Teichmann KD. Correction of severe upper eyelid entropion. Int Ophthalmol 1988;12:37-9.

[49] Dhaliwal U, Monga PK, Gupta VP. Comparison of three surgical procedures of differing complexity in the correction of trachomatous upper lid entropion: a prospective study. Orbit 2004;23:227-36.

[50] Sadiq MN, Pai A. Management of trachomatous cicatricial entropion of the upper eye lid: our modified technique. J Ayub Med Coll Abbottabad. 2005;17:1-4.

[51] Dhaliwal U, Nagpal G, Bhatia MS. Health-related quality of life in patients with trachomatous trichiasis or entropion. Ophthal. Epidemiol. 2006;13:59–66.

[52] Thylefors BA global initiative for the elimination of avoidable blindness. *American Journal of Ophthalmology.* 1998; 125:90-93.

[53] Knirsch C, MeCaskey J, Chami-Khazraji Y, Kilima P, West S, Cook J. Trachoma elimination and a public private partnership: the International Trachoma Initiative (ITI). In: Chlamydial Infections: Proceedings of the 10th international symposium on human chlamydial infections (Schachter J *et al*, eds), 2002. pp 485 - 494, published by International Chlamydia Symposium San Francisco CA 94110.

[54] Bailey RL, Arullendran P, Whittle HC, Mabey DC. Randomised controlled trial of single-dose azithromycin in treatment of trachoma. *Lancet.* 1993;342:3453-3456.

12

Ocular Symptoms (Conjunctivitis, Uveitis) in Reactive Arthritis

Brygida Kwiatkowska and Maria Maślińska
Department of Early Diagnosis of Arthritis, Institute of Rheumatology
Poland

1. Introduction

The reactive arthritis (ReA) is an autoimmune disorder usually induced by the prior infection. Conjunctivitis, urethritis and arthritis emerging after the prior onset of diarrhea were first described by Stoll in 1776. In 1818, Benjamin Brodie described 5 cases of conjunctivitis, urethritis and arthritis with a history of venereal diseases. In 1916, Fiessinger and Leroy described 4 patients with an oculo-urethro-synovial syndrome following a diarrhea caused by Shigella. In the same year, Hans Reiter described a triad of symptoms: nongonococcal urethritis, conjunctivitis and arthritis suffered by a young officer with bloody diarrhea and linked these symptoms to the Treponema infection. Until modern times, many researchers used the term Reiter's syndrome for this triad of symptoms. In 1969, the use of the term reactive arthritis (ReA) was proposed, and in 1977, following the disclosure of the war crimes committed by Hans Reiter, it was recommended not to use the name of Reiter's syndrome due to ethical reasons. Based on the analysis of the literature the proportion of authors who use Reiter's name to describe the syndrome has decreased from 34% in 1998 to 18% in 2003 and to 9% in 2007 (Keyan & Rimar, 2008).
Reactive arthritis belongs to a group of diseases known as autoimmune seronegative spondyloarthropathy that is associated with a high incidence of HLA antigen B 27. Reactive arthritis is a disease with diverse clinical manifestations affecting the peripheral joints, spine, skin, eyes, digestive and other systems. The variety of symptoms means that patients, especially in the initial stage of the disease, are treated by the specialists of other fields than rheumatology.

2. Definition

The reactive arthritis is an asymmetric, non septic inflammation of several joints, mainly of the lower limbs, associated with the occurrence of a change called "enthesitis" (inflammation of the tendon), preceded by an extraarticular manifestation and by a documented infection (with or without symptoms present) with: Salmonella, Campylobacter, Yersinia, Shigella flexneri, Chlamydia trachomatis, Chlamydia pneumoniae; rarely with: Clostridium difficile, Mycobacterium bovis BCG, Mycoplasma species (e.g. Ureoplasma urealyticum), and very rarely with: Giardia Cryptospotidium, Shigella sonnei, Chlamydia psitacci, Hafnia alvei, Vibrio parahaemolyticus or other microorganisms. The reactive arthritis often has an acute onset. ReA may also take an atypical course, as inflammation can affect a single joint only, with the concurrent presence of classic symptoms preceded by the diarrhea or urethritis / cervicitis with no infection detected.

3. Pathogenesis

The key role in the pathogenesis of reactive arthritis is assigned to the presence of bacteria or their products in the joint structures and the local immune response to the bacterial antigens. The presence of Chlamydia trachomatis has been demonstrated not only in reactive arthritis, but also in the synovial fluid of approximately 30% of patients with undifferentiated arthritis of few joints (the same situation takes place in the case of Chlamydia pneumoniae). In the case of Enterobacteriaceae (with the exception of Campylobacter jejuni and Yersinia) PCR (Polymerase Chain Reaction) testing often reveals DNA of these bacteria in the articular structures, while the ribosomal RNA is detected in Yersinia infections. The Yersinia penetrate into the M cells of the Peyer's patches, where the reaction between the invasive bacterial proteins and integrin SS1 takes place. Yersinia can be transferred by phagocytes through the mucosal barrier and enters into the joint via blood pathway. The lymph nodes may constitute a reservoir of live Yersinia bacteria for many months following the manifestation of the first symptoms of reactive arthritis, which leads to a high level of long-lasting antibodies against these bacteria, while only bacteria fragments are detected in the joints.

The emergence of reactive arthritis following the infection with Yersinia can be attributed to the presence of the bacteria derived arthritogenic peptide, which epitope is presented to T-cells by the phagocytes in the synovial tissue. The HLA B27 + T cells respond to the 60kDa heat shock protein epitope and beta-subunit of the Yersinia's urease, which can be detected in the joint. The Yersinia infection may be persistent in the lymph nodes or in the mucosa and the bacteria can be transported to the joint by the monocytes (Gaston et al. 1999). A similar mechanism applies to the development of reactive arthritis induced by Salmonella, in which the persistent presence of the bacterial lipopolysaccharide (LPS) in the synovium has been demonstrated.

In the case of Chlamydia trachomatis, which is an intracellular pathogen, the epithelial cells are the primary location of the bacterial colonization. Chlamydia trachomatis can later infect other types of cells such as macrophages and other phagocytic cells.

A replication of Chlamydia trachomatis in monocytes leads to the recognition of the Chlamydia antigen and induces the process of complex forming with class I and II HLA antigens that are presented on the CD4+ and CD 8+ T cells. The persistence of Chlamydia trachomatis can be long standing, as it is confirmed by the presence of bacterial mRNA, rRNA and DNA (PCR detected) in the synovium and in the peripheral blood (Gerard et al.1998, Kuipers et al., 1998, Zeidler et al.2004). The persistence of the infection is probably aided by the state of imbalance between cytokines such as tumor necrosis factor-α (TNF-α) and interleukin-10 (IL-10) - this imbalance being confirmed in vivo. Th1 cytokines such as: interleukin-12 (IL-12), interferon-γ (IFN-γ) and tumor necrosis factor-α (TNF-α) participate in the elimination of bacteria. The reduction of the activity of these cytokines or increase in Th2/Th3 cytokine production (especially of IL-10) reduces the capability of bacteria elimination from the organism. In patients with persistent infection high levels of IL-10 in the intestine, urogenital and respiratory systems has been demonstrated (Yin et al.1997).

IL-6, IL-1 beta and IL-17 and IL-21 (Singh et al. 2011) play the key role in the formation of synovitis in ReA.

An important role in the pathogenesis of reactive arthritis and other spondyloartroaties is assigned to HLA B27 antigen. According to the arthritogenic peptide theory, it is believed that certain subtypes of HLA-B27 containing unique amino acid may be associated with the bacterial arthritogenic peptide and can be recognized by CD8 + T cells. This causes the response to the bacterial peptide, autoreactivity of T lymphocytes which recognize this peptide similar to the host's and activated by the host's peptides in the joints. HLA-B 27 antigens are present in high proportion of patients with ReA induced by: Shigella (80-90%) Yersinia (70-80%), Chlamydia (40-50%) and Salmonella (20-33%) (Nicholis 1975). According to the recently most popular ReA pathogenesis model, called "multi-hit theory" the activation of the immune response in the reactive arthritis and other spondyloartropathies is a result of many circumstances such as: the effect of bacterial arthritogenic products (including lipopolisaccharides), HLA B-27 antigen presence, the extension of bacteria elimination time and other genetic or biomechanical factors. It was also reported that there is a link between HLA B 51 antigen, not only with the Behcet's disease, but also with the ReA - in particular in Japanese population (Shimamoto et all 2000). In HLA B 27 antigen negative patients the presence of HLA B 7, Bw22,B40,B42, B60 antigens – cross-reactive with HLA B27 antigen - may be also found.

4. Clinical symptoms

4.1 The beginning of the disease

The onset is preceded by the symptoms of infection manifesting themselves approximately 4 weeks before the articular symptoms. In the case of Chlamydia trachomatis and Chlamydia pneumoniae the symptoms of infection can go unnoticed, since 70% of infections may be asymptomatic or proceed with minor symptoms only. Infection caused by Chlamydia trachomatis is characterized by the onset of disuric symptoms, urethritis, prostatitis in men and cervitis and / or adnexitis in women. Chlamydia pneumoniae infections usually lead to symptoms of upper respiratory tract infection, cough, pharyngitis, otitis media and sinusitis. In patients infected with Enterobacteriacae e.g Shigella a short episode of joint symptoms may precede the diarrhea. The abdominal pain in the case of Yersinia may be periodically recurrent with enlargement of abdominal lymph nodes and, in some cases, proceeds with appendicitis symptoms. As reactive arthritis is a systemic disease, it may manifest itself with the systemic illness symptoms such as malaise, weakness and fever.

4.2 Symptoms of the musculoskeletal system

Joint symptoms may vary, ranging from arthralgia to the severe inflammation of several joints. Typically inflammation of a single or asymmetric inflammation of several joints is observed. Most commonly the lower extremities joints, such as knees, ankle and foot joints are affected. Inflammation can affect the fingers (dactilitis). This condition is known as „sausage digit" and is attributed to the inflammatory changes in the articular capsule, tendon sheath, periarticular structures and periosteum of the bone. Inflammation of the sacroiliac or spine joints occurs in approximately 50% of patients, manifesting itself as an inflammatory back pain (IBP) with back stiffness and buttock pain. Recurrent arthritis occurs in about 15% of patients and affects mainly patients with reactive arthritis with a history of Chlamydia infection. Inflammation of the tendon (enthesitis) is a common symptom of reactive arthritis. Very characteristic and helpful in identifying the enthesitis are changes involving the attachments of the bottom surface of the calcaneus, Achilles tendon and plantar attachments - resulting in heel pain and difficulty in walking.

4.3 Changes in skin and mucosa

Inflammation of the mucous membrane of the urogenital tract manifests through the symptoms of urethritis /cystitis and cervitis/ colpitis. In some patients changes may involve the genitals beginning with the vesicular lesions evolving into erosion lesions or macular lesions. These affect the external opening of the urethra, glans and shaft of the penis and may precede joint symptoms. The described changes are referred to as "balanitis circinata" (serpiginous annular dermatitis of the penis). These changes are painless unless subject to secondary infection and after treatment and recovery leave no scars. In women annular changes in the external genital organs are rare and are called "circinate vulvitis".
In reactive arthritis, various changes in the oral cavity may appear, such as painless, shiny aphthae on the palate, tongue or on the mucosa of the cheeks and mouth. Delicate red spots may also rarely occur in the palatal tonsils and lingula. Skin lesions in the course of reactive arthritis may be characteristic of this disease and are referred to as "keratoderma blenorrhagica." There are characteristic maculopapular scaly patches with excessive keratosis occurring on the plantar skin of the feet. They may also appear on the big toe, toes and hands. They appear less commonly on the scrotum, penis, trunk and scalp. Histologically, these changes are identical to psoriatic. Often changes called "palmoplantaris pustulosis"(pustular inflammation of the planta and hands) are observed occurring on the plantar side of hands and feet. Changes in nails occur mainly in chronic reactive arthritis, as yellowish or gray discoloration of the nails, bumps, hollow lines and nail keratosis are observed. "Thimble-pitting" of the nails, characteristic of psoriasis, is rarely observed.
Although erythema nodosum often occurs post Yersinia infection, it is not associated with the course of reactive arthritis and has no connection with the presence of HLA-B27 antigen.

4.4 Symptoms concerning the urogenital tract

In addition to the above described inflammatory changes affecting the mucous membrane of the urogenital tract and the skin of sex organs, pathologies of the urinary system in course of ReA may include prostatitis, testitis and / or epididymitis in men and cervicitis and adnexitis in women (both being often asymptomatic in women and diagnosed incidentally during a pelvic gynecological control). Proteinuria caused by IgA nephropathy and amyloidosis due to chronic ReA may also occur, as well as cases of microhaematuria. Pyuria is observed in patients with sexually acquired reactive arthritis (SARA) mainly and occurs usually in Chlamydia trachomatis infections (42-69% of SARA cases), but also in Ureaplasma urealiticum, Gardnerella vaginalis and rarely in recurrent E. coli infections.
Symptoms associated with urinary tract are usually asymptomatic.

4.5 Ocular changes

Uveitis	Scleritis	Conjuntivitis
Common - mainly anterior (AU)	Rare	Keratitis; rare

Table 1. Eye involvement in reactive arthritis.

4.5.1 Conjunctivitis

Conjunctivitis can occur in all types of reactive arthritis, often as an early symptom. It is predominant pathology of the sight organ in reactive arthritis and especially in patients with reactive arthritis caused by Chlamydia. Conjunctivitis affects 1 in 3 patients with ReA caused by Chlamydia, but it can also be observed in reactive arthritis resulting from Enterobacteriacae infection (usually post Shigella, Salmonella and Campylobacter infections, while only in 10% of Yersinia cases patients suffer from conjunctivitis). Symptoms can be bilateral, mild and progressive. In Chlamydia trachomatis induced reactive arthritis conjunctivitis occurs within a few days of the first symptoms of urethritis and usually withdraws within a week. Conjunctivitis can relapse and take a severe course. Conjunctivitis is often painless and non-septic, but it may also cause burning sensation and irritation of the eyes. In the initial period of ReA conjunctivitis is observed in 2% of patients and in 96% patients with the chronic ReA.

4.5.2 Uveitis

In 10 to 20% of reactive arthritis patients with the HLA-B27 antigen present, one or more episodes of acute anterior uveitis occur. The main symptoms present are unilateral eye pain with redness, lacrimation, photophobia, and blurred vision. 13% of patients hospitalized in ophthalmology departments due to uveitis reveal spondyloarthropathies, with 7.2% diagnosed with reactive arthritis and 5.5% with ankylosing spondylitis.

There are case reports of posterior uveitis involving choroid and retina in ReA. The macular degeneration of retina was also described in literature as emerging during post-dysenteria reactive arthritis (Sawhney, Parihar 2006).

Scleritis is rare in patients with ReA but most common in other rheumatic diseases like rheumatoid arthritis.

Anterior uveitis Iritis/irydocyclitis	Intermediate uveitis Vitreous humor	Posterior uveitis Choroid and retina
Acute, unilateral	Incidous onset,unilateral or bilateral	Incidous onset
red eye, pain , photophobia, visual loss (macular oedema)	floaters, haziness of vision	floaters, blurred vision, scotomata, visual loss

Table 2. comparison of uveitis symptoms

In chronic ReA with recurrent ocular symptoms anterior uveitis (92%) and posterior uveitis (64%) are frequently observed, as well as other ocular changes, such as keratitis (64%), cataract (56%), intermediate uveitis (40%), scleritis (28%), cystoid macular edema (28%), papillitis (16%) and glaucoma (16%) (Kiss et al.2003).

4.6 Other symptoms

Inflammatory changes in the aortic arch and ascending aorta and aortic valve regurgitation may also appear (Deer et al. 1991).

5. Morphological changes

5.1 Morphological changes in the joints

The main change which occurs in the joints of reactive arthritis patients is an inflammation of the synovial tissue and presence of inflammatory fluid, leading to the reduction of complement level in the joint due to local utilization of the complement. In the histological assessment the picture of the inflamed synovium is uncharacteristic and similar to other rheumatic diseases with synovitis. The microscopic examination reveals swelling, vascular lesions with infiltration of lymphocytes and granulocytes as well as plasma cells. In reactive arthritis, in contrast to the synovitis in rheumatoid arthritis, the emergence of pannus rarely takes place. The destructive changes of the bone are unspecific and occur only in patients with chronic inflammatory process. Another characteristic feature of reactive arthritis (as well as of other spondyloartropaties) is the infiltration of macrophages and lymphocytes in ligament trailers and bone tendons (enthesitis), bone resorption and its remodeling, resulting in subchondral hyperostosis and subperiosteal bone formation.

5.2 Morphological changes in the skin and mucous membranes

The skin lesions show infiltration of inflammatory cells such as lymphocytes and plasma cells, causing abnormal thickening and keratinization of the horny layer (stratum corneum), similar to psoriasis. The mucosal changes in the urogenital tract are similar, but keratosis is not observed.

5.3 Morphological changes in the organ of sight

In rheumatic diseases all anatomical parts of eye can be involved. In ReA conjunctiva , iris and cilliary body or both (anterior uveitis), vitreus body (intermediate uveitis), choroid and retina (posterior uveitis) are most commonly affected. ReA rarely concerns sclera (scleritis). In some cases of ReA panuveitis occurs. Changes in the eyes in the course of conjunctivitis are typical of follicular conjunctivitis and occur mainly in infection caused by Chlamydia, Salmonella, Shigella, Campylobacter and Yersinia. In Chlamydia infection , in case of direct autoinfections from the genitourinary tract, typical changes of yellow-white papules (trachoma) frequently occur. Such changes are present in spite of Chlamydia trachomatis serotypes D-K being involved in the pathogenesis of ReA and not serotypes A-C responsible for trachoma forming. Recently, the contribution of Chlamydia trachomatis A-C serotypes to the pathogenesis of ReA with coexisting ocular symptoms has been demonstrated (Gerard et al.2010) as well as the simultaneous presence of chronic inflammatory changes in other tissues and organs.

The histopathology assessment reveals the presence of the chronic inflammation cells localized in submucosal layer, with the predominance of lymphocytes. In addition, extensive fibrynogen deposits in the basal membrane of conjunctiva, infiltration of lymphocytes and macrophages around small blood vessels and lymphocytic infiltrate of the larger vessel walls of conjunctiva have been observed (Purcell & Tsai et al. 1982).

In reactive arthritis, as in other spondyloarthropaties, anterior uveitis occurs. The incidence of anterior uveitis is more common than intermediate or posterior uveitis in ReA patients. The uveitis is more frequent in cases with HLA A-9 and HLA B 40 antigen presence than in cases in which HLA B 27 antigen is present.

Pathomechanism of anterior uveitis development involves humoral and cellular response to retinal antigens (S-antigen) and to interphotoreceptor retinoid binding protein (IRBP) (De Smet et al. 1990). IRBP has been shown to induce posterior uveitis.

The eye is considered as immunologically privileged organ. Some portions of the eye are avascular, and an immunosuppressive factors (such as TGF ß) are present in ocular fluids. In some cases deviated regulation of the cellular response to the exogenous antigen in anterior chamber of the eye (anterior chamber associated immune deviation- ACAID) occurs. In ACAID phenomenon Ts lymphocytes impair the delayed hypersensitivity and complement dependent antibody production. This leads to suppressed cellular immunological response. The specifity of the eye immune environment is therefore important in immune and inflammatory diseases with eye involvement.(Wilbanks GA 1991).

5.4 Morphological changes in the gastrointestinal tract

In the course of reactive arthritis inflammatory bowel disease is observed. It concerns: the ileocecal valve area (22%), terminal ileum (12%) and the colon (3%). In 49% of cases abundant infiltration of inflammatory cells to the lining of the lamina propia of the mucosa is being observed along with the partial flattening of intestinal villi, hyperplasia of the cript epithelial cells, infiltration of cripts' epithelium by neutrophils and cripts abscesses. In 18% erosions of intestinal epithelium with or without granuloma are present (Cuvelier et all, 1987).

5.5 Morphological changes in the circulatory system

The presence of inflammatory changes concerning the aortic arch and ascending aorta (aortitis) often leads to aorta enlargement and aortic valve regurgitation.

6. Diagnostic criteria of reactive arthritis

The reactive arthritis belongs to the spondyloarthropathies and thus must meet the classification criteria for this group of diseases, such as Amor criteria and criteria of the European Spondyloartrhopathy Study Group (ESSG). In 1996 during the Third International Workshop on Reactive Arthritis a group of experts proposed diagnostic criteria for ReA based on the presence of asymmetric peripheral arthritis (predominantly of the lower limbs) concomitant with evident prior infection and diarrhea or urethritis preceding by 4 weeks the emergence of the arthritis. In case of the lack of history of evident infection, the diagnosis should be confirmed after the exclusion of other diseases that cause inflammation of one or a few joints (Sieper et al.1999).

There are no proper criteria for ReA recognition. ACR criteria for ReA diagnosis (1981) are defined as follows: an episode of arthritis lasting more than 1 month with concurrent urethritis and /or cervitis (84,3% of sensitivity and 98,2% specificity of diagnosis); episode of arthritis lasting more than 1 month and one of: urethritis or cervicitis, *or* bilateral conjunctivitis (85.5% of sensitivity and 96.4% of specificity); the episode of arthritis, conjunctivitis and urethritis with no time limits of the episode set (50.6% of sensitivity and 98.8% of specificity), an episode of arthritis lasting more than a month with conjunctivitis and urethritis (48.2% of sensitivity and 98.8% of specificity) [Willkens et al. 1981].

7. Diagnostic tests in reactive arthritis

There is no single diagnostic test to recognize ReA. Thus it is necessary for proper diagnosis to confirm previous infection and recognize characteristic symptoms of spondyloarthropathy such as e.g. enthesitis. It is also required to perform laboratory tests confirming the infection with one of the bacteria responsible for ReA induction.

7.1 Diagnosis of Chlamydia infection

On the basis of serological tests it has been shown that Chlamydia trachomatis is a pathogen detected in 50% of ReA patients with a history of urinary tract infections, including 12-22% of cases in which the infection was asymptomatic. Often mixed infections of Chlamydia trachomatis, Chlamydia pneumoniae and Chlamydia psittaci takes place, being found in 35% of patients with conjunctivitis (Dean et al.2008). ReA develops in 7-10% of patients infected with Chlamydia pneumoniae. Serological tests used to confirm Chlamydia trachomatis infections are often difficult to interpret, as they detect high levels of antibodies in healthy individuals and cross-react with Chlamydia pneumonia antibodies. Moreover, the diagnosis cannot be based on the presence of IgG antibodies, as they may persist for many months after the infection. Serological diagnosis should therefore be based also on the determination of IgM and IgA antibodies levels, which confirm acute or chronic infection. (Bas et al 1998)

The Chlamydia infection can also be confirmed by DNA or RNA presence in urogenital system tested with PCR or LCR (ligand chain reaction). Another diagnostic possibility is detection of Chlamydia trachomatis DNA in synovial fluid.

7.2 Diagnosis of infections of Yersinia, Salmonella, Campylobacter and Shigella

Bacteriological stool examination in Yersinia and Salmonella induced ReA is useful only in case of coexisting diarrhea, as within 4 weeks of the onset of arthritis only in 9% of patients with previous diarrhea symptoms these tests yield positive results (Fendler et al. 2000). Diagnosis of these infections is based mainly on serological tests. In Yersinia-induced ReA IgG and IgA antibodies are found in 100% of patients. In 84% of ReA patients IgA antibodies against Yersinia antigen prevail from 14 up to 16 months from the first signs of infection and the increase in their level correlates with the exacerbation of arthritis. In patients with no arthritis, these antibodies disappear after 5 months. In patients with Yersinia-induced ReA as well as in patients with no arthritis, IgG antibodies may persist for a long time after the onset of the infection, but in patients with no arthritis coexisting IgA antibodies are not present. IgM antibodies persist in the body only from 1 to 3 months after the beginning of the infection. It is recommended, therefore, to determine the level of IgG, IgM and IgA antibodies in acute Re, while only the level of IgG and IgA antibodies should be determined in chronic ReA (Granfors et al. 1980).

In Salmonella-induced ReA stool culture tests prove to be not very useful and yield positive results in only 4% of patients - both with and without persistent diarrhea. In Salmonella-induced ReA all classes of antibodies may persist for a long time - from 9 to 14 months in serum (Maki-Ikola et al. 1991). Yersinia and Salmonella can survive in the body for many months and years (being detected in the peripheral blood), stimulating the production of antibodies IgA and / or IgM. The DNA of these bacteria is very rarely detected within the joint, which confirms that the mucosa and lymph nodes constitute reservoir for these organisms. Therefore the determination of bacterial DNA presence in the synovium or synovial fluid is irrelevant to ReA (Granfors et al. 1998).

Currently a well-developed diagnostic methods for Campylobacter and Shigella infections do not exist. In the case of Campylobacter infections diagnosis can be based on bacteriological (in the presence of abdominal symptoms) or serological tests. For diagnosing infection, the presence of IgA antibodies has a greater specificity than presence of IgM antibodies (Locht & Krogfeld 2002).

7.3 Determination of the presence of HLA B27 antigen

In case of symptoms which suggest ReA – and with the exclusion of other diagnosis – the determination of the HLA-B27 antigen presence increases the likelihood of correct diagnosis from 40 to 69%. The use of the serological methods and HLA-B27 typing increases the possibility of correct diagnosis to about 80% (Sieper et al.2002).

8. Occurrence

The ability of a proper assessment of the reactive arthritis incidence is limited due to: the lack of appropriate classification and diagnostic criteria, constant mobility of young people population and poor registration of venereal diseases as well as underdiagnosis of mild course ReA. Summary of data from various developing countries shows that the incidence of the reactive arthritis in the world is 100-200 per 100 000 inhabitants. Reactive arthritis is observed post Chlamydia trachomatis in 1-4 % of cases, while post Salmonella, Yersinia and Shigella infections it is observed in 2 - 4% of cases, with incidence growing to over 20% of patients with HLA-B27 antigen present. In the case of Campylobacterjejuni reactive arthritis develops in 1 - 5% of those infected.

9. Physical examination

It is necessary to control parameters of all vital signs. The physician performing the examination should pay particular attention for the signs of joint involvement (arthritis), skin and mucosal changes, eye involvement and symptoms suggesting lung pathologies (sarcoidosis).In case of patients presenting symptoms of the increased blood pressure or results of the urinanalysis deviated from the reference values, the renal involvement has to be considered.

10. Ocular examination

A basic observation may reveal red eye symptomatic for conjunctivitis, scleritis and uveitis anterior. Performing the direct ophtalmoscopy (fundoscopy) allows the detection of hyperemia of the conjunctiva adjacent to the cornea and the detection a hypopyon of the anterior chamber (inflammation in vitreous humor) - typical signs of an acute anterior uveitis. The direct ophtalmoscopy is also a basic examination in the case of the complications of uveitis, such as glaucoma or in case of any retinal changes.

If the lens is clouded by a cataract, indirect ophtalmoscopy is a useful tool as it allows the better view of the fundus of the eye.

Slit lamp examination is very important method for the evaluation of changes in the course of uveitis. This test allows assessment of iris stroma for formation of ulcers and edema, and corneal epithelium for abrasions, edema, ulcers and foreign bodies. Slit lamp findings can reveal presence of cells (leukocyte clumps) and flare (haze) in anterior chamber (evidence of protein presence) and posterior synechiae. In intermediate and posterior uveitis slit lamp examination can detect the condensations of the vitreous inflammatory cells occuring over the pars plana and ora serrata, forming "snowballs" and neovasularisation of the retinal periphery.

Of other methods used in ocular examination, ocular coherence tomography (OCT) is used in detection of cystoid macular edema in uveitis (CMO) and fluorescein angiography is

useful in diagnosis of uveitis with macular oedema and in vasculitis. To control intraocular pressure in patient with uveitis, tonometry is used.
In cases of eye pain and suspicion of sinusitis the nasoscopy and bacteriological exam of the nasal secretions are indicated.

11. Results of laboratory tests

The laboratory test results are nonspecific for the ReA and thus not useful to confirm the diagnosis, yet necessary to monitor the course of the disease. The deviations from the norm include: normocytic anemia, moderate leukocytosis with an increase in the number of neutrophils, the increase of ESR and CRP values. In general, urine test can reveal sterile pyuria with concomitant urethritis present. Antinuclear antibodies and rheumatoid factor are not present. An examination of the synovial fluid shows changes non-specific to the ReA with inflammatory fluid characteristic for other arthritis types as well. Synovial fluid is sterile without crystal presence. Synovial biopsy is nondiagnostic and shows inflammatory changes as in other arthritis.
In some cases carrying out a differential diagnosis employing serology methods to exclude other infections - viral e.g. HIV or bacterial e.g. borrelia burgdorferi - is necessary. TPHA test is used for exclusion of syphilis, while the serum Angiotensin Converting Enzyme Assay (ACE) is used in cases of suspected sarcoidosis.

12. ECG

ECG changes occur in 5 - 14% of patients with chronic ReA and most of these changes take the form of prolonged PQ segment of I- degree AV block type.

13. X-ray examinations

Radiographic changes are seen in more than 70% of patients with chronic reactive arthritis and are characterized by the picture of swelling soft tissues (especially characteristic is so-called "sausage finger"), periosteal ossification with exostosis, erosions on the articular surfaces and periarticular osteopenia. Less frequently erosions in small joints of the feet, hands, knees and sacroiliac joints are observed. The presence of enthesitis can be demonstrated on x-ray, tough ultrasound examination can reveal a much earlier stages of the erosions. In the reactive arthritis, bone proliferation develops in many places, including the periosteum and takes a linear or feathery arrangement adhering to the cortical edge, particularly along the shaft of the metacarpal and metatarsal bones, toes, distal femoral end and the ankle. Smilar changes are seen in calcaneal, ischial and femoral trochanter tendon attachments, giving a picture of feathery ossifications. The presence of enthesitis changes may suggest reactive arthritis, but cannot determine the diagnosis, because such changes may occur in other diseases (sensitivity of 30%). Radiographic evidence of the spine in reactive arthritis is associated with disease duration and its nature. 50% of patients with chronic reactive arthritis have radiographic evidence of sacroilitis. Sacroilitis is observed more frequently in patients with Chlamydia trachomatis induced reactive arthritis (32%). Erosions are most often observed at the hip bone. In the later course of the disease pseudo-dilatation of the joint, bone proliferation, sclerosis and ankylosis are observed (Martel et al.1979, Colmegna et al. 2004).

Chest x-ray is important in suspected tuberculosis or sarcoidosis and with other cases with symptoms of respiratory tract involvement. In some cases a hight resolution CT scan chest is needed.

14. Differential diagnosis

14.1 Arthritis

The differential diagnosis of reactive arthritis should be based on the exclusion of other causes of arthritis, including other forms of spondyloarthropathies, arthritis in the course of other rheumatic diseaseas, systemic diseases, such as cancer, post-infectious arthritis e.g. in Lyme disease or in the course of viral or streptococcal infections. Changes of enthesopathy - type, which are typical of reactive arthritis, may also occur in other spondyloarthropaties and other rheumatic diseases.

14.2 Differential diagnosis in patients with ReA and eye involvement

Anterior uveitis
Idiophatic anterior uveitis Spondyloarthropaties other than ReA Sarcoidosis Juvenile idiopathioc arthritis Behcet disease Relapsing polychondritis Vasculitis (Cogan syndrome, Kawasaki disease, Wegeners' syndrome) SLE Sjogren syndrome Infections (Whipple disease, Lyme disease) Others eg. Sweets' syndrome Familal granulomatous synovitis Neonatal onset multisystem inflammatory
Posterior uveitis
Sarcoidosis Eale's disease Bridshot choirodoretinopathy Behcet disease CMV Toxoplasmosis Herpes infection Tuberculosis Histoplasmosis Syphilis

Table 3. Examples of the diseases in differentiation of uveitis (Enzenauer Sterling G.West 2002)

15. The course of the disease

The duration of reactive arthritis is considered to be chronic when it extends over 6 months (Braun et al. 2000). As many as 75% of ReA patients achieve complete remission within one year of the first symptoms and in 15% of patients the disease becomes a chronic spondyloarthropathy. The chronic ReA is induced by: Yersinia - 4%, Salmonella – 19%, Shigella – 19% and Chlamydia – 17% (Leirisalo-Repo et al. 1997, Leirisalo-Repo, 1998). Sacroiliitis is reported in 14-49% of patients, while 12% to 26% of patients with ReA develop ankylosing spondylitis (van der Linden, 2000). In patients with no negative prognostic features the course of the disease can lead to spontaneous recovery or is usually benign.

16. Prognosis

The course of the reactive arthritis depends on the type of inducing bacteria, the presence of HLA-B27 antigen, gender and recurrence of arthritis. The worst prognosis is in Chlamydia induced reactive arthritis. Recovery occurs only in 30% of cases, joint pain persists in 68% of patients, recurrent arthritis occurs in 68% of patients, changes in the sacroiliiac joints are found in 49% of patients and 26% of patients develop AS - ankylosing spondylitis (Leirisalo-repo 1998, Inman 2000). Patients with HLA-B27 antigen presence have more severe course of the disease, more frequently sacroiliac joints are involved and more frequently the disease manifests itself in other organs. Male gender, positive family history of occurrence of spondyloarthropathies (including AS) and the presence of inflammation of the hip are also negative prognostic factors. In these patients the inflammation of the spine, destructive changes in the hip and the involvement of sacroiliac joints are frequent. In the first 2 years of the disease an elevated ESR (> 30 mm after 1 h), the lack of improvement after non-steroidal anti-inflammatory drugs, inflammation of the hip, reduction in spinal mobility, the occurrence of "sausage finger" in the feet, inflammation of several joints and the onset of the disease before the age of 16 – all are considered to be negative prognostic factors (Kelley et al. 2001).

Patients with eye involvement in chronic ReA may develop ocular complications such as: secondary cataract and glaucoma, cystoid macular oedema (CMO), impairment of visual function (to the extent of the complete blindness).

17. Treatment

17.1 Treatment of extraarticular changes

The extraarticular changes should be treated in parallel with general treatment of the disease carried out by the specialists in proper field of medicine.

17.1.1 Ocular symptoms

Aims of treatment include: pain relief and easing photophobia, elimination of inflammation, prevention of complications and preservation of proper visual function (Agrawal, 2010). Conjunctivitis in reactive arthritis should be treated with locally administered antibiotics. In Chlamydia infection the local antibiotic therapy should be simultaneous with general antibiotic therapy. It is recommended to use topical 1% azithromycyn in drops 2 - 3 times daily for 2 - 3 weeks or 0.5% erythromycin ointment 3-3 times daily for 2-3 weeks. Tetracycline and quinolones can also be used locally (Chen et al. 2010).

In anterior uveitis it is recommended to use corticosteroids locally in the form of eye drops or periocular injections or systemic administration, the latter in severe cases. Systemic Glucocorticosteroids can be used in the cases when the local treatment of uveitis is not sufficient or the diseases is recurrent and bilateral. In intermediate and posterior uveitis corticosteroids in subtenon's injection may be administered.

Drugs extending pupils (mydriatics) are recommended as well to relieve pain and prevent posterior synechiae. In the case of the eye being affected in the course of the ReA, it is sometimes necessary not only to use glucocorticosteroides and non-steroidal anti-inflammatory drugs (NSAIDs), but also immunosuppressive agents like methotrexate , cyclosporine, azathiopryne . Immunosuppessive therapy is recommended in cases resistant to corticosteroids. In complications of uveitis e.g. cataract a surgery treatment should be considered. In cases of uveitis associated glaucoma the local or systemic antiglaucoma medications are used.

In CMO the local administration of NSAIDs or corticoids in posterior subtenon's injections may be employed.

The lack of response to uveitis therapy implies that we might be dealing with the masquerade syndromes of diseases such as leukemia, lymphoma, retinoblastoma, malignant melanoma, antiphospholipid syndrome and thus these illnesses should be excluded.

17.1.2 Skin lesions

Skin lesions in the course of reactive arthritis can be treated locally with keratolytic agents (e.g. used locally with salicylates), corticosteroids or calcipotriol in the form of cream or ointment. Balanitis circinata may be treated with corticosteroids such as Hydrocortisone ointment.

17.2 Treatment of arthritis and tendon attachments

17.2.1 General recommendations for treatment of reactive arthritis

In patients with reactive arthritis the limitation of physical activity is recommended, especially walking in cases with lower limbs joints affected. It is important to use physio- and kinesitherapy, together with pharmacological treatment. The treatment of reactive arthritis should be based on reducing pain, anti-inflammatory treatment and – if possible – on the infection eradication.

17.2.2 Non-steroidal anti-inflammatory drugs

The use of NSAIDs is a basic therapy in the initial diagnostic period, while prolonged therapy with these drugs is recommended only in cases with persistent inflammation. 20-25% of patients with reactive arthritis do not feel improvement after non-steroidal anti-inflammatory drugs.

17.2.3 Glucocorticoids

The use of glucocorticoids is recommended intraarticularly only (after excluding purulent arthritis), with such administration reducing the symptoms of synovitis. Oral systemic glucocorticoid treatment may prolong the elimination of the infection, while it does not affect clinical and laboratory activity of the disease. There have been no studies so far assessing the indication for the use of steroids in high dose intravenous injections (pulses) in reactive arthritis.

17.2.4 Disease-modifying drugs

In case of ineffectiveness of NSAIDs in ReA the use of disease-modifying drugs is recommended. The most commonly used drugs in this group include sulfasalazine, methotrexate, azathioprine, cyclosporine, leflunomide.

The use of sulfasalazine in 2g/24 hours dose is very effective in reactive arthritis in case of concomitant mucositis.

Sulfasalazine presents some antibacterial activity as well (Egsmose et al. 1997), being quite effective and well tolerated (Clegg et al.1996). Comparative studies have demonstrated greater efficacy of sulfasalazine in the treatment of peripheral joint involvement in reactive arthritis than in the treatment of ReA axial involvement form (Clegg et al. 1999). Methotrexate treatment is also very effective in ReA, although there are no randomized studies to evaluate its effectiveness. It has been demonstrated however, that in patients with arthritis of the spine joints the methotrexate treatment prevents the emergence of the ossification of the spine and of the erosive lesions of peripheral joints (Ritchelin et al. 2001). Azathioprine, in dose of 1 - 2 mg / kg of body weight, is effective in the treatment of ReA with peripheral joint involvement (Calin1986).

17.2.5 Biological treatment

There are no randomized trials evaluating the efficacy and safety of biological agents of anti-TNF-alpha group in the treatment of ReA. Individual publications about etanercept and infliximab treatment in ReA point to high efficacy of these drugs (Abdelmoulaet al.2008, Gill et al. 2008, Schafranski 2009, Flagg et al.2005). The use of biological agents from the anti-TNF-alpha group is restricted to the chronic form of the disease, in which disease-modifying drugs were ineffective. Such restriction in use of agents result from the risk of extending the latent infection and Chlamydia and Yersinia, associated with the administration of these drugs.

17.2.6 Antibiotic therapy

The use of antibiotics in reactive arthritis still raises controversy. Eradication of bacteria causing reactive arthritis should improve prognosis or prevent the development of reactive arthritis. Studies have shown various effects of antibiotic use for ReA induced by genitourinary infections and different effects in Enterobacteriacae-induced ReA cases.

17.2.6.1 The use of antibiotics in Chlamydia-induced ReA

A study performed on the Greenland population, in which the high incidence of HLA-B27 antigen exists, showed that the use of antibiotics in genitourinary tract infections of patients with HLA B-27 antigen significantly reduces the number of patients who develop ReA - from 37% to 10% (Bardin, 1992). It was also shown that it is vital that the sexual partner of a person who has Chlamydia infection is treated in parallel with the patient. Another study documented the use of limecycline for 3 months in patients with acute Chlamydia-induced ReA, revealing a beneficial therapeutic effect on arthritis, with an ESR reduction and normalization of C reactive protein (CRP) levels in the group treated with antibiotic (Lauhio et al. 1991).

Good results of application of tetracycline or ciprofloxacin for a period from 4 to 12 weeks in acute Chlamydia-induced ReA were also reported (Schumacher et al. 1999). Recent in vitro studies showed high efficacy of using a combination of antibiotics (azithromycin + rifampicin) in eradicating Chlamydia infection (Dreses-Werringloer et al.2001), later confirmed in clinical studies performed with rifampicin and doxycycline (Carter et al. 2004). The therapy with rifampicin and azithromycin has been demonstrated in experimental studies to be very effective in the eradication of chronic Chlamydia pneumoniae infection (Bin et al. 2000). Eradication of Chlamydia infections affects the further course of chronic ReA, resulting in reducing inflammatory activity and pain. In some cases such treatment leads to complete remission.

17.2.6.2 The use of antibiotics in the Enterobacteriacae induced ReA

The use of antibiotics in the Enterobacteriaceae-induced ReA raises a lot of controversy. Many studies have shown no effect of antibiotic therapy used in acute or chronic ReA on the course of the disease (Sieper et al. 1999, Toivanen 2000, Yli-Kerttula, 2000). On the other hand 4-7 year-long observations of patients with Enterobacteriacae induced ReA treated with three-months course of ciprofloxacin revealed the influence of the therapy on the distant course of ReA, particularly in patients with HLA B-27 antigen and may prevent the development of chronic ReA (Yli-Kerttula, 2003). However, this requires further research.

18. References

Abdelmoula LC, Yahia CB, Testouri N, et al. 2008. Treatment of reactive arthritis with infliximab. Tunis Med. Dec 86(12):1095-1097.

Agrawal RV, Murthy S et al Current approach in diagnosis and management of anterior uveitis. 2010 Indian Journal of Ophtalmology 58(1):11-19

Bardin T., Enel C., Cornelis F. et al. 1992. Antibiotic treatment of veneral disease and Reiter's syndrome in a Greenland population. Arthritis Rheum. 35: 190-194.

Bas S., Vischer TL. 1998. Chlamydia trachomatis antibody detection and diagnosis of reactive arthritis. Br J Rheumatol. 37: 1054-1959.

Bin XX., Wolf C., Schaffner T. et al. 2000. Effect of Azithromycin plus Rifampin versus Amoxicillin Alone on Eradycation and Inflammation in the Chronic Course of Chlamydia pneumoniae pneumonitis in Mice. Antimicrob Agents Chemother. 44 (6): 1761-1764.

Braun J., Kingsley D., van der Heijde et al. 2000. On the difficult of establishing a consensus on the definition of and diagnostic investigations for reactive arthritis. Results and discussion of a quesyionaire prepared for the 4th International Workshop on Reactive Arthritis, Berlin, Germany, July 3-6.1999. J. Rheumatol. 27: 2185-2192.

Calin A. 1986. A placebo controlled, crossover study of azathioprine in Reiter's syndrome. Ann Rheum Dis. 45(8): 653-655.

Carter JD., Valeriano J., Vasey FB. 2004. A prospective, randomized 9-month comparison of doxycycline and fifampin in undifferentiated spondyloerthritis – with special reference to Chlamydia-induced arthritis. J Rheumatol. 31(10): 1973-1980.

Chen Y-M., Hu F-R., Hou Y-C. 2010. Effect of oral azithromycin in the treatment of chlamydial conjunctivitis. Eye. 24: 985-989.

Clegg D.O., Reda D.J., Weisman M.H. et al. 1996. Comparison of sulphasalazine and placebo in the treatment of reactive arthritis (Reiter's syndrome): a Department of Veterans Affairs cooperative study. Arthritis Rheum. 39: 2021-2027.

Clegg D.O., Reda D.J., Abdellatif M. 1999. Comparison of sulfasalazine and placebo for the treatment of axial and peripheral articular manifestation of the seronegative spondyloarthropathies. Arthritis Rheum. 42: 2325-2329.

Colmegna I., Cuchacovich R., Espinoza LR. 2004. HLA-B27-Associated Reactive Arthritis: Pathogenetic and Clinical Considerations. Clinical, Microbiology Reviews.17(2): 348-369.

Cuvelier C, Barbatis C, Mielants H, et al. 1987.Histopathology of intestinal inflammation related to reactive arthritis. Gut. 28(4): 394-401.

Dean D., Kandel RP., Adhikari HK et al. 2008. Multiple Chlamydiaceae Species in Trachoma: Implications for Disease Pathogenesis and Control. PLoS Medicine. 5(1): 57-68.

Deer T., Rosencrance G., Chillag S. 1991. Cardiac conduction manifestations of Reiter's syndrome. South. Med. J. 84: 799-800.

De Smet MD., Yamamoto JH., Mochizuki M, et al. 1990. Cellular immune responses of patients with uveitis to retinal antigens and their fragments. Am J Ophtalmol. 15; 110(2): 135-142.

Dreses-Werringloer U., Padubrin I., Zeidler H. et al. 2001. Effects of azithromycin and rifampin on Chlamydia trachomatis infection in vitro. Antimicrob Agents Chemother. 45(11): 3001-3008.

Egsmose C., Hansen T.M., Andersen L.S. et al. 1997. Limited effect of sulphasalazine treatment in reactive aryhritis: a randomized double blind placebo controlled trial. Ann. Rheum. Dis. 56: 32-36.

Enzenauer RJ 2002 Autoimmune eye and ear disorders. Rheumatology secrets 2nd ed Hanley& Belfus inc. Philadelphia 79: 527-537

Fendler C., Laitko S., Sorensen G. et al. 2000. Frequency of triggering bacteria in patients with reactive arthritis and undifferentiated oligoarthritis and the relative importance of the tests used for diagnosis. Ann Rheum. Dis. 60: 337-343.

Flagg SD., Meador R., Hsia E. et al. 2005. Decreased pain and synovial inflammation after etanercept therapy in patients with reactive and undifferentiated arthritis: an open-label trial. Arthritis Rheum. 53(4): 613-617.

Gaston JS., Cox C., Granfors K.1999. Clinical and experimental evidence for persistent Yersinia infection in reactive arthritis. Arthritis Rheum. 42: 2239-2242.

Gérard HC., Stanich JA., Whittum-Hudson JA. et al. 2010. Patients with Chlamydia-associated arthritis have okular (trachoma), not genital, serowar of C. trachomatis in synovial tissue. Microb Pathog. 48(2): 62-68.

Gérard HC., Whittum-Hudson JA., Carter JD et al. 2010. The pathogenic role of Chlamydia in spondyloarthritis. Curr Opin Rheumatol. 22 (4): 363-367.

Gérard HC., Branigan PJ., Schumacher HR et al. 1998. Synovial Chlamydia trachomatis in patients with reactive arthritis/Reiter's syndrome are viable but show aberrant gene expression. 25: 734-742.

Gill H, Majithia V. 2008. Successful use of infliximab in the treatment of Reiter's syndrome: a case report and discussion. Clin Rheumatol. 27(1):121-123.

Granfors K., Merilahti-Palo R., Luukkainen R. et al. 1998. Persistence of Yersinia antigens in peripheral blood cells from patients with Yersinia enterocilitica):3 infection with ot without reactive arthritis. Arthritis Rheum. 41: 855-862.

Granfors K., Viljanen M., Tiilikainen A et al. 1980. Persistance of IgM, IgG and IgA antibodies to Yersinia in Yersinia arthritis. J. Infect. Dis. 141: 432-429.

Inman R.D., Whittum-Hudson J.A., Schumacher H.R. et al. 2000. Chlamydia and associated arthritis. Curr. Opin. Rheumatol. 12: 254-262.

Kelley W.N., Ruddy S., Harris E.D. 2001. Kelley's textbook of rheumatology, 6th ed. The W.B. Saunders Co., Philadelphia, Pa.

Keyan Y., Rimar D. 2008. Reactive Arthritis – The Appropriate Name. IMAJ. 10:256-258

Kiss S., Letko E., Qamruddin S et al. 2003. Long-term progression. Prognosis, and treatment off patients with recurrent ocular manifestation of Reiter's syndrome. Ophtalmology. 110(9): 1764-1769.

Kuipers JG., Jurgens-Saathoff B., Bialowons A et al. 1998. Detection of Chlamydia trachomatis in peripheral blood leukocytes of reactive arthritis patients by polymerase chain reaction. Arthritis Rheum. 41: 1894-1895.

Lauhio A., Leirisalo-Repo M., Lahdevirta J. et al. 1991. Double-blind, placebo controlled study of free month treatment with limecycline in reactive arthritis, with special reference to Chlamydia arthritis. Arthritis Rheum. 34: 6-14.

Leirisalo-Repo M. Helenius T., Hannu T et al. 1997. Long-term prognosis of reactive Salmonella arthritis. Ann. Rheum. Dis. 56: 516-520.

Leirisalo-Repo M. 1998. Prognosis, course of disease and treatment of the spondyloarthropaties. Rheum.Dis. Clin. North. Am. 24: 737-753.

Leirisalo-Repo. 1998. Therapeutic aspects of spondyloarthropaties – a review. Scan. J. Rheumatol. 27: 323-328.

Locht H., Krogfeld KA. 2002. Comparison of rheumatological and gastrointenstinal symptoms after infection with Campylobacter jejuniu/coli and enteroxigenic Escherichia coli. Ann Rheum Dis. 61: 448-452.

Maki-Ikola O., Leirisalo-Repo M., Kantele P. et al. 1991. Salmonella-specific antibodies In reactive arthritis. J. Infect. Dis. 164: 141-148.

Nicholis A. 1975. Reiter's disease and HLA B27. Ann Rheum Dis. 34 (suppl): 27-8.

Purcell JJ., Tsai CC., Baldassare AE. 1982. Conjunctival Immunopathologic and Ultrastructural Alterations. Arch Ophtalmol.100: 1618-1621.

Ritchelin C.T., Daikh B.E. 2001. Recent advances in the treatment of seronegative spondyloarthropathies. Curr. Rheumatol. Rep. 3: 299-403.

Sawhney MPS, Parihar JKS.2006 Macular degeneration in a case of Reiter's disease Indian J Dermatol Venereol Leprol 72: 227-230

Schafranski MD. 2009. Infliximab for reactive arthritis secondary to Chlamydia trachomatis infection. Rheumatol Int. 30(5): 679-680.

Schumacher H.R., Arayssi Jr.S., Crane M. et al. 1999. Chlamydia trachomatis nucleic acids can be found in thesynovium of some asymptomatic subject. Arthritis Rheum. 42: 1281-1282.

Sieper J., Braun J. 1999. Problems and advances in the diagnostic of reactive arthritis. J. Rheumatol.26: 1222-1224.

Sieper J.,Fendler S., Laitko S. et al. 1999. No benefit of long-term ciprofloxacin treatment in patients with reactive arthritis and undifferentiated oligoarthritis. Arthritis Rheum. 42: 1386-1396.

Sieper J., Rudwaleit M., Braun J et al. 2002. Diagnosing Reactive Arthritis. Arthritis & Rheumatism. 46(2): 319-327.

Singh AK., Misra R., Aggarwal A. 2011. Th-17 associated cytokines in patients with reactive arthritis/undifferentiated spondyloarthropathy. Clin Rheumatol. 30(6):771-776.

Shimamoto Y, Sugiyama H, Hirohata S. 2000 Reiter's syndrome associated with HLA B 51. Internal Medicine . 39(2): 182-4

Raymond J. Enzenauer Autoimmune eye and ear disorders 2002 Rheumatology Secrets 2 ed. Hanley&Belfus, INC Philadelphia 527-537

Toivanen P. 2000. Managing reactive arthritis. Rheumatology. 39:117-121.

van der Linden S., van der Heijde D. 2000. Clinical aspects, outcome assessment, and management of ankylosing spondylitis and postenteric reactive arthritis. Curr. Opi. Rheumatol. 12: 263-268.

Wilbanks GA, Mammolenti M,Streilein JW. 1991 Studies on the induction of anterior chamber-associated immune deviation (ACAID). II. Eye-derived cells participate in generating blood-borne signals that induce ACAID The Journal of Immunology, 146 (9): 3018-3024

Willkens RF., Arnett FC., Bitter T. et al. 1981. Reiter's sundrome: evaluation of preliminary criteria for definite disease. Arthritis Rheum. 24: 844-849.

Yin Z., Braun J., Neure L. et al. 1997. Crucial role of interleukin-10/interleukin-12 balance in the regulation of the type 2 T helper cytokine response in reactive arthritis. Arthritis Rheum. 40: 1788-1797.

Yli-Kerttula T., Luukkainen R., Yli-Kerttula U. et al. 2000. Effect of a three month course of ciprofloxacin on the outcome of reactive arthritis. Ann. Rheum. Dis. 59: 656-570.

Yli-Kerttula T., Luukkainen R., Yli-Kerttula U. 2003. Effect of a three month course of ciprofloxacin on the late prognosis of reactive arthritis. Ann. Rheum. Dis. 62: 880-884.

Zeidler H., Kuipers J., Kohler L. 2004. Chlamydia- induced arthritis. Curr Opin Rhaumatol. 16: 380-392.

13

Thelazia Species and Conjunctivitis

Soraya Naem
Urmia University
Iran

1. Introduction

Thelazia nematodes (Spirurida: Thelazioidea), are commonly known as eyeworms and cause ocular infections in animals and humans (Anderson 2000; Soulsby 1986). This genus of spirurids represents one of the most specific taxon among nematodes because of its very close relationship with its intermediate and final hosts (Otranto and Traversa 2005). *Thelazia* Bosc, 1819 should be considered an "endoparasite". However, the immature and mature stages occur in the anterior chamber of the eye, thereby being exposed to the external environment. Therefore, it could be considered an "ectoparasite". The sixteen species of this genus have been reported from canids, felids, ruminants, equids and humans (Skrjabin et al. 1971; Yamaguti 1961). They have been documented in Europe (Italy, France, Switzerland and Germany), Asia (China, Japan, Korea and Taiwan), North America (Canada and U.S.A.), South America (Peru) and South Africa. The adult worms live under the eyelids, nictitating membranes and lacrimal ducts. However, they are also found in the nose and pharynx. They are milky-white worms, with males measuring up to 12 mm in length and females up to 18 mm in length. The numbers of pre-cloacal and post-cloacal papillae in males differ among species. Usually, the spicules are unequal. Also, the location of the vaginal opening and the number of cuticular transverse striations differ among species. The worms are viviparous, and the first-stage larvae are passed by females into the lachrymal secretions where they are ingested by non-biting Diptera flies. Larval development takes place in the thorax and abdomen of the vector, and infective stages are present in 18–25 days. Development to the adult stage takes place without migration, and the prepatent period is between 3 and 6 weeks. The first stage larva of *Thelazia* is very short-lived in the lachrymal secretions, only surviving a few hours, and transmission depends upon the continuous presence of the vectors. For this reason, thelaziasis has a seasonal occurrence according to the seasonality of the intermediate hosts (Dunn 1978). The two species known to cause human thelaziasis are *T. callipaeda* and *T. californiensis. T. callipaeda* is commonly found in humans and animals (dogs, cats, foxes, wolves and rabbits) in the former Soviet Union, China, South Korea, Japan, Indonesia, Thailand Taiwan, and India (Anderson 2000), while *T. californiensis* is found in the United States (YJ Yang et al. 2006). Although human ocular parasitic infestation is rare, additional case studies are needed to fully understand the route of infestation and pathogenic mechanism. In final hosts, both the larval stages and adults of *Thelazia* spp. cause clinical signs such as excessive lacrimation, epiphora, conjunctivitis, keratitis and corneal ulcers (Hong et al. 1995; Kim, 2010; Otranto and Dutto, 2008; Singh and Singh 1993; CH Yang et al. 2005). A definitive diagnosis is made by the detection of the parasites in the conjunctival sac. Examination of lacrimal secretions may reveal eggs or first-stage larvae. Also, morphological differentiation has been done on some *Thelazia* species using scanning electron microscopy (WY Choi et al. 1989; Naem 2005, 2007a,b,c). Molecular characterization and phylogeny of some *Thelazia* species have been studied by Nadler et al. (2007), Otranto et al. (2001, 2005b), and Traversa et al. (2005). Due to the localization of the nematode, thelaziasis can be treated topically by direct application of drugs into the eyes. Removal of the adult parasites with fine forceps, using local anasthesia, is also helpful. Patients with an intraocular infestation with *T. callipaeda* have been successfully treated with a pars plana vitrectomy. Michalski (1976) found that two ml of levamisole injected into the subconjunctival sac was more effective than levamisole given orally. Treatment of dog thelaziasis, caused by *T. callipaeda,* using a topical formulation of 10% imidacloprid and 2.5% moxidectin has been studied by Bianciardi and Otranto (2005). Also, the prophylactic use of a monthly treatment with milemycin oxime showed a 90% efficacy against *T. callipaeda* in naturally exposed dogs (Ferroglio et al., 2008). In this chapter, both human and animal thelaziasis will be discussed.

2. Etiologic agent: *Thelazia* Bosc, 1819

Thelazia Bosc is parasite of the conjunctival sac or lacrimal ducts of mammals and birds. The presence of the nematodes in these particular sites is usually sufficient for a generic diagnosis. The adult worms are small, thin and milky-white in color. Females measure up to 20 mm in length, and males measure up to 12 mm in length. The mouth has no lips and the anterior border of the buccal cavity is everted and divided by indentations into six festoons, of which four appear to be occupied by a small refractile papilliform organ. There are two lateral and four submedian cephalic papillae. The body may be transversely striated. The male's tail is blunt, and has no caudal alae. There are many pre-cloacal papillae, one of which is unpaired and located in front of the anal pore and three or four pairs are post-cloacal. The spicules are unequal. The posterior end of the female is bluntly rounded, with a pair of lateral papillae near its end. The females are larviparous or viviparous and the vulva is in the esophageal region (Dunn 1978; Soulsby 1986). *Thelazia* species found in canids, felids, ruminants, equids, birds, and humans (Anderson 2000; Skrjabin et al. 1971; Yamaguti 1961).

3. Human thelaziasis

Very few cases of human thelaziasis are reported worldwide. There are two species of the genus *Thelazia* that have been found in the human eye,*Thelazia callipaeda* (Railliet and Henry 1910) and, more rarely, *Thelazia californiensis* (Price 1930). The former species occurs under the nictitating membrane of the eye in canids, cats, rabbits, rats, monkeys and, rarely, humans in China, Japan, India, Burma, Korea, Taiwan, Thailand, Indonesia, Russia, Italy, Switzerland, Germany, and France (Anderson 2000; Otranto and Eberhard 2011; Ruytoor et al. 2010; YJ Yang et al. 2006). *T. californiensis* is mainly a parasite of dogs, but it has also been reported in sheep, deer, coyotes, cats, bears, and rarely humans in western North America. Most ocular *T. californiensis* infestations in humans have occurred in California, particularly in the Sierra Nevada Mountains. However, this worm's habitat is also located within areas of New Mexico, Nevada, Arizona and Oregon (Anderson 2000; Levine 1968).

3.1 *Thelazia callipaeda* and *T. californiensis*

3.1.1 Morphology

T. callipaeda is nicknamed the "oriental eyeworm" because of its widespread prevalence in the Far East. Adult worms look like creamy white threads. Light and scanning electron microscopy have been used to study the surface of adult worms of this nematode (Arizono et al. 1976; DK Choi and Choi 1979; WY Choi et al. 1989; Kagei et al. 1983; Min and Chun 1988; Miyazaki 1991). The morphological identification of *T. callipaeda* has been reviewed by Otranto et al. (2003a). In both sexes, the mouth opening has a hexagonal profile. The internal margins of the buccal capsule are everted and subdivided by excavations into 6 festoons. SEM observations on the female *T. callipaeda* showed only one pocket-shaped amphid at the anterior end (WY Choi et al. 1989). On the mouth opening of male *T. callipaeda,* two large head papillae were observed, which were absent in the females and were distinct from the cephalic papillae in both their morphology and orientation (WY Choi et al. 1989). Adult female *T. callipaeda* measure 12–18.5 mm in length and 370–510 mm in width. The vulva, which has a short flap, is located in the anterior region of the body, whereas the anal opening is 70–102 mm from the caudal end. The vagina opens at 62.0–162.2 mm (mean 108.7 619.6 mm) anterior to the esophagus–intestinal junction. Two phasmids are present on the tip of the tail. The number of cuticular transverse striations was 400~650/mm on the head region, 250/mm on the middle region and 300~350/mm on the tail region. *T. callipaeda* is ovoviviparous rather than viviparous (Hong et al. 1988; Nagada 1964). Adult *T. callipaeda* males measure 7.7–12.8 mm in length and 338–428 mm in width at the mid-portion of the body. The caudal end is ventrally curved, without caudal alae. There are 15 pairs of papillae on the ventral surface of the caudal end, 10 of which are pre-cloacal and 5 post-cloacal. The first 3 of the 5 post-cloacal pairs are situated behind the cloaca near the anus, 1 pair in the middle, and another pair in the posterior–terminal position. The two dissimilar spicules are characterized by the well-defined shape of the anterior extremity of the longer left spicule and the typical crescent shape of the shorter right spicule (Otranto et al. 2003a).

T. californiensis can infect humans and cause ocular thelaziasis. The females are 12-18.8 mm long, with a vulva 800-1000 μ from the anterior end. The eggs in vitro are 51 by 29 μ, and are embryonated when laid. The males are 7.7-13 mm long, with unequal spicules 1.5-1.7 mm and 150-187 μ long, respectively. A small gubernaculum may or may not present (Levine 1968). Also, 6-7 pairs of pre-cloacal papillae are seen at the posterior end of the male worm. *T. californiensis* is different morphologically from *T. callipaeda* based on the numbers of pre- and post-cloacal papillae in the male and the position of the vulva in the female (Bhaibulaya et al. 1970).

3.1.2 Life cycle

T. callipaeda was originally reported from Asian countries (Bhaibulaya et al. 1770; Shi et al. 1988), where human infections with this nematode are considered to be emerging over the last two decades, particularly in poor rural communities (JL Shen et al. 2006). *T. callipaeda* requires a vector which also acts as an intermediate host to accomplish its life cycle (Otranto et al. 2006a). Species of the dipteran family Drosophilidae (fruit flies, subfamily Steganinae) have been incriminated as vectors. *Amiota variegata,* recently taxonomically reclassified as *Phortica variegata* (Maca 1977), was first identified as the intermediate host and vector. However, *A. okadai* is also considered to be a vector of this parasite in China (summarized in Ortanto et al. 2006a). *Phortica* spp. and, to a lesser extent, *Amiota* spp. display a zoophilic behavior , i.e. they feed on ocular secretions of animals and humans in addition to feeding on fruits and on fermenting tree sap (Bachli et al. 2005). Interestingly, only males of *P. variegata* were found to be infected with *T. callipaeda* under natural conditions in Italy (Otranto et al. 2006a,b), whereas both male and female flies were positive in dissection and/or molecular assays under experimental conditions (Otranto et al. 2003c) (Fig. 1). An efficient method for trapping high numbers of such drosophilid flies under natural conditions and determining the presence and the population dynamics of *Phortica* and *Amiota* spp. in Switzerland was designed by Roggero et al. (2010). In this metheod, a large polyethylene terephthalate (PET) container was used, oriented horizontally, with a single aperture covered by a net (mesh 0.4 mm) and narrowing through a funnel towards the brighter side of the trap. The traps were installed close to each other (maximum distance 40 cm). All traps were baited with sliced fresh apples and peeled bananas, the bait being changed once per week, after collection of the flies. In another study which was carried out by Ortanto et al. (2005a), the results clearly suggested that *Musca domestica* is not a vector of *T. callipaeda* under experimental or natural conditions. Also, local transmission of *T. callipaeda* in southern Germany was investigated by Magnis et al. in 2010. Transmission of *T. callipaeda* occurs when the intermediate host and vector *P. variegata* feeds on lachrymal secretions from an infected animal and/or human and ingests *T. callipaeda* first stage larvae (L1) produced by adult female nematodes in the conjunctival sac of the final host. First stage larvae penetrate the gut wall in a few hours. They remain in the abdominal haemocoel for about 2 days. On the third day, larvae invade the fat body of the female and the testes of the male, where they subsequently become encapsulate, grow and moult twice to third stage larvae ~ 14-21 days after infection. After migrating through the body cavity of the vector, the L3s of *T. callipaeda* emerge from the labella of infected flies, after which they feed on the lachrymal secretions from infected hosts and develop into the adult stage in the conjunctical sac and prebulbar tear film within ~ 35 days (Otranto et al. 2005c). The existence of a seasonal periodicity in the reproductive cycle of female nematodes, coinciding with the presence/absence of the vector/s, has been demonstrated by Otranto et al. (2004).

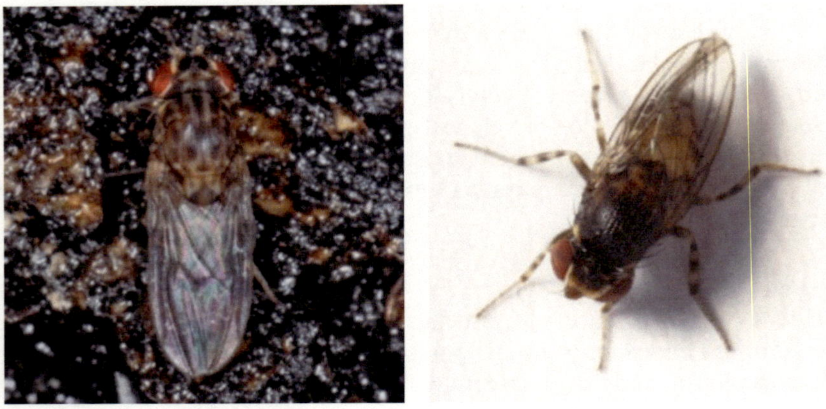

Fig. 1. *Phortica variegata*, female (Left), *Phortica variegata*, male (Right), (Courtesy Jorge Almeida, Viseu , Portugal).

Adult *T. californiensis are* commonly found in the tear ducts and conjunctival sacs of its hosts. Burnett et al. (1957) allowed laboratory-reared flies to feed on the sheathed larvae and discovered developmental stages in *Fannia canicularis* (Fig. 2). Similar larvae were found in wild-caught *F. benjamini* collected in an enzootic area in California.

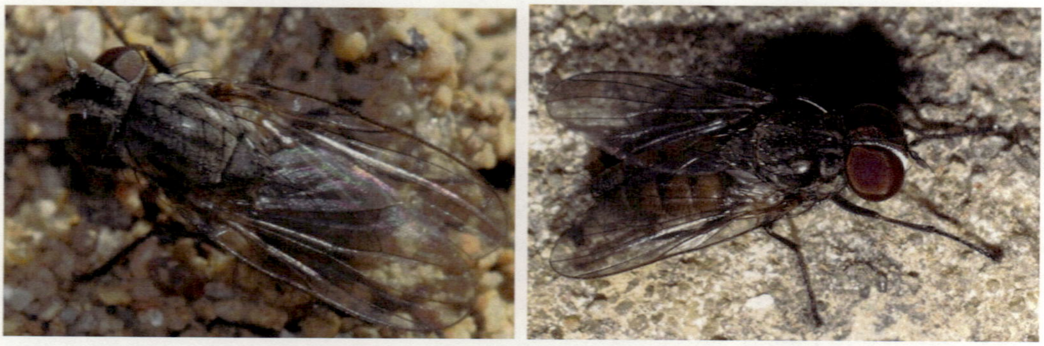

Fig. 2. *Fannia canicularis*, female (Left), *Fannia canicularis*, male (Right) , (Courtesy Nikita E. Vikhrev, Moscow, Russia).

3.1.3 Epidemiology

T. callipaeda is prevalent in dogs, cats, and humans in the former Soviet Union and in countries of the Far East, including China, Korea, Myanmar, Japan, Indonesia, Thailand, Taiwan, and India. The parasite's distribution explains the use of the name, oriental eyeworm (Anderson 2000). However, the main final reservoir hosts of *T. callipaeda* seem to be farm dogs, as they often live in areas populated by a large hematophagous fauna. In an investigation carried out by Seo et al. (2002) in Korea, military dogs were found to be acting as reservoir hosts. Experimentally implanted adult worms of *T. callipaeda* have adapted to dogs, rabbits, cats and monkeys but not to goats and sheep, perhaps due to their different susceptibilities (Faust 1928).

The climate of the countries in which *T. callipaeda* has been reported varies from tropical (e.g. Indonesia) and subtropical (e.g. Japan) in the Far East, to temperate in the Russian Federation. In a study which was carried out in two distinct areas of Italy (the Piedmont region, North Western Italy and the Basilicata region, Southern Italy), dogs, cats and foxes were examined. *T. callipaeda* has been reported with high prevalence in dogs (60%), and foxes (49.3%) in southern Italy (Otranto et al. 2003b). The oropraphy of the Basilicata region is characterized by the presence of a ring of sandstone mountains surrounding a woodlands bordering the study municipalities. These results confirm the hypothesis that the vectors of *T. callipaeda* need a mountainous environment for their survival and biological cycle, and the high prevalence in dogs and foxes indicates that *T. callipaeda* infection is hyper-endemic in this area (site B). Of the dogs examined from site A, 23.07% were found to be infected with eyeworms (Otranto et al. 2003b). Cats are less frequently in contact with the vector (i.e. dipteran flies), moreover it may be assumed that reports of thelaziosis from practitioners are rare due to difficulties in inspecting cats' eyes (Otranto et al. 2003b).

Canine thelaziasis has also been reported in France and Germany (Chermette et al. 2004; Hermosilla et al. 2004). In southern Switzerland (Ticino), the first case of *T. callipaeda* in a dog was detected in 2000 (Malacrida et al. 2008). *Thelazia* infection was also diagnosed in 5.6% of foxes shot in Ticino during the winter of 2005-2006. Affected foxes, dogs and cats originated from the same regions. The cats and 57.9% of the infected dogs had never crossed the Swiss border. In addition, five cats with thelaziasis were registered. Infected animals harbored 1-23 eye worms. The most common symptoms were conjuctivitis and epiphora, while keratitis was present only in a few animals. Young and small sized dogs were significantly less involved than larger dogs over 3 years of age (Malacrida et al. 2008). There is little information on the role of wild carnivores as hosts of this nematode. Otranto et al. (2009) reported, for the first time, the infection of beech martens, wildcats, and brown hares by *T. callipaeda*. In addition, the retrieval of *T. callipaeda* in one of two wolves examined supported the previous report of nematodes in this animal species (Otranto et al. 2007). The finding of adult worms of *T. callipaeda* in the eyes of wildlife species indicates their competence as final hosts of this parasite, since it implies that third stage larvae, released by the intermediate host, developed to adults in their ocular cavity. From a parasitological viewpoint, these results are interesting because *T. callipaeda* has the broadest spectrum of final hosts among *Thelazia* species, while *T. lacrymalis* parasitizes only horses and *T. rhodesi* and *T. gulosa* mainly infect cattle (Anderson 2000).

The eyeworm,*T. californiensis* is confined to the Western United States (Dozie et al. 1996; Skrjabin et al. 1971; Soulsby 1965). It is a parasite of dogs and can infect cats, foxes, coyotes, sheep, deer, horses, rabbits and black bears. Humans can become infected, but it is extremely rare and thought to be accidental.

Both *T. callipaeda* and *T. californiensis* are responsible for human thelaziasis. The first report of human thelaziasis was from Beijing, China, where adult nematodes were removed from the eyes of a man (Stuckey 1917). In subsequent years, the number of human thelaziasis cases has increased in China (Chen and Zhang 1954), the Soviet Union (Miroshnichenko et al. 1988), Indonesia (Kosin et al. 1989), Thailand (Bhaibulaya et al. 1970; Yospaiboon et al. 1989), India (Singh and Singh 1993), Taiwan (Cheung et al. 1998; YJ Yang et al. 2006), Japan (Koyama et al., 2000), and Korea (Min et al. 2002; Youn 2009). Human thelaziasis occurs mostly in rural communities with poor living and socioeconomic standards, and mainly affects children and the elderly. It seems that the prevalence and relevance of human thelaziasis have increased in China in the last 2 decades. By October 2005, a total of 371 human cases were reported from different provinces in China (JL Shen et al. 2006). Epidemiological investigations of 179 human cases in China revealed that 51% of cases were females and 49% of cases were males; the majority of individuals were children less than 6 years of age (64.2%) (Jiang et al. 1991). The remainder was comprised of young people between 7 and 18 years of age (7.8%) and adults of >19 (19.0%) years of age; host age was not reported for 9.0% of the samples. The ocular infection was unilateral in 88.1% of patients. Furthermore, the parasites were detected in the anterior eye chamber in 4 patients from the provinces of Anhui, Jiangsu, and Guangxi, and in the vitreous body and on the retina in 1 patient from Sichuan province (CC Chen and Zhang 1954; YJ Wang et al. 2002). In China, cases of human thelaziasis have been reported mainly in rural areas (ZX Wang et al. 2002a), particularly where domestic dogs and other animals, for example, cats and foxes, are heavily infected (ZX Wang et al. 2002b; ZX Wang et al. 2003). For instance, the prevalence of thelaziosis in dogs in Guanghua county, Hubei province, was 95%, with as many as 52 nematodes recovered from a single dog. In Anhui province, more than 190 nematodes were isolated from a single dog (ZX Wang et al. 1998). Recently, human thelaziasis has been reported from China by W Chen (2010). Meanwhile, most clinical reports have been published in Chinese, Russian or Korean and have not been accessible to a large part of the international scientific community (JL Shen et al. 2006).

In 2008, Otranto and Dutto reported human infection by *T. callipaeda* in Italy and France in the same area where canine thelaziasis had already been reported. From a clinical viewpoint, these infections indicate the importance of this parasitic disease in differential diagnoses from bacterial or allergic conjunctivitis. All cases of human thelaziasis were reported during the summer months, which is the period of *T. callipaeda* vector activity (Otranto et al. 2006a,b). Also, concurrence of human thelaziasis and allergic conjunctivitis (e.g. caused by pollens) in the spring and summer seasons may impair correct etiologic diagnosis of this disease (Otranto and Dutto 2008).

3.1.4 Pathogenesis and clinical signs

Human infections with *T. callipaeda* have received little attention, despite the high prevalence recorded in some Asiatic countries (reviewed in JL Shen et al. 2006), and human infections by *T. californiensis* have only been reported occasionally in the USA (Doezie et al. 1996). To our knowledge, with the exception of Japan, 157 cases have been reported worldwide (China, 124; Korea, 24; Thailand, 5; India, 2; Russia and Indonesia, 1 each). In Japan, approximately 100 cases have been reported, mostly (66 cases) in western regions, and especially in Kyushu (Koyama et al. 2000).

One human case, reported by Howard (1927), in which larvae of *T. callipaeda*, in an advanced stage of development, was found in a papilloma of the skin of the lower right eyelid near the internal canthus, may possibly have a bearing on the early stage of the mature infective larvae of this species present in mammalian infections. The patient, from whom the papilloma was excised, gave a history of having played with a pet dog which had an irritation of both eyes, although "eye worms" were not actually observed in the dog. There was no evidence that the patient himself had ever been parasitized by adult *Thelazia*. The papilloma, which had been present for many years, developed a persistent itching several months prior to Dr. Howard's examination of the case. The patient was conscious of having frequently rubbed the wart during the period when the dog was being played with. Scratching resulted in the development of an indurated scab-like encrustation around the lesion. Microscopic slides of the excised papilloma, showing the worms in position in the tissue, were referred for diagnosis. The nematodes were directed head-inward into pockets produced by the infolding of the epithelium, or had migrated into the ducts of the sebaceous glands. In another case, the epithelial folds were strongly cornified and the tissue just beneath the epithelium was characterized by a marked lymphocytic infiltration. Two or more worms were found in each focus (Faust 1928; Faust et al. 1975).

In an experimental infection conducted by ZX Wang and Yang (1985) the clinical signs induced by thelaziasis were studied and it was demonstrated that adult parasites transplanted into the eyes of rabbits induced an inflammatory reaction within 3– 5 hr. Swelling of the eyelids, congestion of the conjunctiva, and yellow secretions from affected eyes indicated a purulent inflammation; the extent of symptoms gradually decreased after 1 wk of infection. The results of another study showed that heavy experimental infection (with 40–50 worms) led to blindness in 3 of 20 rabbits, as a consequence of leukoma (ZX Wang et al. 2002b; ZX Wang et al. 2006).

The most common clinical manifestations in natural infections are mild conjunctivitis, follicular hypertrophy of the conjunctiva, excessive lachrimation, ocular secretions, itchiness, congestion, swelling, hypersensitivity to light, and keratitis, depending on the number of nematodes present in the eye, their location, and the host response (ZX Wang and Yang, 1985; KC Wang et al. 1999). In some cases, patients show redness of the eye, discharge, photopsia, decreased vision and "floaters" within the eye chamber, a partially blocked field of vision, or even complete vision loss (Zakir et al. 1999). Follicles, ulcers, nubecula, swelling, paralysis of the eye muscles, ectropion, and papilloma, have also been reported in some patients (Ohira 2000). In addition, the presence of the nematodes causes infants to rub their eyes, and symptoms become more serious upon secondary infection with bacteria (*Pasteurella, Chlamydia,* and/or *Staphylococcus*). localization to the anterior chamber, the vitreous body, or the retina are often associated with the development of fibrous tissue, inducing more serious clinical manifestations, for example, black spots in the visual field, ocular congestion, and sometimes purulent exudation under the anterior chamber (CC Chen and Zhang, 1954; YJ Wang et al. 2002). Compared with the eye ball of the host, the adult worm is a fairly large, live foreign body. It is generally noticed at an early stage and usually examination of the patient reveals the adult and/or larval nematodes (Fig. 3), mostly in the conjunctival sac or medial or lateral canthus of the eye (JL Shen et al. 2006).

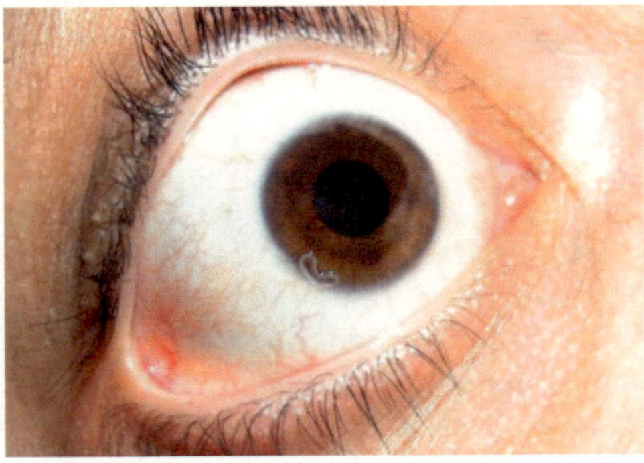

Fig. 3. Conjunctivitis in a human patient infected by adult *Thelazia callipaeda* (Courtesy Domenico Otranto, Bari, Italy).

In Taiwan, a 62-year-old woman presented with unilateral eye swelling and itching (YJ Yang et al. 2006). Subsequent examination showed *T. callipaeda* infection. Although this is a known form of ocular infection, especially in Asia, this is one of few reported cases in Taiwan.

In a study from Italy, a case of ocular thelaziasis was reported in a man living in Piedmont (northern Italy). The patient first complained of hyperlacrimation and conjunctivitis. After a series of treatments with eye drops, the nematode responsible for the symptomatology was identified (Dutto 2008). These parasites are rather rare in Italy especially in the north of the country. Otranto and Dutto (2008) reported *T. callipaeda* infection in 4 human patients in Italy and France in the same area where canine thelaziasis had been reported. The 4 male patients (37–65 years of age) lived in northwestern Italy and southeastern France, where infections had been reported in dogs, cats, and foxes (Dorchies et al. 2007; Rossi and Bertaglia 1989). All patients showed exudative conjunctivitis, lacrimation, and foreign body sensation for a few days to weeks before referral.

In 2010, Kim et al. reported a case of intraocular infestation with *T. callipaeda* in a patient who was successfully treated by a pars plana vitrectomy in South Korea. A 74-year-old woman came to the hospital complaining of visual disturbance and floaters in the left eye. She had redness but no pain. A white, thread-like, live and mobile worm was observed in the vitreous cavity, and identified as an adult male *T. callipaeda* (Fig. 4). In 2006, the left eye of a 50-year-old man from Seoul, Korea was injured by shattered glass from the broken lens of his spectacles. Clinical examination of the eye revealed a 6mm-sized peripherally located, single, full thickness corneal laceration with iris incarceration and traumatic lens opacity. The corneal wound was repaired. Two days after the operation, a 15 mm live thread-like worm was found inside the vitreous cavity. Trans pars plana vitrectomy for removal of the worm was performed, and the worm was identified as *T. callipaeda* (Lee et al., 2006). There have been only a few case reports about intraocular infestation by *T. callipaeda*. In these reports, all of the parasites were found in the anterior chamber except in one case where the worm was found in the vitreous cavity (Mukherjee et al. 1978; Zakir et al. 1999).

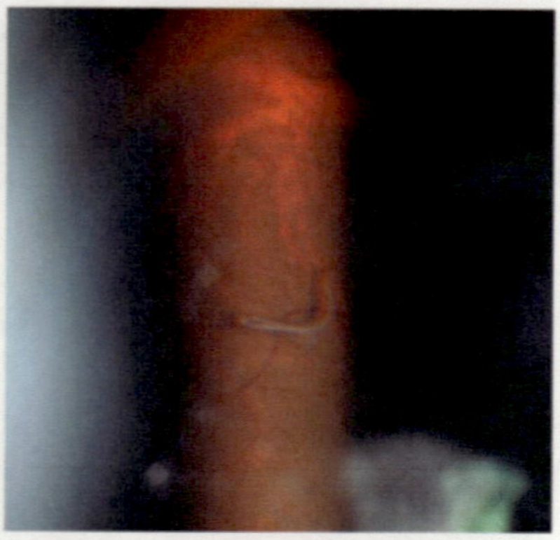

Fig. 4. A live *Thelazia callipaeda* worm in the vitreous cavity was clearly observed (Courtesy Hyun Woong Kim, South Korea).

Recently, the first case of human thelaziasis was reported from Bangladesh (Hossain et al. 2011). A 58 year old man was admitted with itching, redness, foreign body sensation, lacrimation and filamentary discharge from the right eye. He had conjunctival congestion and advanced bi-headed pterygium of the right eye. After exposure of the right eye ball with a universal eye speculum, a thin white nematode was found in the right lower conjunctival fornix. The nematode was identified as an adult *T. callipaeda*. In a previous report, small, white, thread-like, motile worms were recovered from the conjunctival sac of a 13-year-old girl and a 50-year-old woman from Dibrugarh district, Assam, India. They were identified as *thelazia* species (Nath et al., 2008). In another investigation, *T. callipaeda* was isolated from the conjunctival sac of a 32 year-old woman residing in the Himalaya Mountains (Sharma et al., 2006). Also, more intraocular infestations with *T. callipaeda* were reported from China (W Chen et al. 2010; Leiper 1917; Lv et al., 2009; Xue et al. China 2007).

T. callipaeda infects dogs, cats, foxes, rabbits (Kozlov 1962; Skrjabin et al. 1971), and wolves (Otranto et al. 2007). In affected wild animals, *T. callipaeda* adult and larval stages (Fig. 5) may cause mild ocular manifestations (conjunctivitis, epiphora, and ocular discharge) to severe disease (keratitis and corneal ulcers) (Otranto and Traversa 2005). In dogs and cats, however, chronic conjunctivitis will usually result, with manifestations such as photophobia and sometimes accompanied by blepharitis marginalis, lacrimation, corneal opacity, ulceration of the cornea, or even corneal perforation. The most common symptoms in affected dogs and foxes in Switzerland were conjunctivitis and epiphora, while keratitis was present only in a low number of animals. Young and small sized dogs were significantly less involved than large animals over 3 years of age (Dorchies et al. 2007; Malacrida et al. 2008).

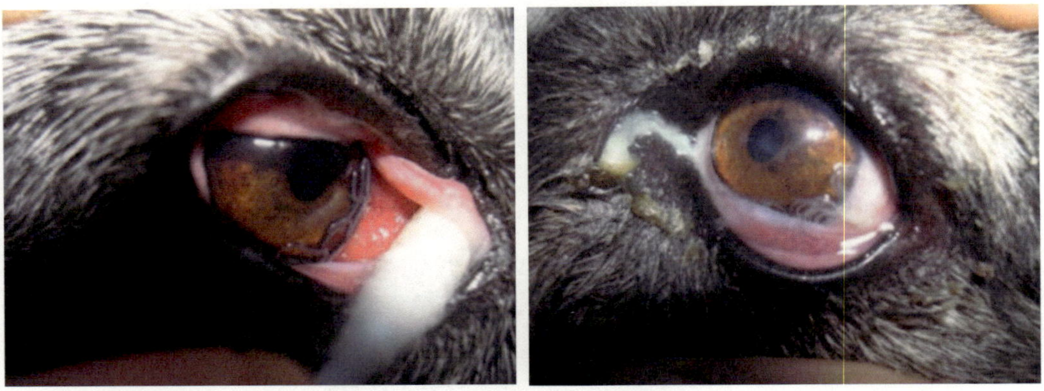

Fig. 5. Both adult and larval stages of eyeworms are responsible for eye disease with symptoms ranging from mild e.g. lacrimation, ocular discharge, epiphora (Left) to severe e.g. conjunctivitis, keratitis and, corneal opacity or ulcers (Right) (Courtesy Domenico Otranto, Bari, Italy).

In humans, *T. californiensis* worms tend to reside in the superior and inferior fornices of the eye (Fig. 6). The most common clinical findings in infected patients include a mild conjunctival inflammation, foreign body sensation, follicular hypertrophy of the conjunctiva and possibly excessive lacrimation. The worms may occasionally migrate across the ocular surface, eventually causing corneal scarring, opacity and blindness. Human infection is extremely rare and thought to be accidental (Knierim and Jack 1975; Krischner et al. 1990).

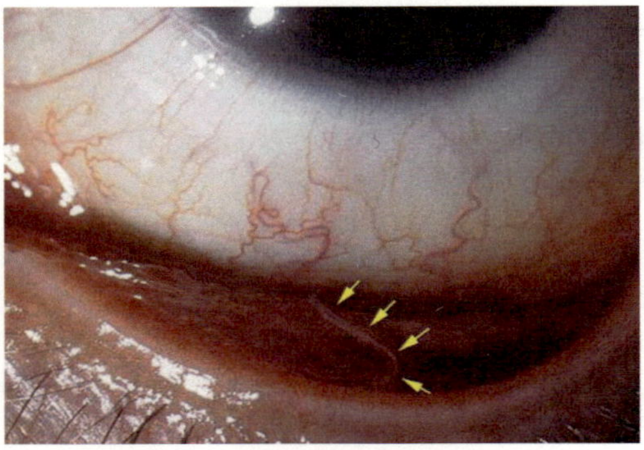

Fig. 6. Adult specimens of *Thelazia californiensis* on the eye of a man (Courtesy Yan Peng, Dallas, USA).

T. californiensis was found on the conjunctivas of six of seven deer from Zion National Park, Utah. Based on field observations, adults appeared to be affected clinically at a higher incidence during both years of the study (1992-1994) as opposed to juveniles. Corneal opacity was the most apparent clinical sign from 1992 to 1993. However, in the following year, blepharospasm and epiphora were noted often (Knierim and Jack 1975; Taylor et al. 1996). Also, *T. californiensis* was found in 15% of hunter-harvested deer in Utah in 1994 and in 8% in 1995. Three live animals showed clinical signs of infectious keratoconjunctivitis (IKC) in 1996, but pathogenic bacteria were not isolated from these individuals (Dubay et al. 2000).

3.1.5 Diagnosis

The clinical diagnosis of thelaziosis in animals and humans may be difficult if only small numbers of nematodes are present, because clinical signs relate to an inflammatory response linked predominantly to the presence of developing third-stage larvae (L3) and/or fourth-stage larvae (L4), similar to an allergic conjunctivitis (Otranto and Dutto 2008).

A definitive diagnosis is made by the detection of the parasites in the conjunctival sac. Examination of lacrimal secretions may reveal eggs or first-stage larvae. However, morphological differentiation between *T. callipaeda* and *T.californiensis* is based on the numbers of pre- and post-cloacal papillae in the male and the position of the vulva in the female (Bhaibulaya et al. 1970; WY Choi et al. 1989; Miyazaki 1991; Otranto et al. 2003a). Also, in a study which was carried out on molecular characterization of *Thelazia callipaeda* (Otranto et al. 2005b), the results for the SSCP (single-strand conformation polymophism) analysis and sequencing were concordant, indicating that the mutation scanning approach provides a useful tool for investigating the population genetics and molecular ecology of *T. callipaeda*.

3.1.6 Treatment, prevention and control

Due to the localization of the nematode, thelaziasis can be treated topically by direct application of drugs into the eyes. Mechanical removal of the adult parasites with fine forceps or cotton swabs using local anesthesia, is helpful. The clinical signs, excluding secondary infections with other pathogens, usually resolve rapidly after the removal of the worms (KC Wang et al. 1999). Patients with an intraocular infestation with *T. callipaeda* had a successful recovery after a pars plana vitrectomy. Untimely or incorrect treatment of the infection may result in a delay in recovery, mainly in children and the elderly, who are most likely to be exposed to infection by the fly. Thus, prevention of human thelaziasis should include control of the fly vector by use of bed nets to protect children while they are sleeping and by keeping their faces and eyes clean. Genetic identification of haplotype 1 has shown that this is the only haplotype circulating in animals (dogs, cats, and foxes) in Europe (Otranto et al. 2005b). This finding confirms the metazoonotic potential of *Thelazia* spp. infection and the need to treat infected domestic animals, which may act as reservoirs for human infection (Otranto and Dutto 2008).

The treatment for canine infection with *T. callipaeda* is to remove the worm. In the case of dogs having numerous worms, they must be eliminated under general anesthesia by turning up the third eyelid. Michalski (1976) found 2 ml of levamisole injected into the subconjunctival sac was more effective than levamisole given orally. Also, application of organophosphates (Rossi and Peruccio 1989) or 1% moxidectin (Lia et al. 2004) is effective. Meanwhile, the treatment of dog thelaziasis caused by *T. callipaeda* using a topical formulation of 10% imidacloprid and 2.5% moxidectin was studied by Bianciardi and Otranto in 2005. A clinical trial of ivermectin against eyeworm in German Shepherd militray working dogs carried out by Fudge et al. (2007). Although ivermectin does not prevent dogs from being infected with eyeworms, the study suggests that ivermectin administered orally at a dose of 0.2 mg/kg every 3 weeks significantly reduces the prevalence of *Thelazia* species eyeworms in dogs. The efficacy of the prophylactic use of a monthly treatment with milbemycin oxime showed 90% efficacy against *T. callipaeda* in naturally exposed dogs (Ferroglio et al. 2008).

The treatment of human *T. californiensis* conjunctival infestation is fairly straight forward. The symptoms usually resolve immediately after removal of the worms. Therefore, *T. californiensis* infestation should be included in the differential diagnosis of patients with chronic conjunctivitis following hiking or camping in the mountains or back-country. Irrigation with Lugol's iodine or 2-3% boric acid is recommended immediately after worm removal or for parasites that are in the lacrimal ducts where they cannot be removed manually. Levamisole, either orally or parenterally, at 5mg/kg or 2ml injected into the conjunctival sac has also been recommended. A dose of 1mg/lb of Ivermectin given subcutaneously has been shown to cure similar infestations in Asia and Europe. There is no vaccine for thelaziasis (Doezie et al. 1996; Kirschener et al. 1990; Peng et al. 2001).

4. Animal thelaziasis

As *T. callipaeda* and *T. californiensis* infect both humans and animals, they were already discussed in the section of human thelaziasis. Thus, in the following section, the other *Thelazia* species, which only infect animals, will be discussed.

4.1 *Thelazia rhodesi* Desmarest, 1822

T. rhodesi occurs on the surface of the cornea, under the nictitating membrane, in the conjunctival sac and in the lachrymal duct of cattle, buffalo, zebu, bison, and less commonly horses, sheep and goats.

The body is milky-white, with thick, prominent transverse striations. The cephalic region is similar in both sexes. The stoma is short and broad, widest at the middle, and has no lips. Around the mouth, four pairs of sub-median small, conoidal cephalic papillae and two lateral amphidal apertures are seen (Fig. 7, Top, Left). Nematode amphids exist in a variety of forms and sizes, some probably purely chemosensory, some photoreceptive, with an associated gland (McLaren 1974). Also, there are two lateral cervical papillae, one on each side, 350–384 µm from the anterior end (Fig. 7, Top, Right). These organs determine whether the nematode can pass through a small space (McLaren 1976). At the anterior end of both sexes, an excretory pore is seen (Naem 2007a).

The females are 12.5–20.5 mm long and 300–500 µm wide. At the anterior end of the body, the vulva is located in the esophageal region, 505.2–536.3 µm from the cephalic region. The pattern of the cuticle around the vulva is different from the rest of the body (Fig. 7, Bottom). At the posterior end, the anal pore is seen, and the tail end is stumpy with two phasmids near its extremity (Naem 2007a). The eggs are 26-29 µ long at first, but later when stretched by developing larvae they are 207 by 4 µ (Levine 1968). The males are 7.5–14.5 mm long and 420–475 µm wide. The tail is blunt, and without caudal alae, with dissimilar and unequal spicules 624-850 µ and 100-130 µ long, respectively, and no gubernaculum. There are 14 paired pre-anal papillae, one single papilla directly anterior to the cloaca, one paired post-anal papilla, and two nipple shaped phasmids at the posterior end (Naem 2007a).

The females are viviparous. The first-stage larvae are passed by females into the lachrymal secretions where they are ingested by non-biting Diptera flies. It has been confirmed that *Musca autumnalis* and *Musca larvipara* are suitable intermediate hosts (Anderson 2000; Giangaspero et al. 2004). The first stage of *Thelazia* is very short-lived in the lachrymal secretion, only surviving a few hours, and transmission depends upon the continuous presence of the vectors. For this reason, thelaziasis has a seasonal occurrence according to the seasonality of the intermediate hosts (Dunn 1978).

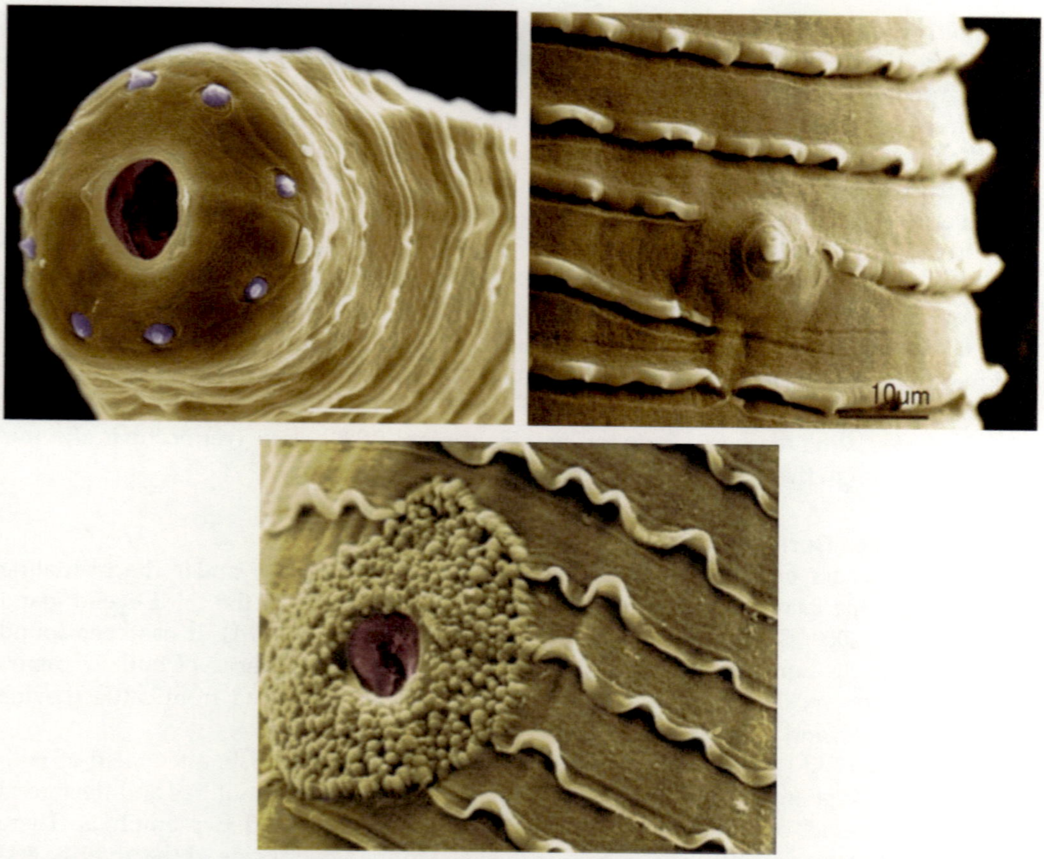

Fig. 7. SEM of adult female's mouth, *Thelazia rhodesi* (Top, Left); SEM of cuticular sensory papillae of *T. rhodesi* (Top, Right); SEM of adult female's vulva, *T. rhodesi* (Bottom), (Courtesy Soraya Naem, Urmia, Iran), "With kind permission of Springer Science+Business Media."

T. rhodesi is particularly common in the Old World. Bovine thelaziasis was first reported in Iran by Ebadi in 1951. Other investigations indicate the presence of bovine thelaziasis in Japan, Ghana, Afghanistan, USA, Canada, UK, Italy, and Zambia (Arbuckle and Khalil 1978; Barus et al. 1976; Genden and Stoffolano 1980; Ghirotti and Iliamupu 1989; Krafsur and Church 1985; Okoshi and Kitano 1966; O'Hara and Kennedy 1991; Munangandu et al., 2011; Turfrey and Chandler 1978; Vohradsky 1970). In a study conducted at an abattoir located in Cagayan de Oro City, Philippines, 23% of examined animals were infected with *T. rhodesi*. In nearly half of the animals, both eyes were infected. *T. rhodesi* infection was significantly more common in cattle of more than 3 years of age (25%) than in younger animals (15%). Ocular lesions were observed in 73 (11%) of examined cattle (Van Aken et al. 1996). This eyeworm was also reported in southern regions in Italy and the ecology of *Thelazia* spp. in cattle and their vectors has been documented by Giangaspero et al. (2004). In another survey, change in the prevalence of *Thelazia* species in bovine eyes was studied in England (Tweedle et al.,2005).

The adult and larval stages live in eyes causing conjunctivitis, keratitis, lacrimation, ocular discharge, and ulcers (Ikeme 1967; Otranto and Traversa 2005).

A definitive diagnosis is made by the detection of the nematode in the conjunctival sac. Examination of the lacrimal secretions may reveal eggs or first stage larvae (Soulsby 1986). The morphological descriptions (Guttekova 1987; Kikuchi 1976) and molecular findings (Otranto et al. 2001; Otranto et al. 2003c; Otranto and Traversa 2004; Tarsitano et al. 2002) already discussed have demonstrated the differences among *Thelazia* species.
Removal of the adult nematodes with fine forceps, using local anesthesia is helpful. The use of "nilverm" (tetramisole) in the control of clinical signs of *T. rhodesi* infection in cattle has been studied by Aruo in 1974. Halpin and Kirkly (1962) have reported that methyridine produces rapid recovery from *Thelazia* infection, as do tetramisole and levamisole given orally or parenterally. Eye salves containing 4% morantel tartrate or 1% levamisole have also been used with success. A case of eye infection in a heifer was reported with bilateral blindness, cornea opacity, excessive lachrimation and nasal discharge. Treatment with 6-10 drops of a 10% solution of levamisole resulted in a complete recovery, with a total of 127 adult *T. rhodesi* being recovered from the eyes (Salifu et al. 1990). Also, ivermectin is effective against *T. rhodesi* in the eyes of cattle (Kennedy 1994; Soll et al.1992).

4.2 *T. lacrymalis* Gurlt, 1831

T. lacrymalis occurs on the surface of the cornea and conjunctiva, under the nictitating membrane, in the lacrymal gland and its ducts and in the ducts of the third eyelid gland (Dongus et al. 2000; Giangaspero et al. 1999, 2000a; Lyons et al. 1981). It has been found occasionally in the aqueous humor of the eye. *T. lacrymalis* is a parasite of buffalo, camel, dog, and equine species, especially horses. It has also been reported from cattle (Levine 1968; Moolenbeek and Surgeoner 1980).
According to an SEM study, the body of the female was thin, whitish, attenuated at both ends, 12.5 mm long and up to 279 μm in width. The mouth was without lips and the buccal opening was round, and surrounded by four cephalic papillae and two amphids. There were two lateral cervical papillae, one on each side. On the ventral side of the anterior end of the body, the vulva was located 493 μm from the anterior end (Naem 2005). In a study carried out on *T. lacrymalis* obtained from a naturally infected horse, the vulva was situated 593 μm from the anterior end (Beelitz et al. 1997). The anal pore was located on the ventral side of the posterior end of the body, and there was one button-like sub-terminal phasmid on each lateral side of the female's tail (Naem 2005). These phasmids are involved in evaluating the intensity of a given stimulus and helping the worm to maintain itself in a suitable environment (McLaren, 1976). The males are 8-12 mm long, with spicules 170-190 and 130-140 μ long, respectively (Levine, 1968).
Thelazia spp. are generally described as being viviparous (Dunn 1978; Fiebiger 1947; Lohrer and Horning 1967; Tretjakowa 1960; Yamaguti 1961) or ovoviviparous (Anderson 1992). *T. lacrymalis* can be described as ovoviviparous (Craig and Davies 1937; Dongus et al. 2003; Ivashkin et al. 1979; Lyons et al. 1980; Skrjabin 1971). Transmission occurs by means of non-biting dipteran flies of the genus *Musca* (Muscidae) which feed on animal ocular secretions, tears and conjunctiva. The intermediate host in the USSR is *M. osiris* (Barker 1970). In the fly body, the parasite goes through further larval development (Anderson 2000; Ivashkin et al. 1979; Lyons et al. 1997; O'Hara and Kennedy 1991).
T. lacrymalis has so far been documented in Europe, Asia, North Africa, and North and South America (Anderson 1992; Barker 1970; Beelitz et al. 1997; Eckert 1992; Ladouceur and Kazacos 1981; Lohrer and Horning 1967; Lyons et al. 1986). In a survey, which was

performed on the occurrence of internal parasites in 461 horses (1-30 years old) slaughtered at the Linköping abattoir in central Sweden, 3.1% of examined horses were infected with *T. lacrmalis* (Hoglund et al. 1997). The results of another study indicated that *T. lacrymalis* has greatly increased in prevalence and intensity in central Kentucky (Dougherty and Knapp 1994; Lyons et al. 1976; Lyons et al. 1997).

Thelaziasis in horses is primarily a summer problem, comparable to the condition in cattle (Dunn 1969; Soulsby 1965). In a survey, which was carried out in Normandy, France,*T. lacrimalis* was recovered from 10.3% of examined horses (Collobert et al. 1995). Another survey evaluated the prevalence of *Thelazia* spp. in slaughtered native horses in the province of Bari, Italy (Giangaspero et al. 1999). Sixty horses (14.7%) were found parasitized by *T. lacrymalis.* This is the first report of *T. lacrymalis* infection in a horse in Italy (Giangaspero et al. 1999). In the following year, another similar survey was done in the Abruzzo region of Italy, where 39.06% of examined horses were found infected with *T. lacrymalis* (Giangaspero et al. 2000a).

The importance of *T. lacrymalis* in causing follicular conjunctivitis, ulcerative keratitis and ophthalmia has been documented (Giangaspero et al. 1999; Skrjabin et al. 1971). Occasionally the anterior chamber may be invaded, causing extensive endophthamitis and blindness (Grant et al. 1973; Skrjabin et al. 1971; Stewart 1940). Schebitz (1960) described a complicated case in an Egyptian horse which progressed from conjunctivitis to severe ulceration and granulation of the eye. However, in many cases, eyeworms have no pathogenic effect on the host, especially in larger animals (Soulsby 1986).

Diagnosis of the disease may be accomplished by irrigating the eyes with saline and examining centrifuged sediment for the first stage larvae. Schebitz (1960) also described finding larvae in the blood of infected horses and donkeys. *Post mortem* diagnosis may be accomplished by placing the lacrymal glands in warm saline, permitting larvae and adults to emerge (Skrjabin et al. 1971). Besides the potential implications for studies on vectors, a PCR-RFLP based assay on the first and/or second internal transcribed spacer (ITS1 and ITS2) of ribosomal DNA was developed for the detection of *T. lacrymalis* DNA in its putative vector/s (Traversa et al al. 2005). Thus, it could be used for diagnosis of equine thelaziasis at the species level especially considering that horses can be occasionally infected by *T. skrjabini* (Lyons et al. 1976).

Treatment generally includes mechanical removal of worms under local anesthesia, irrigation of the eye with dilute solutions of topical antiseptics such as iodine or boric acid, and treatment of any corneal ulceration to suppress the development of opacity (Soulsby 1965). Activity of 15 compounds, given alone or in mixtures was evaluated in 102 equids. None of the compounds appeared to be active against *T lacrymalis* (Lyons et al. 1981).

4.3 *T. gulosa* Railliet and Henry, 1910

T. gulosa is a parasite mainly of cattle, and occurs on the surface of the cornea, under the nictitating membrane, and in the conjunctival sac and lachrymal duct. The mouth is without lips, surrounded by four cephalic papillae and two amphids. There are two lateral cervical papillae, one on each side (Naem 2007b). Gibbons (1986) included one scanning electron micrograph of the anterior end of *T. gulosa* in her atlas. An electron microscopic study of the cuticle of two *T.gulosa and T. rhodesi*, carried out by Guttekova (1987), revealed very interesting architectonics of the body surface of these nematodes.

According to an SEM study, the body of the female was thin, whitish, attenuated at both ends, 8.0–11.5 mm long, and of 350–460 µm wide at the maximum body width. The vulva was located 460– 610 µm from the cephalic region. The anal pore was located 70–120 µm from the posterior end of the body. There was one button-like sub-terminal phasmid on each lateral side of the female's tail (Naem 2007b). The males were 7.5–8.0 mm long and 300–370 µm wide at the maximum body width. The tail was blunt without caudal alae and curved ventrally. The number of pre-anal papillae was 35–40 (Fig. 8). These papillae were unpaired, and one single papilla directly anterior to the cloaca was also seen. Three pairs of post-anal papillae were present. The spicules were unequal (608-1025 µm and 120-125 µm long, respectively), dissimilar and showed a groove-like structure (Naem 2007b). There was no gubernaculum (Levine 1968).

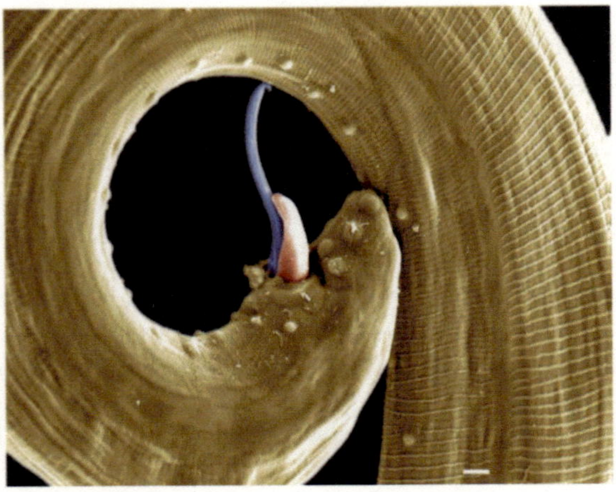

Fig. 8. Coiled posterior pole of a *Thelazia gulosa* male, showing the 2 different spicula (Courtesy Soraya Naem, Urmia, Iran), "With kind permission of Springer Science+Business Media."

Like *T. lacrymalis* of horses, *T.gulosa* is now widely distributed in North America where it is transmitted by the face fly, *Musca autumnalis*, which was introduced to the continent in the early 1950s and has spread widely in the northern USA and the Canadian provinces (Chitwood and Stoffolano 1971; Chirico 1994; Greenberg 1971). Also, other *Musca* species act as intermediate hosts in the Ukraine, the Far East of CIS, the Crimea, and Europe (Branch et al. 1974; Krastin 1950a,b; Genden and Stoffolano 1981, 1982; Moolenbeek and Surgeoner 1980; Skrjabin et al. 1971; Vilagiova 1967). Kennedy and MacKinnon (1994) noted that the distribution of *T. gulosa* differed from that of *T. skrjabini* in the orbits of cattle. The two lachrymal ducts associated with the Harderian gland contained 58% of the *T. skrjabini* whereas the large ventral duct of the orbital glands contained 58% of the *T. gulosa*. The eyeworms were found more often in a lachrymal duct as a single species (90%) than as a mixed infection of two species (10%).

T. gulosa has been reported in the CIS, Asia, Australia, North America and Europe (Anderson 2000; Genden and Stoffolano 1980; Giangaspero et al. 2000 b; Gutierres et al. 1980; Lyons and drudge 1975; Overend 1983; Patton and Marbury 1978). It occurs on rare occasions in England (Fitzsimmons 1966). *T. gulosa* found in cows in Poland and southeast Kazakhstan (Levine 1968). In another study, *T. gulosa* was reported in an imported giraffe in California and *T. lacrymalis* was identified in a native horse in Maryland (Walker and Becklund 1971). An eight month survey of bovine eyes from an abattoir in southern Ontario revealed the presence of *T. gulosa* and *T. lacrymalis* in 32% of the cattle (Moolenbeek and

Surgeoner 1980). In the aforementioned study (Moolenbeek and Surgeoner 1980), a total of 2,191 adult female face flies (*M. autumnalis*) were examined. Sixty-five (3%) of these harbored larvae of *Thelazia* spp. The prevalence of *Thelazia* spp. in cattle has been reported in southern Italy. *T. rhodesi, T. gulosa* and *T. skrjabini* were found in 80%, 34.5% and 1.8% of examined animals, respectively. This was the first report of *T. gulosa* and *T. skrjabini* in Southern Europe (Giangaspero et al. 2000b).

Oakley (1969) described a group of calves showing signs of lacrimation, keratitis and corneal opacity in which the presence of *T. gulosa* was demonstrated. Also, keratoconjunctivitis has been reviewed by Baptista (1979). Examination of histological sections of two heavily infected lacrimal ducts revealed evidence of chronic follicular conjunctivitis although this was considered not to be specific to *Thelazia* spp. (Moolenbeek and Surgeoner 1980).

Diagnosis of T. *gulosa* is made by the detection of the nematode in the conjunctival sac. Examination of the lacrimal secretions may reveal eggs or first stage larvae (Soulsby 1986). The morphological descriptions, and molecular findings (Guttekova 1987; Kikuchi 1976; Naem 2007b; Otranto et al. 2001; Tarsitano et al. 2002) demonstrate the differences among *T. gulosa*, *T. skrjabini*, and *T. rhodes*.

The anthelmintic efficacy of doramectin was assessed for the control of *T. gulosa* and *T. skrjabini* in two studies using 44 naturally or experimentally infected calves (Kennedy and Phillips 1993). No eyeworms were found in any doramectin-treated animal. Also, the efficacy of ivermectin (pour-on) against the eyeworms *T. gulosa* and *T. skrjabini* in naturally infected cattle was studied by Kennedy et al. (1994).

4.4 *T. leesei* Railliet and Henry, 1910

T. leesei, is a parasite of the dromedary and the Bactrian camel in India, Europe (France), the USSR (Turkemenistan), and Africa (Kenya). The females are 14-21 mm long and 400 µm wide, with a vulva 425-440 µm from the anterior end. The males are 12 mm long and 210 µm wide, with unequal spicules 340 and 105 µm long, respectively (Anderson 2000; Aypak 2007; Levine 1968). *T. leesei* is transmitted by *M. lucidula* in Turkmenistan, and Infected flies were found around the eyes of dromedaries from the end of May to the beginning of October (Anderson 2000).

4.5 *T. alfortensis* Railliet and Henry, 1910

T. alfortensis occurs in the conjunctival sac of cattle in Europe, but is considered to be a synonym of *T. gulosa* (Soulsby 1986).

4.6 *T. skrjabini* Erschow, 1928

T. skrjabini is normally found within the lacrimal ducts of the third eyelid in cattle, and less frequently is found beneath the third eyelid or lacrimal ducts leading from the orbital lacrimal gland opening into the conjunctiva near the fornix. The cephalic region is similar in both sexes. The mouth is orbicular and has no lips with its anterior edge turned over and has six grooves. Around the mouth, two circles of cephalic papillae are seen: the inner circle with six papillae and the outer circle with four sub-median cephalic papillae. At both lateral sides of the head, two amphids are observed. The cuticle shows fine, scarcely visible transverse striations and two lateral cervical papillae (Naem 2007c).

The females are 11–19 mm long and 178–378 µm wide. The protruded vulva is located 410–710 µm from the cephalic region. The anal pore is located at the posterior end of the body and the tail has two phasmids near the tip (Naem 2007c). The males are 5–9 mm long and 178–260 µm wide. The tail is blunt without caudal alae and curved ventrally. There are 31 to 38 unpaired pre-anal papillae, two paired post-anal papillae, and two nipple-shaped phasmids at the posterior end. The pattern of the cuticle around the cloaca is different from the rest of the body (Naem 2007c).

The mature females are viviparous. According to Krastin (1952) and Skrjabin et al. (1971), the intermediate hosts are *Musca amica* and *M. vitripennis*. O'Hara and Kennedy (1989,1991) orally inoculated *M. autumnalis* with first-stage larvae of *T. skrjabini*, which was recently introduced to North America.

T. skrjabini is common in cattle in Alberta, Canada (Kennedy et al., 1993) and is occasionally reported from other mammals including horses in the United States (Lyons et al.m 1976), and buffalo in India (Bhopale et al. 1970; Pande et al. 1970). Also, this nematode occurs in cattle in, Denmark, Poland, USSR, and Australia (Anderson, 2000; De Chaneet 1970; Kolstrup 1974). Kennedy and Mackinnon studied site segregation of *T. skrjabini* and *T. gulosa* in the eyes of cattle (1994). Eyeworms occurred 90% of the time in a duct as a single species compared to 10% of the time as a mixed species infection. The data suggest that *T. skrjabini* and *T. gulosa* are more site specific than previously believed (Kennedy and Mackinnon 1994).

The adult and larval stages of *T. skrjabini* live in eyes, causing conjunctivitis, keratitis, lacrimation, and ocular discharge (Ikeme 1967; Otranto and Traversa 2005; Soulsby 1986). Diagnosis is made by the detection of the nematode in the conjunctival sac. Examination of the lacrimal secretions may reveal eggs or first stage larvae (Soulsby 1986). The morphological descriptions (Guttekova 1987; Kikuchi 1976; Naem 2007c) and molecular findings (Otranto et al. 2001; Otranto et al. 2003a; Tarsitano et al. 2002) indicate the differences among *Thelazia* species.

The efficacy of doramectin against *Thelazia* spp. in both naturally and experimentally infected calves was 100%, and no worms were found in any doramectin-treated animal (Kennedy and Phillips 1993; Marley et al. 1999). In another investigation, the efficacy of ivermectin was 97.02% and 100% against adults of *T. skrjabini* and *T. gulosa*, respectively (Kennedy et al. 1994).

4.7 *T. ershowi* Oserskaja, 1931

T. ershowi occurs in the tear ducts and the conjunctiva of pigs in the USSR. Oserskaja (1931) found the parasite in 7 of 350 pigs in the Ural area. The females are 5.0-8.7 mm long and 188-207 µm wide, with a tail 65-105 µm long and a vulva 395-489 µm from the anterior end. The males are 4.9-5.5 mm long and 176-188 µm wide, with a left spicule 152-155 µm long and a right spicule 114-115 µm long (Levine 1968).

4.8 *T. bubalis* Ramanujachari and Alwar, 1952

T. bubalis is a nematode of the conjunctival sac of the water buffalo in India. The females are 6.5-7.8 mm long and 250 µm wide, with a vulva 900 µm from the anterior end. The males are 6 mm long, with a left spicule 800 µm long and a right spicule 150 µm long (Levine 1968; Soulsby 1986).

4.9 *T. anolabiata* Molin, 1860

Twenty-two *Thelazia* species have been reported from wild birds (Anderson 2000). *T. anolabiata* occurs in the orbits of birds, which can cause lacrimation, keratitis, conjunctivitis, and corneal ulcers. This species was reported for the first time from an Andean Cock-of-the-rock (*Rupicola peruviana*) from a zoo in Lima, Peru (Elias et al. 2008). The nematodes were identified as *T. anolabiata* based on the lengths of spicules (1770 μm) and other morphologic characteristics such as the number of anal papillae of the males (8 pairs of pre-anal papillae), and the appearance of the first annulations on the anterior part of the body (45 mm posterior to the buccal capsule). There is some controversy about the number of *Thelazia* spp. in South American birds. Although Anderson and Diaz-Ungria (1959) believed that both *T. anolabiata* and *T. digitata* were valid species, Rodrigues (1992) lists *T. digitata* and *T. lutzi* as synonyms of *T. anolabiata*. However, molecular assays would be of great use in validating the avian species of *Thelazia* (Elias et al. 2008). In the Peruvian study, clinical signs of the infected bird (keratoconjunctivitis) were resolved with treatment with ivermectin and ciprofloxacin. Other studies have documented avian thelaziasis in Israel, Senegal and Japan (Brooks et al. 1983; Murata and Asakawa 1999; Wertheim and Giladi 1977).

5. Conclusion

Among *Thelazia* species causing ocular infections in animals, *Thelazia callipaeda* and, more rarely, *Thelazia californiensis* have also been found in human eyes. Human and animal thelaziasis have been documented in Europe, Asia, North America, South America and South Africa. The adult nematode lives in the eyes and associated tissues, including under the lids and in the conjunctiva and lacrimal glands and ducts. The transmission of eyeworms occurs when flies acting as intermediate hosts, feed on lachrymal secretions from an infected animal and/or human and ingest first-stage larvae of *Thelazia* spp. produced by female nematodes in the conjunctival sac of the final host. The larvae develop into the third-stage larvae in the fly, and emerge from the labella of an infected fly, when it feeds on the ocular secretions of a new host. Larvae develop into the adult stage in the conjunctival sac within ~ 35 days. Disease caused by *Thelazia* spp. is characterized by a range of subclinical and clinical signs, such as lacrimation, epiphora, conjunctivitis, keratitis, and corneal ulcers. Diagnosis is made by the detection of eggs or first-stage larvae in lacrimal secretions or by finding the adult worms in the conjunctival sac. Species identification is confirmed on the basis of microscopic examination with reference to keys. Thelaziasis can be treated topically by direct application of drugs into the eyes, and removal of the adult parasites with fine forceps, using local anesthesia. An integration of medical and veterinary expertise is needed to improve scientific knowledge to control eyeworm disease.

6. Acknowledgements

The author expresses her sincere gratitude to Professor Domenico Otranto, Department of Veterinary Public Health, Faculty of Veterinary Medicine, University of Bari, Italy for sharing his valuable experienes in writing this chapter. The author is particularly indebted to Dr. Christine M. Budke of Texas A&M University, USA, whose comments greatly increased the clarity of the manuscript. Many thanks are given to Dr. Hamed Seifi for the critical reading of the references. Lastly, the author is grateful to Dr. Ako Shabrandi for editing one of SEM images (Fig. 7, Bottom).

7. References

Anderson, RC. (1992). Nematode parasites of vertebrates: their development and transmission. CABI, ISBN 978-0851-987996, Wallingford, UK

Anderson, RC. (2000). Nematode parasites of vertebrates: their development and transmission. (2nd ed.) CABI, ISBN 978-0851-994215, Wallingford, UK

Anderson, RC. & Diaz-Ungria, C. (1959). Revision preliminar de las especies de *Thelazia* Bosc (Spiruroidea: Thelaziidae), parasitas de Aves. Mem Soc Cienc Nat La Salle , Vol.19, No.52, pp.37–75, ISSN 0037-8518

Arbuckle, JB. & Khalil, LF. (1978). A survey of *thelazia* worms in the eyelids of British cattle. *Vet Rec* Vol.102, No.10, (Mars 1978), pp.207-210, ISSN 0042-4900

Arizono, N.; Yoshida, Y.; Konodo, K.; Kurimoto, H.; Oda, K.; Shiota, T.; Shimata, Y. & Ogino, K. (1976). *Thelazia callipaeda* from man and dogs in Kyoto and its scanning electron microscopy. Japanese J Parasitol, Vol.25,. p.402–408 ISSN 0021-5171

Aruo, SK. (1974). The use of "nilverm" (tetramisole) in the control of clinical signs of *Thelazia rhodesii* (eyeworm) infection in cattle. Bull Epizoot Dis Afr Vol.22, No.3 (Sep 1974), pp. 275-277, ISSN 0007-487X

Aypak, S. (2007). Develerin Helmint Enfeksiyonları. Türkiye Parazitol Dergisi, Vol.31, No.3, (2007), pp. 225-228, ISSN 1300-6320

Bächli, G.; Vilela, CR.; Escher, SA. & Saura, A. (2005). The Drosophilidae (Diptera) of Fennoscandia and Denmark, vol. 39. (In: Series: Fauna Entomologica Scandinavica), Brill, ISSN 978-9004-140745, Leiden, Netherlands

Baptista, PJ. (1979). Infectious bovine keratoconjunctivitis: a review. *Br Vet J*, Vol.135, No.3, (May-June1379), pp.225-242, ISSN 0007-1935

Barker, IK. (1970). Case report. *Thelazia lacrymalis* from the eyes of an Ontario horse. Can Vet J, Vol.11, No.9, (Sept 1970), pp.186–189, ISSN 0008-5286

Barus, V.; Amin, A.; Blazek, K. & Moravec, F. (1976). Nematodes parasitizing domestic ruminants in Afghanistan. Folia Parasitol (Praha), Vol.23, No.3, (1976) pp. 207–216, ISSN 0015-5683

Beelitz, P.; Dongus, H.; Schöl, H.; Gerhards, H. & Gothe, R. (1997). *Thelazia lacrymalis* (Nematoda, Spirurida, Thelaziidae): report in a horse in Germany and contribution to the morphology of adult worms. *Parasitol Res,* Vol. 83, No.6, (May1997) pp627-631, ISSN *0932-0113*

Bhaibulaya, M.; Prasertsilpa, S. & Vajrasthira, S. (1970). *Thelazia callipaeda* Railliet and Henry 1910, in man and dog in Thailand. Am J Trop Med Hyg, Vol.19, No.3, (May1970) 476–479, ISSN 0002-9637

Bhopale, KK.; Joshi, SC.; Jain, PC.; & Kamalapur, SK. (1970). *Thelazia skrjabini* Erschow, 1928 from an Indian buffalo (*Bubalus bubalis*). *Indian Vet J*, Vol.47, No.7, (July 1970), pp.564-566, ISSN 0019 - 6479

Bianciardi, P. & Otranto, D. (2005). Treatment of dog thelaziosis caused by *Thelazia callipaeda* (Spirurida, Thelaziidae) using a topical formulation of imidacloprid 10% and moxidectin 2.5%. Vet Parasitol, Vol.129, No.1-, (April 2005), pp.89–93, ISSN 0304-4017

Branch, J.; Stoffolano, G. & Stoffolano, JR. (1974). Invertebrate vector and host of mammalian eye worms in Massachusetts. J Econ Entomol, Vol.67, No.2, (Apr 1974), pp.304-305 ISSN 0022-0493.

Brooks, DE.; Greiner, EC. & Walsh, MT. (1983). Conjunctivitis caused by *Thelazia* sp in a Senegal parrot. J Am Vet Med Assoc, Vol.183, No.11, (December 1983), pp.1305-1306, ISSN 0003-1488

Burnett, HS.; Parmelee, WE.; Lee, RD. & Wagner, ED. (1957). Observation on the life cycle of *Thelazia californiensis* Price, 1930. J Parasitol, Vol.43, No.4, (Aug 1957), p.433 ISSN 0020-7519

Chen, CC. & Zhang, YM. (1954). A case report of human thelaziosis in the eye anterior chamber. Chinese J Ophthalmol, Vol.4, p.466

Chen, W.; Zheng, J.; Hou P.; Li, L. & Hu, Y. (2010). A case of intraocular thelaziasis with rhegmatogenous retinal detachment. Clin Exp Optom, Vol.93, No.5, (Sep 2010), pp.360-362, ISSN 0816-4622

Chermette, R.; Guillot, J. & Bussie'ras, J. (2004). Canine ocular thelaziosis in Europe. Vet Rec, Vol.154, No.8, (Feb 2004), p.248, ISSN 0042-4900

Cheung, WK.; Lu, HJ.; Liang, CH.; Peng, ML. & Lee, HH. (1998). Conjunctivitis caused by *Thelazia callipaeda* infestation in a woman. J Formos Med Assoc, Vol.97, No.6, (Jun 1998), pp.425-427, ISSN 0929-6646

Chirico, J. (1994). Prehibernating *Musca autumnalis* (Diptera: Muscidae); an overwintering host for parasitic nematodes. Vet Parasitol, Vol.52, No.3-4,(Apr 1994), pp.279-284, ISSN 0304-4017

Chitwood, MB.; & Stoffolano, JG. (1971). First report of *Thelazia* sp. (Nematoda) in the face fly, *Musca autumnalis,* in North America. J Parasitol, Vol.57, No.6, (Dec 1971), pp.1363-1364, ISSN 0022-3395

Choi, DK. & Choi, SY. (1979). A case of human thelaziasis concomitantly found with a reservoir host. Korean J Ophthalmol, Vol.19, No.1, pp.125-129, ISSN 1011-8942

Choi, WY.; Youn, JH.; Nam, HW.; Kim, WS.; Kim, WK.; Park, SY. & Oh, YW. (1989). Scanning electron microscopic observations of *Thelazia callipaeda* from human. Korean J Parasitol, Vol.27, No.3, (Sep 1989), pp.217-223, ISSN 0023-4001

Collobert, C.; Bernard, N. & Lamidey, C. (1995). Prevalence of *Onchocerca* species and *Thelazia lacrymalis* in horses examined post mortem in Normandy. Vet Rec Vol.136, No.18, (May 1995), pp.463–465, ISSN 0042-4900

Craig, JF. & Davies, GO. (1937). *Thelazia* lacrymalis in a horse. Vet Rec, Vol.49, p.1117, ISSN 0042-4900

De Chaneet, G. (1970). *Thelazia* in a cow in western Australia. Aust Vet J, Vol.46, No5, (Mar 2008), p.240, ISSN1751-0813 / P: 0005-0423

Doezie, AM.; Lucius, RW.; Aldeen, W.; Hale, DV.; Smith, DR. & Mamalis, N. (1996). *Thelazia californiensis* conjunctival infection. Ophthalmic Surg Laser, Vol.27, No.8, (Aug 1996), pp.716–719, ISSN 1082-3069

Dongus, H.; Beelitz, P. & Schol, H. (2003). Embryogenesis and the first-stage larva of *Thelazia lacrymalis*. J Helminthol Vol.77, No.3, (Sep 2003), pp. 227–233, ISSN 0022-149X.

Dongus, H.; Beelitz, P.; Wollanke, B.; Gerhards, H. & Gothe, R. (2000). Occurrence of *Thelazia lacrymalis* (Nematoda, Spirurida, Thelaziidae) in horses in Germany. Tieraerztliche Umschau, Vol.55, pp.599–602, ISSN 0049-3864

Dorchies, P.; Chaudieu, G.; Siméon, LA.; Cazalot, G.; Cantacessi, C. & Otranto, D. (2007). First reports of autochthonous eyeworm infection by *Thelazia* callipaeda (Spirurida,

Thelaziidae) in dogs and cat from France. Vet Parasitol, Vol.149, No.3-4, (Nov 2007), pp.294-297. ISSN 0304-4017

Dougherty, CT. & Knapp, FW. (1994). Oviposition and development of face flies in dung from cattle on herbage and supplemented herbage diets. Vet Parasitol, Vol.55, No.1-2, (Oct 1994), pp.115-127, ISSN 0304-4017 b

Dubay, SA.; Williams, ES.; Mills, K. & Boerger-Fields, A. (2000). Association of *Moraxella ovis* with keratoconjunctivitis in mule deer and moose in Wyoming. J Wildl Dis, Vol.36, No.2, (Apr 2000),pp 241–247, ISSN 0090-3558

Dunn, AM. (1978). Veterinary helminthology, (2nd ed.), William Heinemann Medical Books, ISBN 0-433-07951-7 London, UK

Dutto, M. (2008). Ocular thelaziasis in man in Northern Italy. Bull Soc Pathol Exot, Vol.101, No.1, (Feb 2008), pp.9-10, ISSN 0037-9085

Ebadi, A. (1951). A survey on *Thelazia* spp. in cattle in Tehran, Iran. DVM thesis No. 428, College of Veterinary Medicine, Tehran University, Tehran, Iran

Eckert, J. (1992). Parasiten der Einhufer. Helminthen, in: Veterinarmedizinische Parasitologie, Eckert J, Kutzer E., Rommel, M., Burger, H.-J. & Korting, W. (eds.), pp. 375–431, Parey Verlag, ISBN 3-489-52916-2, Berlin, Germany

Elias, R.; Mamani, J.; Hermoza, C. & Kinsella, J. (2008). First report of thelaziosis (*Thelazia anolabiata*) in an Andean Cock of the Rock (*Rupicola peruviana*) from Peru. Vet Parasitol Vol.158, No.4, (Dec 2008), pp.382–383, ISSN 0304-4017

Faust, EC. (1928). Studies on *Thelazia callipaeda* Railliet and Henry, 1910. J Parasitol, Vol.15, No.2, (Dec 1928), pp.75-86, ISSN 0022-3395

Faust, EC.; Beaver PC.; Jung, RC. (1975). Animal Agents and Vectors of Human Disease, (4th ed.), Lea and Febiger, IBSN 0-8121-0503-6, Philadelphia, USA

Ferroglio, E.; Rossi, L.; Tomio, E.; Schenker, R. & Bianciardi, P. (2008). Therapeutic and prophylactic efficacy of milbemycin oxime (intereceptor) against *Thelazia callipaeda* in naturally exposed dogs. Vet Parasitol, Vol.154, No.3-4, (Jul 2008), pp.351-353, ISSN 0304-4017

Fiebiger, J. (1947). Die tierischen Parasiten der Haus- und Nutztiere, sowie des Menschen, (4th ed.), Urban & Schwarzenberg, Wien, Austria

Fitzsimmons, WM. (1966). Ophthalmia due to *Thelazia* infection in British cattle. Vet Rec , Vol.78, No.7, (Feb 1966), pp.257-258 ISSN 0042-4900

Geden, CJ. & Stoffolano, JG. (1980). Bovine thelaziasis in Massachusetts. *Cornell Vet*, Vol.70, No.4, (Oct 1980), pp.344-359, ISSN 0010-8901

Geden, CJ. & Stoffolano, JG. (1981). Geographic range and temporal patterns of parasitization of *Musca autumnalis* De Geer by *Thelazia* spp. in Massachussets with observation on *Musca domestica* as an inusuitable host. J Med Entomol Vol.18, No.6, (Nov 1981), pp.449–456, ISSN 0022-2585

Geden, CJ.; & Stoffolano, JG (1982). Development of the bovine eyeworm, *Thelazia gulosa* (Railliet and Henry) in experimentally infected female *Musca autumnalis* de Geer. J Parasitol Vol.68, No.2, (Apr 1982) pp.287–292, ISSN 0022-3395

Ghirotti, M. & Iliamupu DS. (1989). *Thelazia rhodesii* (Desmarest, 1828) in cattle of Central Province, Zambia. Parassitologia, Vol.31, No.2-3, (Aug-Dec 1989), pp.231-237, ISSN 0048-2951

Giangaspero, A.; Lia R.; Vovlas, N. & Otranto, D. (1999). Occurrence of *Thelazia lacrymalis* (Nematoda, Spirurida,Thelaziidae) in native horses in Italy. Parassitologia, Vol.41, No.4, (Dec 1999), pp.545–548 ISSN 0048-2951

Giangaspero, A.; Otranto, D.; Vovlas, N. & Puccini, V. (2000b). *Thelazia gulosa* Railliet & Henry, 1910 and T. skrjabini Erschow, 1928 infection in southern Europe (Italy). Parasite. Vol.7, No.4, (Dec 2000), pp.327–329, ISSN 1252-607X

Giangaspero, A.; Tieri, E.; Otranto, D. & Battistini, ML. (2000a). Occurrence of *Thelazia lacrymalis* (Nematoda, Spirurida, Thelaziidae) in native horses in Abruzzo region (central eastern Italy). Parasite, Vol.7, No.1, (Mar 2000), pp.51–53, ISSN 1252-607X

Giangaspero, A.; Traversa, D. & Otranto, D. (2004). Ecology of *Thelazia* spp. in cattle and their vectors in Italy. Parassitologia, Vol.46, No.1-2, (Jun 2004), pp.257-259, ISSN 0048-2951

Gibbons LM (1986) SEM guide to the morphology of nematode parasites of vertebrates. CABI, ISBN 9780-8519-85695 Wallingford, UK

Grant, B.; Slatter, DH. & Dunlap, JS. (1973). *Thelazia* sp. (Nematoda) and dermoid cysts in a horse with torticollis. *Vet Med Small Anim Clin,* Vl.68, No.1, (Jan 1973), pp.62-4, ISSN 0042-4898

Greenberg, B. (1971). Flies and disease. Volume I. Ecology, classification and biotic associations. Princeton University Press, ISBN 978-0691080710 Princeton , USA

Gutierres, VC.; Onama, RK. & Todd AC (1980). Prevalence of the eyeworms *Thelazia gulosa* (Railliet and Henry, 1910) and *T. skrjabini* (Erschow, 1928) in Wisconsin dairy cattle. *J Parasitol,* Vol.66, No.2, (Apr 1980), p.304, ISSN 0022-3395

Gutteková, A. (1987). Ultrastructure of the surface sculpture of the nematodes *Thelazia gulosa* and *Thelazia rhodesi*. Vet Med (Praha) Vol.32, No.2, (Feb 1987), pp.113-120, ISSN 0375-8427

Halpin, RB. & kirkly, WW. (1962). Experience with an anthelmintic. Vet Rec, Vol.74, p.495, ISSN 0042-4900

Hermosilla, C.; Herrmann, B. & Bauer, C. (2004). First case of Thelazia callipaeda infection in a dog in Germany. Vet Rec 154, No.18, (May 2004), pp.568–569, ISSN 0042-4900

Höglund, J.; Ljungström, BL.; Nilsson, O.; Lundquist, H.; Osterman, E. & Uggla, A. (1997). Occurrence of *Gasterophilus intestinalis* and some parasitic nematodes of horses in Sweden. Acta Vet Scand, Vol.38, No.2, pp.157-165, ISSN 0065-1699

Hong, ST.; Lee, SH. & Han, H. (1985). A human case of Thelaziasis in Korea. Korean J Parasitol Vol.23, No.2, (Dec 1985), pp.137-139 ISSN 0023-4001

Hong, ST.; Lee, SH. & Kim, SI. (1988). A human case of *Thelazia callipaeda* infection with reference to its internal structures. Korean J Parasitol, Vol.26, pp.137-139, ISSN 0023-4001

Hong, ST.; Park, YK.; Lee, SK.; Yoo, JH.; Kim, AS.; Chung, YH. & Hong, SJ. (1995). Two human cases of *Thelazia callipaeda* infection in Korea. *Korean J Parasitol,* Vol.33, No.2, (Jun 1995), pp.139-144 ISSN 0023-4001

Hossain, MI.; Hossain, MA.; Nahar, L.; Hossain, MM.; Mondal, AS.; Alim, MA.; Mahmud, MC. & Islam, A. (2011). Human thelaziasis in Bangladesh. Mymensingh Med J, Vol.20, No.1, (Jan 2010), pp.128-130, ISSN 1022-4742

Howard, HJ. (1927). Thelaziasis of the eye and its adnexa in man. Am J Ophthalmol, Vol.10, pp.807-809, ISSN 0002-9394

Jiang, ZX.; Xu, LQ. & Yu, LQ. (1991). Human thelaziasis in China. Chinese J Parasitic Dis Control, Vol.4, pp. 48–51

Kagei, N.; Uga, S. & Kugi, G. (1983). On the caudal papillae of the male of *Thelazia callipaeda* Railliet and Henry, 1910. Jpn J Parasitol Vol.32, No.5, pp.481-484, ISSN 0021-5171

Kennedy, MJ. (1994). The effect of treating beef cattle on pasture with ivermectin on the prevalence and intensity of *Thelazia* spp. (Nematoda: Thelazioidea) in the vector, *Musca autumnalis* (Diptera: Muscidae). J Parasitol Vol.80, No.2, (Apr 1994), pp.321-326, ISSN 0022-3395

Kennedy, MJ.; Holste, JE.; & Jacobsen, JA. (1994). The efficacy of ivermectin (pour-on) against the eyeworms, *Thelazia gulosa* and *Thelazia skrjabini* in naturally infected cattle. Vet Parasitol, Vol.55, No.3, (Nov 1994), pp.263-266 ISSN 0304-4017

Kennedy, MJ. & MacKinnon, JD. (1994). Site segregation of *Thelazia skrjabini* and *Thelazia gulosa* (Nematoda: Thelazioidea) in the eyes of cattle. J Parasitol, Vol.80, No.4, (Aug 1994), pp.501-504, ISSN 0022-3395

Kennedy, MJ.; Moraiko, DT. & Treichel, B. (1993). First report of immature *Thelazia skrjabini* (Nematoda: Thelazioidea) from the eye of a white-tailed deer, *Odocoileus virginianus*. J Wildl Dis Vol.29, No.1, (Jan 1993), pp.159-160, ISSN 0090-3558

Kennedy, MJ. & Phillips, FE. (1993). Efficacy of doramectin against eyeworms (Thelazia spp.) in naturally and experimentally infected cattle. Vet Parasitol, 49, No.1, (Jul 1993), pp.61-66, ISSN 0304-4017

Kikuchi, S. (1976). Scanning electron microscopy of nematodes of mammals and birds. *Thelazia* and *Gnathostoma*. J Vet Med 655:73–79

Kim, HW.; Kim, JL. & Kho, WG. (2010). Intraocular Infestation with *Thelazia callipaeda*. Jpn J Ophthalmol Vol.54, No.4, (Jul 2010), pp.370-372 ISSN 0021-5155

Kirschner, BI.; Dunn, JP. & Ostler, HB. (1990). Conjunctivitis caused by Thelazia californiensis. Am J Ophthalmol, Vol.110, No.5, (Nov 1990), pp.573-574, ISSN 0002-9394

Knierim, R. & Jack, MK. (1975). Conjunctivitis due to Thelazia californiensis. Arch Ophthalmol, Vol.93, No.7, (Jul 1975), pp.522-523, ISSN 0003-9950

Kolstrup, N. (1974). *Thelazia skrjabini* in Danish cattle. *Nord Vet Med*, Vol.26, No.7-8, (Jul-Aug 1974), pp.459-462, ISSN 0029-1579

Kosin, E.; Kosman, ML.; Depary, AA. (1989). First case of human Thelaziasis in Indonesia. *Southeast Asian J Trop Med Public Health*, Vol.20, No.2, (Jun 1989), pp.233-236, ISSN 0125-1562

Koyama, Y.; Ohira, A.; Kono, T.; Yoneyama, Y. & Shiwaku, K. (2000). Five cases of thelaziasis. Br J Ophthalmol Vol.84, No.4, (Apr 2000), p.441, ISSN 0007-1161

Kozlov, DP. (1963). The life cycle of nematode *Thelazia callipaeda* parasitic in the eye of the man and carnivores. Doklady Akademy Nauk SSSR, Vol.142, pp.732–733, ISSN 0869-5652

Krafsur, ES. & Church, CJ. (1985). Bovine thelaziasis in Iowa. *J Parasitol.* Vol.71, No.3, (Jun 1985), pp.279-286 ISSN 0022-3395

Krastin, NI. (1950b). Determination of the cycle of development of *Thelazia gulosa*, parasite of the eye of cattle. Dokl Akad Nauk SSSR, Vol.70, No.3, pp.549-551, ISSN 0002-3264

Krastin, NI. (1950a) The biology of two nematode of the genus *Thelazia Bose* 1819, parasites of the eye of cattle. Dokl Akad Nauk SSSR, Vol.75, No.4, pp.591-594, ISSN 0002-3264

Krastin, NI. (1952). The life cycle of the nematode *Thelazia skrjabini* Ershov, 1928 ocular parasite in cattle. Dokl Akad nauk SSSR, Vol.82, pp.829–831, ISSN 0002-3264

Ikeme, MM. (1967). Kerato-conjunctivitis in cattle in the plateau area of Northern Nigeria. A study of *Thelazia rhodesi* as a possible aetiological agent. Bull Epizoot Dis Afr , Vol.15, No.4, (Dec 1967), pp.363-367, ISSN 0007-487X

Ivashkin, VM.; Khromova, LA. & Baranova, NM. (1979). The development cycle of *Thelazia lacrymalis*. Veterinariya, Vol.7, No.7, (Jul 1979), pp.46–47, ISSN 0042-4846

Ladouceur, CA. & Kazacos, KR. (1981). Eye worms in cattle in Indiana. *J Am Vet Med Assoc*, Vol.178, No.4, (Feb 1981), pp.385-387, ISSN 0003-1488

Lee, J.; Chung, SH.; Lee, SC. & Koh, HJ. (2006). A technique for removal of a live nematode from the vitreous. *Eye* (Lond), Vol.20, No.12, (Dec 2006), pp.1444-1446, ISSN 0950-222X

Leiper, RT. (1917). Thelaziasis in man: A summary of recent reports on "circumocluar filariasis" in Chinese literature, with a note on the zoological position of the parasite. Br J Ophthalmol, Vol.1, No9, (Sep 1917), pp.546-549, ISSN 0007-1161

Levine, ND. (1968). Nematode parasites of domestic animals and man. (2nd ed.), Burgess, ISBN 9780-0109-84842, Minneapolis, USA

Lia RP.; Traversa, D.; Agostini, A. & Otranto, D. (2004). Field efficacy of moxidectin 1 per cent against *Thelazia callipaeda* in naturally infected dogs. Vet Rec. Vol.154, No.5, (Jan 2004), pp.143-145, ISSN 0042-4900

Löhrer, J. & Hörning, B. (1967). *Thelazia lacrimalis* of the horse. Schweiz Arch Tierheilkd, Vol.109, No.12, (Dec 1967), pp.644-53, ISSN 0036-7281

Lyons, ET. & Drudge, JH. (1975). Two eyeworms, Thelazia gulosa and *Thelazia skrjabini*, in cattle in Kentucky. *J Parasitol*, Vol.61, No.6, (Dec 1975), pp.1119-1122, ISSN 0022-395

Lyons, ET.; Drudge, JH. & Tolliver, SC. (1976). *Thelazia lacrymalis* in horses in Kentucky and observations on the face fly (*Musca autumnalis*) as a probable intermediate host. J Parasitol, Vol.62, No.6, (Dec 1976), pp.877–880 ISSN 0022-395

Lyons, ET.; Drudge, JH. & Tolliver, SC. (1980). Experimental infections of *Thelazia lacrymalis*: maturation of third-stage larvae from face flies (*Musca autumnalis*) in eyes of ponies. J Parasitol . Vol.66, No.1, (Feb 1980), pp.181–182, ISSN 0022-395

Lyons, ET.; Drudge, JH. & Tolliver, SC. (1981). Apparent inactivity of several antiparasitic compounds against the eyeworm *Thelazia lacrymalis* in equids. Am J Vet Res, Vol.42, No.6, (Jun 1981), pp.1046-1047, ISSN 0002-9645

Lyons, ET.; Tolliver, SC.; Collins, SS.; Drudge, JH. & Granstrom, DE. (1997). Transmission of some species of internal parasites born in 1993, 1994, and 1995 on the same pasture on a farm in central Kentucky. Vet Parasitol, Vol.70, No.4, (Jul 1997), pp.225-240, ISSN 0304-4017

Lyons, ET.; Tolliver, SC.; Drudge, JH.; Swerczek, TW. & Crowe, MW. (1986). Eyeworms (*Thelazia lacrymalis*) in one- to four-year-old Thoroughbreds at necropsy in Kentucky (1984 to 1985). *Am J Vet Res* Vol.47, No.2, (Feb 1986, pp.315-316, ISSN 0002-9645

Lv, ZY.; Cao, AL. & Wu, ZD. (2009). Ocular infection of *Thelazia callipaeda* in an infant. Chinese J Parasitol Parasitic Dis, Vol.27, No.1, (Feb 2009), p.86, ISSN 0022-1767

Ma'ca, J. (1977). Revision of Palearctic species of *Amiota* subg. *Phortica* (Diptera, Drosophilidae). Acta Entomol Bohemoslovaca Vol.74 No2, pp.114–130, ISSN 0001-5601

Magnis, J.; Naucke, TJ.; Mathis, A.; Deplazes, P. & Schnyder, M. (2010). Local transmission of the eye worm *Thelazia callipaeda* in southern Germany. Parasitol Res, Vol.106, No.3,(Feb 2010), pp.715–717 ISSN 0932-0113

Malacrida, F.; Hegglin, D.; Bacciarini, L.; Otranto, D.; Nageli, F.; Nageli C.; Bernasconi, C.; Scheu, U.; Balli, A.; Marenco, M.; Togni, L.; Deplazes, P. & Schnyder, M. (2008). Emergence of canine ocular thelaziosis caused by *Thelazia callipaeda* in southern Switzerland. Vet Parasitol, Vol.157, No.3-4, (Nov 2008), pp.321–327, ISSN 0304-4017

Marley, SE.; Illyes, EF.; Keller, DS.; Meinert, TR.; Logan, NB.; Hendrickx, MO. & Conder, GA. (1999). Efficacy of topically administered doramectin against eyeworms, lungworms, and gastrointestinal nematodes of cattle. Am J Vet Res, Vol.60, No.6, (Jun 1999), pp.665-668, ISSN 0002-9645

McLaren, DJ. (1974). The anterior glands of *Necator americanus* (Nematoda: Strongyloides). I. Ultrastructural studies. Int J Parasitol, Vol.4, No.1, (Feb 1974) pp.25–34, ISSN: 0020-7519

McLaren, DJ. (1976). Nematode sense organs. Adv Parasitol. Vol.14, pp.105–265, ISSN 0065-308X

Michalski, I. (1976). The efficacy of levamisole and tetramisole in the treatment of thelaziasis in cattle. Med Weter, Vol.32, pp.417-419, ISSN 0025-8628

Min, HK. & Chun, KS. (1988). A case of human thelaziasis in both eyes. Korean J Parasitol, Vol.26, No.2, (Jun 1988), pp.133-135, ISSN 0023-4001

Min, S.; Jae RY, Hyun YP (2002) Enzooticity of the dogs, the reservoir host of *Thelazia callipaeda*, in Korea. Korean J Parasitol, Vol.40, No.2, (Jun 2002), pp.101–103, ISSN 0023-4001

Miroshnichenko, VA.; Desiaterik, MP.; Novik, AP.; Gorbach, AP. & Papernova, Niu. (1988). A case of ocular thelaziasis in a 3-year-old child *Vestn Oftalmol*, Vol.104, No.2, (Mar 1988), p.64, ISSN 0042-465X

Miyazaki, I. (1991). An illustrated book of helminthic zoonoses. International Medical Foundation of Japan, LC RC119. M58 1991, Tokyo, Japan

Moolenbeek, WJ. & Surgeoner, GA. (1980). Southern Ontario Survey of Eyeworms, *Thelazia gulosa* and *Thelazia lacrymalis* in Cattle and Larvae of *Thelazia* spp. in the Face Fly, *Musca autumnalis*. Can vet J, Vol.21, No.2, (Feb 1980), pp.50-52, ISSN 0008-5286

Mukherjee, PK.; Verma, S. & Agrawal, S. (1978). Intra ocular *thelazia* (a case report). *Indian J Ophthalmol,* Vol.25, No.4, (Jan 1978), pp.41-42 ISSN 0301-4738

Munang'andu, HM.; Chembensofu, M.; Siamudaala, VM.; Munyeme, M. & Matandiko, W. (2011). *Thelazia rhodesii* in the African Buffalo, Syncerus caffer, in Zambia. Korean J Parasitol Vol.49, No.1, (Mar2011), pp. 91-94, ISSN 0023-4001

Murata, K. & Asakawai, M. (1999). First Report of *Thelazia* sp. from a Captive Oriental White Stork (*Ciconia boyciana*) in Japan. Vet Med Sci , Vol.61, No.1, (Jan 1999), pp.93–95 ISSN 0916-7250

Nadler, S.; Hoberg, EP.; Hudspeth, DS. & Rickard, LG. (2000). Relationships of *Nematodirus* species and *Nematodirus battus* isolates (Nematoda: Trichostrongyloidea) based on nuclear ribosomal DNA sequences. J Parasitol, Vol.86, No.3, (Jun 2000), pp.588–601, ISSN 0022-395

Naem, S. (2005). Ultrastructural observations on the surface of *Thelazia lacrymalis* (Nematoda: Spirurida, Thelaziidae). Acta Vet Hung, Vol.53, No.2, (Apr 2005), pp.205-212, ISSN 0236-6290

Naem, S. (2007a). *Thelazia rhodesi* (Spirurida, Thelaziidae), bovine eyeworm: morphological study by scanning electron microscopy. Parasitol Res. Vol.100, No.4, (Mar 2007), pp.855-860 ISSN 0932-0113

Naem, S. (2007c). Fine structure of body surface of *Thelazia skrjabini* (Nematoda: Spirurida, Thelaziidae). Parasitol Res. Vol.100, No2, (Jan 2007), pp.305-310 ISSN 0932-0113

Naem, S. (2007b). Morphological differentiation among three *Thelazia* species(Nematoda: Thelaziidae) by scanning electron microscopy. Parasitol Res. Vol.101, No.1, (Jun 2007), pp.145–151 ISSN 0932-0113

Nagada, Y. (1964). A study on the oriental eyeworm *Thelazia callipaeda*. Jpn J Parasitol, Vol.13, No7, pp.600–602 ISSN 0022-3395

Nath, R.; Narain, K.; Saikia, L.; Pujari BS.; Thakuria, B. & Mahanta, J. (2008). Ocular thelaziasis in Assam: a report of two cases. Indian J Pathol Microbiol, Vol.51, No.1, (Jan-Mar 2008), pp.146-8 ISSN 0377-4929

Oakley, GA. (1969). *Thelazia* infestation of cattle in Cambridgeshire. Br Vet J, Vol 125, No.12 Suppl(Dec 1969), p. xxxix+ ISSN 0007-1935

O'Hara, JE. & Kennedy, MJ. (1989). Prevalence and intensity of *Thelazia* spp. (Nematoda: Thelazioidea) in a *Musca autumnalis* (Diptera: Muscidae) population from Central Alberta. J Parasitol, Vol.75, No.5, (Oct 1989), pp.803-806 ISSN 0022-3395

O'Hara, JE. & Kennedy, MJ. (1991). Development of the nematode eyeworm, *Thelazia skrjabini* (Nematoda: Thelazioidea), in experimentally infected face flies, *Musca autumnalis* (Diptera: Muscidae). J Parasitol, Vol.77, No.3, (Jun 1991) pp.417–425, ISSN 0022-3395

Ohira, A. (2000). Five cases of thelaziasis. Br J Ophthalmol, Vol.84, No.4, (Apr 2000) p.441, ISSN 0007-1161

Okoshi, S. & Kitano, N. (1966). Studies on thelaziasis of cattle I. *Thelazia skrjabini* Erschow, 1928 found in Japan. Jpn J Vet Sci , 28, No.1, (Feb 1966), pp.11–15, ISSN 0021-5295

Otranto, D.; Brianti E, Cantacessi C, Lia RP, Máca J (2006b) The zoophilic fruitfly Phortica variegata: morphology, ecology and biological niche. Med Vet Entomol. Vol.20, No4, (Dec 2006), pp.358-364, ISSN 0269-283X

Otranto, D.; Cantacessi C, Mallia E, Lia RP (2007) First report of *Thelazia callipaeda* (Spirurida, Thelaziidae) in wolves in Italy. J Wildl Dis, Vol.43, No.3, (Jul 2007), pp.508-511, ISSN 0090-3558

Otranto, D.; Cantacessi, C.; Testini, G. & Lia, RP. (2006a). *Phortica variegata* as an intermediate host of *Thelazia callipaeda* under natural conditions: evidence for pathogen transmission by a male arthropod vector. Int J Parasitol , Vol.36, No.10-11, (Sep 2006), pp.1167-1173, ISSN 0020-7519

Otranto, D.; Dantas-Torres, F.; Mallia, E.; DiGeronimo, PM.; Brianti, E.; Testini, G.; Traversa, D. & Lia, RP. (2009). *Thelazia callipaeda* (Spirurida, Thelaziidae) in wild animals: report of new host species and ecological implications. Vet Parasitol, Vol.166, No.3-4, (Dec 2009), pp.262-267 ISSN 0304-4017

Otranto, D. &, Dutto, M. (2008). Human thelaziasis, Europe. Emerg Infect Dis, Vol.14, No.4, (Apr 2008), pp.647-649, ISSN 1080-6040

Otranto, D.; Tarsitano, E.; Traversa D.; Giangaspero A.; De Luca, F. & Puccini, V. (2001). Differentiation among three species of bovine *Thelazia* (Nematoda: Thelaziidae) by polymerase chain reaction-restriction fragment length polymorphism of the first internal transcribed spacer ITS-1 (rDNA). Int J Parasitol, Vol.31, No.14, (Dec 2001), pp.1693-1698, ISSN 0022-7519

Otranto, D.; Ferroglio, E.; Lia, RP.; Traversa, D. & Rossi, L. (2003b). Current status and epidemiological observation of *Thelazia callipaeda* (Spirurida, Thelaziidae) in dogs, cats and foxes in Italy: a "coincidence" or a parasitic disease of the Old Continent? Vet Parasitol , Vol.116, No.4, (Oct 2003), pp.315-325 ISSN 0304-4017

Otranto, D.; Lia. RP.; Buono, V.; Traversa, D. & Giangaspero, A. (2004). Biology of *Thelazia callipaeda* (Spirurida, Thelaziidae) eyeworms in naturally infected definitive hosts. Parasitol, Vol.129, Pt.5, (Nov 2004), pp.627-633, ISSN 0971-7196

Otranto, D.; Lia, RP.; Cantacessi, C.; Testini, G.; Troccoli, A.; Shen, JL. & Wang, ZX. (2005c). Nematode biology and larval development of *Thelazia callipaeda* (Spirurida, Thelaziidae) in the drosophilid intermediate host in Europe and China. Parasitol, Vol.131, Pt.6, (Dec 2005), pp.847-855, ISSN 0971-7196

Otranto, D.; Lia, RP.; Testini, G.; Milillo, P.; Shen, JL.; Wang, ZX. (2005a). *Musca domestica* is not a vector of *Thelazia callipaeda* in experimental or natural conditions. Med Vet Entomol, Vol.19, No.2, (Jun 2005), pp.135-139, ISSN 0269-283X

Otranto, D.; Lia, RP.; Traversa, D. & Giannetto, S. (2003a). *Thelazia callipaeda* (Spirurida, Thelaziidae) of carnivores and humans: morphological study by light and scanning electron microscopy. Parassitologia, Vol.45, (3-4):Dec 2003), pp.125-133 ISSN 0048-2951

Otranto, D.; Tarsitano, E.; Traversa, D.;, De Luca, F.; Giangaspero, A. (2003c). Molecular epidemiological survey on the vectors of *Thelazia gulosa, Thelazia rhodesi* and *Thelazia skrjabini* (Spirurida: Thelaziidae). Parasitol, Vol.127, Pt.4, (Oct 2003), pp.365-373, ISSN 0971-7196

Otranto, D.; Testini, G.; De Luca, F.; Hu, M.; Shamsi, S. & Gasser, RB. (2005b). Analysis of genetic variability within *Thelazia callipaeda* (Nematoda: Thelazioidea) from Europe and Asia by sequencing and mutation scanning of the mitochondrial cytochrome c oxidase subunit 1 gene. Mol Cell Probes, Vol.19, No.5, (Oct 2005), pp.306-313, ISSN 0890-8508

Otranto, D. & Traversa, D. (2004). Molecular characterization of the first internal transcribed spacer of ribosomal DNA of the most common species of eyeworms (Thelazioidea: Thelazia). J Parasitol, Vol.90, No.1, (Feb 2004), pp.185-188, ISSN 0022-3395

Otranto, D.; & Traversa, D. (2005) *Thelazia* eyeworm: an original endo- and ecto-parasitic nematode. Trends Parasitol, Vol.21, No.1, (Jan 2005), pp.1-4, ISSN 1471-4922

Overend, DJ. (1983). *Thelazia gulosa* in cattle. *Aust Vet J*, Vol.60, No.4, (Mar 2008), pp.126-127, ISSN 1751-0813

Pande, BP.; Chauhan, PS.; Bhatia, BB. & Arora, GS. (1970). Studies on bubaline eyeworms with reference to the species composition of *Thelazia* and their pathogenic significance. Indian J Anim Sci, Vol.40, pp.330-345, ISSN 0367-8318

Patton, S. & Marbury, K. (1978). Thelaziasis in cattle and horses in the United States. *J Parasitol*, Vol.64, No.6, (Dec 1978), pp.1147-8 ISSN 0022-3395

Peng, Y.; Kowalski, R.; Garcia, LS. & Pasculle, W. (2001). Case 279—A case of *Thelazia californiensis* conjunctival infestation in human. Department of Pathology, University of Pittsburgh-Columbia 2001, Available from http://www.stanford.edu/class/humbio103/ParaSites2002/thelaziasis/Thelaziasis.html

Railliet, A. & Henry, A. (1910). Nouvelles observations sur les *Thelazies*, nema-todes parasites de l'oeil. Compt Rend Soc Biol, Vol.68, pp.783-785, ISSN 0037-9026

Price, EW. (1930). A new nematode parasitic in the eyes of dogs in the United States. J Parasitol, Vol.17, No.2, (Dec 1930), pp.112-113 ISSN 0022-3395

Rodrigues, HO. (1992). On Thelazia anolabiata (Molin, 1860) Railliet y Henry, 1910 (Nematoda, Thelazioidea)—a new host record and systematic considerations. Mem Inst Oswaldo Cruz, Vol. 87, Suppl.1, pp.217–222, ISSN 0074-0276

Roggero, C.; Schaffner, F.; Bächli, G.; Mathis, A. & Schnyder, M. (2010). Survey of *Phortica* drosophilid flies within and outside of a recently identified transmission area of the eye worm *Thelazia callipaeda* in Switzerland. *Vet Parasitol* Vol.171, No.1-2, (Jul 2010), pp.58-67, ISSN 0304-4017

Rossi, L. & Bertaglia, P. (1989). Presence of *Thelazia callipaeda* Railliet & Henry, 1910, in Piedmont, Italy. Parassitologia, Vol.31, No.2-3, (Aug-Dec), pp.167–172, ISSN 0048-2951

Rossi L, Peruccio C (1989) Thelaziosi oculare nel Cane: Aspetti clinici e terapeutici. Veterinaria, Vol2, pp.47–50

Ruytoor, P.; Déan, E.; Pennant, O.; Dorchies, P.; Chermette, R.; Otranto, D. & Guillot, J. (2010). Ocular thelaziosis in dogs, France. Emerg Infect Dis, Vol.16, No.12, (Dec 2010), pp.1943-1945, ISSN 1080-6040

Salifu, DA.; Haruna, ES.; Makinde, AA. & Ajayi, ST. (1990) A case report of *Thelazia* infection in a 15-month old heifer in Vom, Plateau State, Nigeria. *Rev Elev Med Vet Pays Trop*, Vol.43, No.2, pp.197-198, ISSN 0035-1865

Schebitz, H. (1960). Eine durch *Thelazia lacrimalis* beim Pferd verursachte Conjunctivitis ulcerosa. Dt. tierarztl. Wschr Vol.67, No.20, pp. 564-567, ISSN 0341-6593

Seo, M.; Yu, JR.; Park, HY.; Huh, S.; Kim, SK. & Hong, ST. (2002). Enzooticity of the dogs, the reservoir host of *Thelazia callipaeda* in Korea. Korean J Parasitol, Vol.40, No.2, (Jun 2002), pp.101–103, ISSN 0023-4001

Sharma, A.; Pandey, M.; Sharma, V.; Kanga, A. & Gupta, ML. (2006). A case of human thelaziasis from Himachal Pradesh. Indian J Med Microbiol, Vol.24, No.1, (Jan 2006), pp.67-69, ISSN 0255-0857

Shen, JL.; Gasser, RB.; Chu, D.; Wang, ZX.; Yuan, X. & Cantacessi, C. (2006). Human thelaziosis:a neglected parasitic disease of the eye. J Parasitol. Vol.92, No.4, (Aug 2006), pp.872–875 ISSN 0022-3395

Shen, JL.; Wang, ZX.; Luo, QL.; Li, J.; Wen, HQ. & Zhou YD. (2009). *Amiota magna* as an intermediate host of *Thelazia callipaeda* under laboratory conditions. Chinese J Parasitol Parasitic Dis, Vol.27, No.4, (Aug 2009), pp.375-376, ISSN 0022-1767

Shi, YE.; Han, JJ.; Yang, WY. & Wei, DX. (1988). *Thelazia callipaeda* (Nematoda: Spirurida): Transmission by flies from dogs to children in Hubei, China. Trans R Soc Trop Med Hyg, Vol.82, No.4, p.627. ISSN 0035-9203

Singh, TS. & Singh, KN. (1993). Thelaziasis: Report of two cases. Br J Ophthalmol, Vol.77, No.8, (Aug 1993), pp.528–529 ISSN 0007-1161

Skrjabin, KI.; Sobolov, AA. & Ivashkin, VM. (1971) Essentials of nematodology, Vol.16-Spirurata of animals and man and the diseases caused by them, part 4, Thelazioidea. Israel Program for Translations, ISBN 978-0706511796, Jerusalem, Israel

Soll, MD.; Carmichael, IH.; Scherer, HR. & Gross, SJ. (1992). The efficacy of ivermectin against *Thelazia rhodesii* (Desmarest, 1828) in the eyes of cattle. Vet Parasitol, Vol.42, No.1-2, (Apr 1992), pp.67-71, ISSN 0304-4017

Soulsby, EJL. (1965). Textbook of veterinary clinical parasitology, vol 1 Helminths. Blackwell, Oxford UK

Soulsby, EJL. (1986.) Helminths, arthropods and protozoa of domesticated animals. (7th ed.) Bailliere Tindall, ISBN 9780-8121-07807, London UK

Stewart MA (1940) Ovine thelaziasis. J AmVet Med Ass, Vol.96,No.757, pp.486-490 ISSN 0003-1488

Stuckey, EJ. (1917). Circumocular filariasis.Br J Ophthalmol, Vol.1, No.9, (Sep 1917), pp.542-546 ISBN ISSN 0007-1161, Reprint from: Chinese Med J, Jan 1917

Tarsitano, E.; Traversa, D.; DeLuca, F.; Guida, B. & Otranto, D. (2002) Intraspecific and interspecific differences in the ITS-I (rDNA) of four species of *Thelazia* (Nematoda: Thelaziidae). Parassitologia. Vol.44, No.1, p.181, ISSN 0048-2951

Taylor, SK.; Vieira, VG.; Williams, ES.; Pilkington, R.; Fedorchak, SL.; Mills, KW.; Cavender, JL.; Boerger-Fields, AM. & Moore, R. (1996). Infectious keratoconjunctivitis in free-ranging mule deer (*Odocoileus hemionus*) from Zion National Park, Utah. J Wildl Dis, Vol.32, No.2, (Apr 1996), pp.326-330, ISSN 0090-3558

Traversa, D.; Otranto, D.; Iorio, R. & Giangaspero, A. (2005) Molecular characterization of *Thelazia lacrymalis* (Nematoda, Spirurida) affecting equids: a tool for vector identification. Mol Cell Probes, Vol19, No.4, (Aug 2005), pp.245-249, ISSN 0890-8508

Tretjakowa, ON. (1960). Thelaziasis in horses. Veterinariya, Vol.37, p.58, ISSN 0042-4846

Turfrey, BA. & Chandler, RL. (1978). Incidence of thelazia nematodes in the eyes of cattle at a research institute in Berkshire. *Vet Rec*, Vol.102, No.19, (May 1978), p.23, ISSN 0042-4900

Tweedle, DM.; Fox, MT.; Gibbons, LM. & Tennant, KV. (2005). Change in the prevalence of Thelazia species in bovine eyes in England. Vet Rec, Vol.157, No.18, (Oct 2005), pp.555-556, ISSN 0042-4900

Van Aken, D.; Dargantes, AP.; Lagapa, JT. & Vercruysse, J. (1996). *Thelazia rhodesii* (Desmarest, 1828) infections in cattle in Mindanao, Philippines. Vet Parasitol, Vol.66, No.1-2, (Nov 1996), pp.125-129, ISSN 0304-4017

Vilagiova, I. (1967). Results of experimental studies on the development of pre-invasive stage of worms of the genus Thelazia Bosc 1819 (Nematoda: Spirurata) parasitic in the eye in the cattle. Folia Parasitol (praha), Vol.74, pp.275–280, ISSN 0015-5683

Vohradsky, F. (1970). Clinical course of *Thelazia rhodesii* infection of cattle in the Accra plains of Ghana. *Bull Epizoot Dis Afr*, Vol.18, No.2, (Jun 1970), pp.159-170, ISSN 0007-487X

Walker, ML. & Becklund, WW. (1971). Occurrence of a cattle eyeworm, *Thelazia gulosa* (Nematoda: Thelaziidae), in an imported giraffe in California and *T. lacrymalis* in a native horse in Maryland. *J Parasitol*, Vol.57, No.6, (Dec 1971), pp.1362-3, ISSN 0971-7196

Wang, KC.; Wang, ZX. & Shen, JL. (1999). Canine infection with *Thelazia callipaeda* and human thelaziosis. J Trop Dis Parasitol, Vol.28, pp.216–218

Wang, YJ.; Penia, L.; & Lin, L. (2002). A case of thelaziasis in Guang'an of Sichuan, China. Bull Endemic Dis, Vol.17, No.58, ISBN 0007-4845

Wang, ZX.; Chen, Q. & Jiang, BL. (2002). Epidemiology of thelaziasis in China. Chinese J Parasitic Dis Control. Vol.6, pp.335–337

Wang, ZX.; Du, JS. & Yang, ZX. (1998). The epidemiologic determinants and mechanism of transmission of thelaziosis in China. Chinese J Zoonoses, Vol.4, pp.30–32, ISSN 1002-2694

Wang, ZX.; Shen, JL. & Du, JS. (2003). Studies on the relationship between alternative generation of house dogs and control of human thelaziosis. J Trop Dis Parasitol, Vol.1, pp.204–207, ISSN

Wang, ZX.; Shen, JL.; Wang HY. & Otranto, D. (2006). An update on the research of human thelaziosis. Chinese J Parasitol Parasitic Dis, Vol.24, No.4, (Aug 2006), pp.299-303, ISSN 0022-1767

Wang, ZX.; Wang, KC. & Chen, Q. (2002). Experimental studies on the susceptibility of *Thelazia callipaeda* to Amiota okadai in three provinces of China. Chinese Journal of Zoonoses, Vol.18, pp.61–63. ISSN 1002-2694

Wang, ZX. & Yang, ZX. (1985). Experimental observations on the biological features and pathogenicity of *Thelazia callipaeda* parasitized in rabbits. Chinese J Parasitol Parasitic Dis, Vol.3, No.2, pp.128-130 ISSN 0022-1767

Wertheim, G. & Giladi, M. (1977). Helminths of birds and mammals of Israel. VII. - *Pneumospirura rodentium* n. sp. (Pneumospiruridae - Thelazioidea). Ann Parasitol Hum Comp. Vol.52, No.6, (Nov-Dec 1977), pp.643-646, ISSN 0003-4150

Xue, C.; Tian, N. & Huang, Z. (2007). *Thelazia callipaeda* in human vitreous. Can J Ophthalmol Vol.42, No.6, (Dec 2007), pp.884-885, ISSN 0008-4182

Yamaguti, S. (1961). Systema Helminthum, vol. 3. The nematodes of vertebrates, part 1 and 2. Interscience Publishers, ISBN 978-0470970201, New York, USA

Yang, CH.; Tung, KC.; Wang, MY.; Chan,g SC.; Tu, WC.; Wang, KS.; Shyu, CL. & Lee, WM. (2006). First *Thelazia callipaeda* infestation report in a dog in Taiwan. J Vet Med Sci Vol.68, No.1, (Jan 2006), pp.103-104, ISSN 0916-7250

Yang, YJ.; Liag, TH.; Lin, SH.; Chen, HC.; & Lai, SC. (2006). Human Thelaziasis occurrence in Taiwan. Clin Exp Optom, Vol.89, No.1, (Jan 2006), pp.40–44, ISSN 0816-4622

Yospaiboon, Y.; Sithithavorn, P.; Maleewong, V.; Ukosanakarn, U. & Bhaibulaya, M. (1989). Ocular thelaziasis in Thailand: a case report. *J Med Assoc Thai*, Vol.72, No.8, (Aug 1989), pp.469-73, ISSN 0125-2208

Youn, H. (2009). Review of Zoonotic Parasites in Medical and Veterinary Fields in the Republic of Korea. Korean J Parasitol. Vol.47, Suppl, (Oct 2009), pp.S133-S141, ISSN 0023-4001

Zakir, R.; Zhong-Xia, ZP.; Chiodini, P. & Canning, CR. (1999). Intraocular infestation with the worm, *Thelazia callipaeda*. Br J Ophthalmol, Vol83, No.10, (Oct 1999), pp.1994-1995,. ISSN 0007-1161